Concussion

AF778104

Progress in Neurological Surgery

Vol. 28

Series Editor

L. Dade Lunsford Pittsburgh, Pa.

Concussion

Volume Editors

Ajay Niranjan Pittsburgh, Pa.
L. Dade Lunsford Pittsburgh, Pa.

49 figures, 21 in color, and 26 tables, 2014

KARGER Basel · Freiburg · Paris · London · New York · Chennai · New Delhi · Bangkok · Beijing · Shanghai · Tokyo · Kuala Lumpur · Singapore · Sydney

Ajay Niranjan, MD
L. Dade Lunsford, MD
Department of Radiosurgery
UPMC Presbyterian
200 Lothrop Street
Pittsburgh, PA 15213 (USA)

Library of Congress Cataloging-in-Publication Data

Concussion / volume editors, Ajay Niranjan, L. Dade Lunsford.
p. ; cm. -- (Progress in neurological surgery, ISSN 0079-6492 ; vol. 28)
Includes bibliographical references and indexes.
ISBN 978-3-318-02648-1 (hard cover : alk. paper) -- ISBN 978-3-318-02649-8 (electronic version)
I. Niranjan, Ajay, editor. II. Lunsford, L. Dade, editor. III. Series: Progress in neurological surgery ; v. 28. 0079-6492
[DNLM: 1. Brain Concussion--diagnosis. 2. Athletic Injuries. 3. Brain Concussion--therapy. W1 PR673 v.28 2014 / WL 354]
RC394.C7
617.4'81044--dc23
2014011673

Bibliographic Indices. This publication is listed in bibliographic services, including Current Contents® and Index Medicus.

Disclaimer. The statements, opinions and data contained in this publication are solely those of the individual authors and contributors and not of the publisher and the editor(s). The appearance of advertisements in the book is not a warranty, endorsement, or approval of the products or services advertised or of their effectiveness, quality or safety. The publisher and the editor(s) disclaim responsibility for any injury to persons or property resulting from any ideas, methods, instructions or products referred to in the content or advertisements.

Drug Dosage. The authors and the publisher have exerted every effort to ensure that drug selection and dosage set forth in this text are in accord with current recommendations and practice at the time of publication. However, in view of ongoing research, changes in government regulations, and the constant flow of information relating to drug therapy and drug reactions, the reader is urged to check the package insert for each drug for any change in indications and dosage and for added warnings and precautions. This is particularly important when the recommended agent is a new and/or infrequently employed drug.

All rights reserved. No part of this publication may be translated into other languages, reproduced or utilized in any form or by any means electronic or mechanical, including photocopying, recording, microcopying, or by any information storage and retrieval system, without permission in writing from the publisher.

© Copyright 2014 by S. Karger AG, P.O. Box, CH–4009 Basel (Switzerland)
www.karger.com
Printed in Germany on acid-free and non-aging paper (ISO 9706) by Kraft Druck, Ettlingen
ISSN 0079–6492
e-ISSN 1662–3924
ISBN 978–3–318–02648–1
e-ISBN 978–3–318–02649–8

Contents

Series Editor's Note

Over the last 100 years, the recognition of minimal traumatic brain injury, or concussion, has greatly expanded. Each year, millions of children and adults suffer one or more concussive events, which in years past were often deemed clinically insignificant, unaffected by treatment, and time limited. Our international preoccupation with sports and sport heroes has led to an in-depth analysis of the potential long-term effects of repeated concussion. This volume presents a historical perspective of concussion, possible mechanisms that define the biomechanics and neurophysiology of it, the variation in the clinical picture presented by those who are injured, and methods to diagnose and treat concussive events.

New investigations, neurocognitive tests, and advanced neuroimaging tools have revealed the potential biochemical as well as structural changes associated with concussive events, and new neurophysiological tests may help define the previously unrecognized effects of concussion. As multiple management options including medical, physiatric, pharmacologic, sociologic, and behavioral therapies are needed to treat patients, assessment and care requires a collaborative team that includes physicians, neuropsychologists, and other specialists in order to individualize care for each affected individual.

Sport-related concussion, with well-publicized examples in both hockey and American football, has become a topic of major concern. The publication of *League of Denial*, an analysis of the United States National Football League's assessment of concussion, as well as reports of various important players in the field, has further heightened concerns relative to the deleterious effects of repeated concussive events. Only recently has the recognition of major postmortem proteinopathies been associated with progressive behavioral and cognitive deterioration in patients subjected to multiple minimal brain traumas. In the worst cases, such findings mimic many aspects of Alzheimer's disease. Both emerging knowledge and increasing attention has awakened the world to the important healthcare impact that repeated concussive events may have.

This volume of *Progress in Neurological Surgery* has assembled a number of international authors with special expertise in the diagnosis, recognition, evaluation, and treatment of concussion. It is truly a most topical and timely book.

L. Dade Lunsford, MD, Pittsburgh, Pa.

Niranjan A, Lunsford LD (eds): Concussion. Prog Neurol Surg. Basel, Karger, 2014, vol 28, pp 1–13
DOI: 10.1159/000358746

Cerebral Concussion: A Historical Perspective

Joseph C. Maroon · Christina Mathyssek · Jeffrey Bost
Department of Neurosurgery, University of Pittsburgh Medical Center, Pittsburgh, Pa., USA

Abstract
No topic in sports has gathered more attention and publicity than the diagnosis, management, and long-term effects of cerebral concussion. The relevant history of concussion starts in 1905 when President Theodore Roosevelt drew attention to the football 'death harvest'. Soon after, rules started to change to reduce the amount and severity of head injuries in football. Up until 1980, the primary focus regarding concussions was to diagnose a potentially fatal intracranial hemorrhage. While aware of long-term consequences of concussions, the perception at the time was that virtually all concussions would 'clear' with time and rest. Concussion management guidelines gave way to objective neuropsychological testing in the early 1990s with the development of the ImPACT™ (Immediate Post-Concussion Assessment and Cognitive Testing) neurocognitive test. Led by organized football, in 1994 the National Football League (NFL) formed the Mild Traumatic Brain Injury Committee which began to investigate the cause of concussions, evaluate equipment (particularly helmets), and recommend methods for prevention. In 2005, the first case of chronic traumatic encephalopathy was described in a deceased football player, raising concerns about the long-term consequences of head injuries and concussions. Major advancements in contact sports and the military are underway to reduce the incidence of concussions and subconcussive blows to the head.

© 2014 S. Karger AG, Basel

No topic in sports has gathered more attention and publicity than the diagnosis, management, and long-term effects of traumatic cerebral concussion. Derived from 'concutere', which in Latin means to shake violently, concussion is the most common type of traumatic brain injury (TBI). Mild TBI (mTBI), mild head injury, and minor head trauma are all used interchangeably for concussion. A concussion is defined as a posttraumatic transient impairment of neurological function. It is a complex pathophysiological process that is estimated to occur annually in approximately 1.7 million participants in sports of all kind in the USA alone.

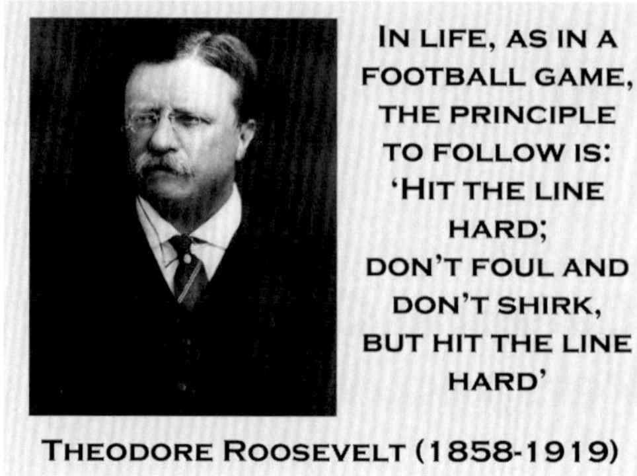

Fig. 1. Roosevelt believed that the football field was a proving ground for the battlefield and for life. In life, as in a football game, the principle he advocated to follow was: 'Hit the line hard; don't foul and don't shirk, but hit the line hard'.

Although concussions have been recognized and diagnosed as a specific entity since the time of Hippocrates, we must only go back to the turn of the 20th century and President Theodore Roosevelt to obtain perspective on current concussion prevention and management. In the early 1900s, American gridirons were considered killing fields. Players locked arms in mass formations and charged helmetless like battering rams into their opponents with bone-crushing force. Many injuries were catastrophic – skull fractures, subdural and epidural hematomas, twisted spinal cords, and broken ribs that pierced the lungs and great vessels were far too common. In 1904 there were 18 football deaths and 159 serious injuries, most of which occurred in prep school or college athletes. Their obituaries were run on a nearly weekly basis in newspapers throughout the country and led to calls from parents, news media, and politicians to banish football as a legal sport. It was at this time that President Theodore Roosevelt, one of the biggest proponents of physical competition, personal fitness, teamwork, and self-discipline, became concerned.

Roosevelt believed that the football field was a proving ground for the battlefield and for life. In life, as in a football game, the principle he advocated to follow was: 'Hit the line hard; don't foul and don't shirk, but hit the line hard' (fig. 1). Because of the carnage and despite his beliefs, Roosevelt realized that reform had to occur, particularly since his son, Theodore Jr., was then a student at Harvard playing the sport!

On October 9, 1905, Roosevelt met with the coaches and representatives of the major Ivy League schools – Harvard, Yale, and Princeton – at the White House. Drawing presidential attention, the schools subsequently condemned the brutality of the sport and took steps to reduce the carnage which the Chicago Tribune referred to as a 'death harvest'.

In 1906, an intercollegiate conference was formed that was the forerunner of the National Collegiate Athletic Association (NCAA). Immediately, the rules were changed to reduce fatalities, which subsequently sharply declined in 1906 and 1907. Many of these early reforms are still in place and set the stage for many of the changes that occurred throughout the rest of the century.

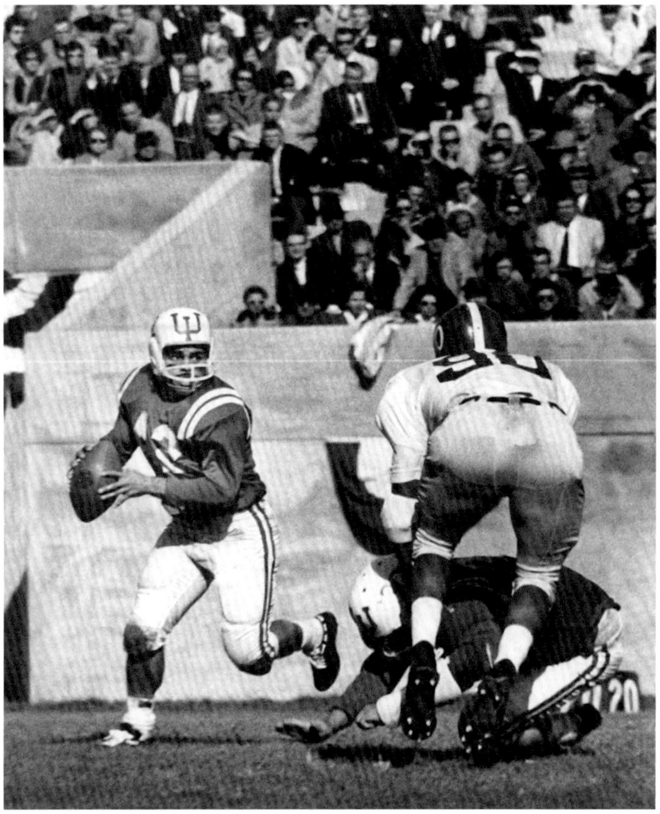

Fig. 2. The first author played college football for Indiana University. As a 5′6″, 160-pound undergraduate on a football scholarship, he personally experienced the violence and brutality of the sport. During his tenure Dr. Maroon experienced at least four concussions, a severe cervical sprain/strain syndrome, and fractured ribs.

Neurosurgery and Concussion Management

As a 5'6", 160-pound undergraduate at Indiana University on a football scholarship, I personally have experienced the violence and brutality of the sport. During my tenure I experienced at least four concussions, a severe cervical sprain/strain syndrome, and fractured ribs – all of which were considered a badge of honor at the time (fig. 2). Despite these injuries, organized football also provided me the underemphasized qualities of teamwork, perseverance, tenacity, and leadership that one acquires from this sport. At the time, however, I had no idea how this experience would affect my subsequent professional interests and future research.

Upon joining the neurosurgical faculty at the University of Pittsburgh in the 1970s with interests in both athletics and neurosurgery, I set out to investigate what appeared to be a constant stream of young football players with spinal cord injuries. To my horror I discovered the incidence of quadriplegia while playing football in Western Pennsylvania was approximately 1 per 12,000, which was markedly higher than the national average of 1 per 150,000. Western Pennsylvania was mostly known for its coal mines and steel mills at that time and many young males saw football as their only

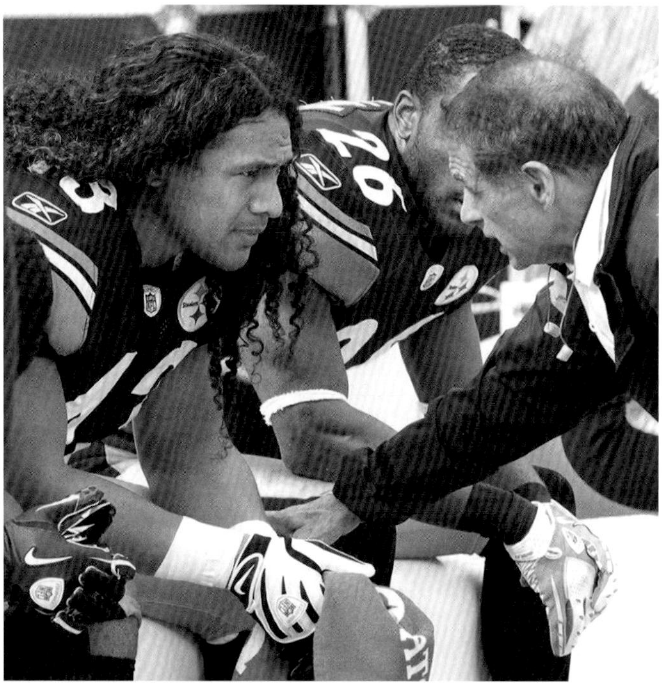

Fig. 3. Dr. Maroon, Pittsburgh Steelers' team neurosurgeon, talking with Troy Polamalu, Pittsburgh Steelers strong safety on the side lines of the football field.

chance to escape that life and get a college education. After publishing these results I embarked on an educational program along with Dr. James McMaster, then team physician for the Pittsburgh Panthers, to reduce and help prevent the incidence of catastrophic head and neck injuries in contact sports, particularly football. Because of these efforts I was subsequently invited to be the team neurosurgeon for the Pittsburgh Steelers in the early 1980s, the first such position for a neurosurgeon in the National Football League (NFL; fig. 3).

At the time, the primary focus regarding concussions was to not fail to diagnose the possibly associated intracranial hemorrhage that would be, while rare, most likely fatal. Although fully aware of the long-term consequences of head injuries, the perception at the time was that virtually all concussions would 'clear' with time and rest, and acutely with ammonium chloride (smelling salts)! There were those occasional athletes with a postconcussion syndrome characterized by headache, nausea, and 'foggy' thinking, but again, for the most part, these symptoms improved with time.

In the late 1980s and early 1990s, however, we became more aware that some athletes did not respond to 'benign neglect'; in other words, time did not sufficiently do its job of healing the injured brain. Indeed, some athletes had prolonged postconcussion syndrome, as documented by others interested in sports concussion at the time. During this time, leaders in the field like Robert Cantu began recommending concussion management guidelines. The Cantu guidelines, first published in 1986 relied heavily on loss of consciousness and posttraumatic amnesia to determine grades I–III. Over 16 different and revised guidelines based on signs and symptoms of concussion were eventually published and reported to aid in the diagnosis and management of concussion.

ImPACT™ (Immediate Post-Concussion Assessment and Cognitive Testing)

In the fall of 1990, I told Coach Chuck Noll, four-time Super Bowl coach of the Pittsburgh Steelers, that his starting quarterback at the time could not play the following week against the Baltimore Ravens. Coach Noll challenged this directive and asked, 'Why not?' I explained that various concussion guidelines stipulated that a minimum of 2 weeks of rest were required before returning to play. He questioned whether or not these guidelines were evidence-based and in frustration stated, 'If you want me to keep an athlete who appears normal in every way from football participation, I need objective data that something is wrong with his brain'. Chagrined but aware that he was correct, I contacted Mark Lovell, PhD, a brilliant neuropsychologist, to discuss the problem. After studying the literature, we constructed a paper-and-pencil neurocognitive test battery that subsequently was approved by Coach Noll and then Steelers President and owner, Dan Rooney. After baseline testing the entire team, we realized that for the first time, we did indeed have an objective test. We called the test Immediate Post-Concussion Assessment and Cognitive Testing, or ImPACT™. This objective testing combined with clinical judgment and a normal neurological examination proved to be an important tool in making safe and defendable return-to-play decisions.

Over the ensuing years, ImPACT™ was continually refined in content and administration, going from a paper-and-pencil to a computer-based test and more recently an Internet-based application. It has been adopted as a standard of care by most major professional (including the NFL), collegiate, and high school athletic organizations, and has been administered for baseline testing to over 4.5 million athletes and to over 60,000 soldiers in the military.

Sideline concussion evaluation has also advanced and several standardized assessment tools are now used that help to identify common signs and symptoms of concussion to remove players who have sustained a concussion from playing. Additionally, new technology is being employed to measure the balance of athletes following a head injury, called Sway Balance, made by Sway Medical LLC. Along with ImPACT™, it can aid in return-to-play decisions. Sway Balance is a software application, which along with a biometric strap placed to the athlete's body, can use the internal gyroscope of a tablet computer device to assess the balance function of athletes following injury. While cognitive testing is the cornerstone of concussion management, the Sway Balance application provides critical balance assessment information in real time to help further assess potential injuries.

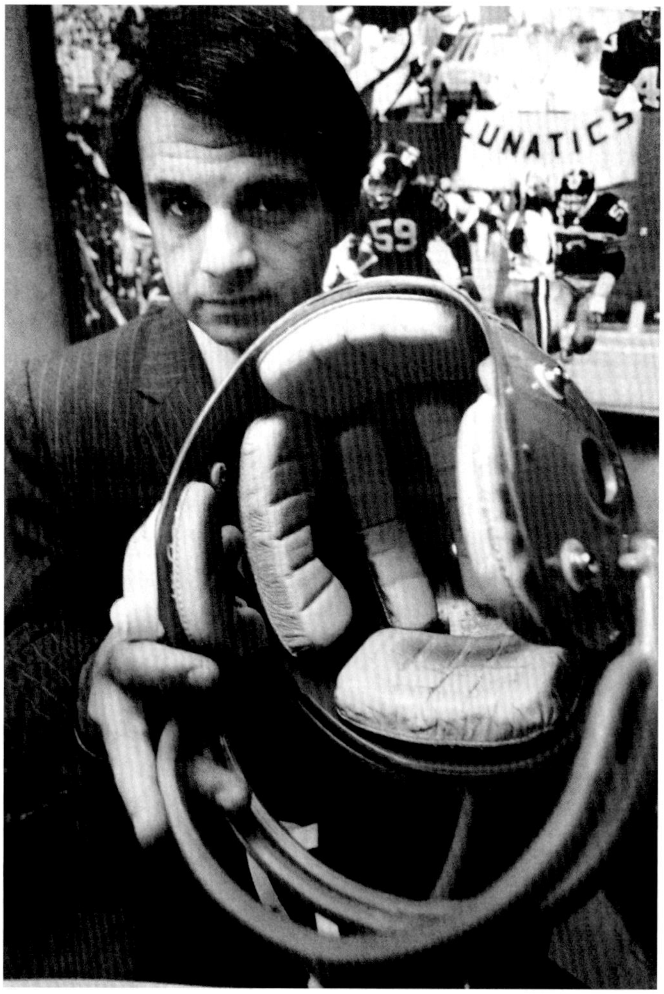

Fig. 4. Helmet evolution in American football.

NFL Concussion Management Advancements

As the objective concussion data improved in the early 1990s, along with several high-profile players like Al Toon of the New York Jets and Merril Hoge from the Chicago Bears retiring due to the postconcussion syndrome, the then NFL Commissioner Paul Tagliabue formed the Mild Traumatic Brain Injury Committee in 1994 to study concussion in the NFL. Dr. Elliott Pellman was selected to chair the committee. The charge of the committee was to investigate the cause of concussions, evaluate equipment (particularly helmets), and recommend methods for prevention [1]. One of the first projects was to conduct fact-finding interviews with helmet manufacturers to gain understanding about the development and evaluation of helmets for head protection. Soon after, the committee also funded biokinetic studies under the direction of Jim Newman, PhD to help design methods to better evaluate head protection and helmets (fig. 4).

In 1996, the commissioner mandated collection of mTBI data specifically to identify the incidence of concussions. In 1997, an education initiative was carried out to inform clubs about neuropsychological testing and concussion management. The following year, mTBI conferences were held in New York and Arizona with mandatory attendance for NFL medical staff.

Between 1998 and 2009 an extraordinary amount of data was compiled that resulted in 17 separate peer-reviewed publications. Issues addressed in these papers included the reconstruction of game day impacts and velocities, the location and direction of helmet impacts, epidemiological features of game injuries, return-to-play timing, and neuropsychological testing. Today, the systems in place to monitor and track NFL player injury are looked to as a model for many other sport organizations and the military.

In 2007, NFL commissioner Roger Goodell hosted a meeting in Chicago for all NFL team physicians and athletic trainers. Presented were the summary of NFL Mild Traumatic Brain Injury Committee research findings, including updated return-to-play criteria, the essential role of neuropsychological testing in mTBI diagnosis, and a comprehensive review of what was known of chronic traumatic encephalopathy (CTE) at that time. Based on that conference, the Mild Traumatic Brain Injury Committee of the NFL reaffirmed that all team physicians and athletic trainers should take a conservative approach in diagnosing and treating concussions. Furthermore, it specified that criteria, which include that concussion return-to-play criteria include the athlete is completely asymptomatic at rest and after a progressive aerobic stress test, has a completely normal neurological examination, and – for the first time – mandated neurocognitive testing as part of the evaluation. The ImPACT™ neurocognitive test was chosen by all 32 NFL teams.

Concussions have not just become a major concern for athletes and NFL teams, as the military has also been battling with an increasing number of concussions in their soldiers due to our two recent wars. To address this, another major conference was held in 2008 with NFL team physicians and trainers as well as medical personnel from the Department of Defense. The purpose of this gathering was to better characterize the mechanisms, long-term effects, and methods of protection from concussive injuries to the brain and to share data derived from athletics and the military.

In 2009, even more stringent guidelines were issued by the NFL. For the first time in NFL history, any player diagnosed with, or suspected of, a concussion was to be immediately removed from the game. This represented a significant change in NFL culture since in previous reports up to 48% of athletes with transient disturbances of neurological function without loss of consciousness would return to the same game. In addition, follow up by an independent 'neurological specialist' was made mandatory before clearance for return to play was possible. Also, an anonymous concussion 'hotline' was instituted for players to report any deviation from these mandatory practices to the NFL.

In 2010, the NFL changed the name of the Mild Traumatic Brain Injury Committee to the 'NFL Head, Neck and Spine Committee' and selected Richard Ellenbogen, MD, Chairman of Neurological Surgery at the University of Washington and former chief at Walter Reed Medical Center, together with Hunt Batjer, MD, Chair of the Department of Neurological Surgery at the University of Texas Southwestern Medical Center, to be the Co-Chairs of this committee. Both had no affiliation with the NFL, received no salary from the organization, and had an in-depth knowledge of TBI.

In 2011, substantial funds were provided by the NFL to the Centers for Disease Control and Prevention (CDC) to promote concussion awareness. Additionally, new rules were instituted relative to kickoffs and kickoff returns, and a new NFL sideline evaluation tool was constructed by the NFL Committee. This tool was distributed to all NFL teams and usage was made mandatory. The NFL instituted athletic trainers as 'spotters' in the press box to aid in the identification of head injuries on the field that may be missed by the on-field physicians. Also to aid in the diagnosis and evaluation of possible concussion, sideline video monitors were placed for medical staff to replay and evaluate play-action videos to determine the mechanism of injuries.

Chronic Traumatic Encephalopathy

Perhaps the most contentious problem today, particularly at the professional football level, is the potential etiology and scope of the neuropathological condition known as CTE. Unfortunately, relatively little is known to date about the neuropathology of the described brain changes or the pathophysiological pathways that lead to this condition. In 2005, pathologist Ben Omalu, MD and colleagues [2] published the first reported case of a former NFL player who had neuropathological changes consistent with CTE. Subsequently, pathologist Ann McKee, MD and neurosurgeon Robert Cantu, MD and others further characterized CTE as both a histological and clinical abnormal behavioral condition related to prior concussion(s) and/or subconcussive trauma to the brain. The typical chain of events so far described in the literature consists of mTBI followed by a prolonged latent period which may be years to decades later. Eventually a clinical syndrome develops that is characterized by early behavioral and emotional changes, such as altered personality, memory loss, and in some cases progressive dementia and suicidality [3, 4].

CTE can only be diagnosed postmortem; histological findings and published case reports thus far have almost exclusively come from high-risk populations such as athletes in contact sports and former combat veterans. There are many disparate scientific reports that speculate on the significance of various contributing factors such as age, the number and intensity of blows, effects of substance abuse, and genetic predisposition. To address this problem of limited knowledge, we recently reviewed the medical literature and summarized all 153 known cases of CTE. This is the largest and most exhaustive review to date. The described cases were primarily boxers, with professional football players as a close second. The following facts were determined from our review. The clinical presentation ranges from asymptomatic to severe depression, substance abuse, dementia, and suicide; there is no specific genetic profile, and there are no agreed upon neuropathological criteria for diagnosis. Yet, the literature is plagued by considerable ascertainment bias in the postmortem selection of cases to be studied, and conclusions drawn therefrom have to be considerate of this limitation. Importantly, reduction of even minor blows to the head may be the primary preventive strategy. Prospective studies in well-described samples are imperative to better understand incidence and specific risk factors for CTE, but have not been done to date.

The Pathophysiology of Traumatic Brain Injury

Is there a central underlying mechanism of concussion and CTE? It has been recognized in recent years that an impact to the head results in a cascade of metabolic and excitotoxic reactions. There is a massive release of glutamate and aspartate, and delayed reuptake of these neurotransmitters, which overstimulate glutamate receptors [5]. Overactivated glutamate receptors allow high levels of calcium ions in the cell, leading to excitotoxicity and subsequent cell death. We also know trauma to the head results in a major perturbation in glucose metabolism and also abnormal ionic changes in sodium, potassium, and calcium. Not so well understood or popularized is the immunoexcitotoxic reaction that occurs. Following a blow to the head, microglial cells become activated. These resident macrophages of the brain and spinal cord are the first line of active immune defense for the central nervous system.

When microglia are activated, they release a series of immune factors including both reactive oxygen and nitrogen species, inflammatory prostaglandins, cytokines, chemokines, proteases, nitric oxide, and trophic factors, as well as additional glutamate, aspartate, and quinolinic acid [6]. Subsequently, the microglia produces neuroreparative agents including neurotropic factors and anti-inflammatory cytokines to 'heal' the brain. Normally, this innate immune response to trauma is protective and meant to remove any inciting pathogens, clear dead and dying neurons, and then assume a phenotype conducive to neural rescue in order to facilitate the healing response. However, if additional traumatic blows to the brain occur before the reparative mode is initiated after the initial blow, the microglia can remain 'active' and a chronic neuroinflammatory state ensues. This neuroinflammation contributes to the postconcussion syndrome and if it fails to reverse, may progress to chronic progressive neurodegeneration. Neuroinflammation may be the underlying mechanism behind the development of CTE. Immunoexcitotoxicity may also explain why in some, but not all, individuals there is a progression to chronic persistent symptoms associated with postconcussion syndrome [7].

Neurosurgeon Julian Bailes, MD has been a major contributor and leader in the field of concussion diagnosis, management, and the long-term potential consequences thereof. In 2013 he published a review on the role of subconcussion in repetitive mTBI [8]. This review of recent biophysics studies utilizing accelerometers placed in the helmets of collegiate and high school athletes demonstrated a surprisingly high number of head impacts, ranging from several hundred to well over 1,000 hits during the course of a season. Although most of these have no discernible symptoms, sophisticated high-definition tractography can now demonstrate significant axonal injury, blood/brain barrier permeability changes, and evidence of neuroinflammation – all in the absence of behavioral changes. Dr. Bailes and his associates suggest that subconcussive level impacts may lead to long-term neurological alterations. He proposed the term 'subconcussion' as a significant emerging concept that requires more consideration and study [8].

Concussion: Politics, Media, and Chronic Traumatic Encephalopathy

In 1906, President Roosevelt felt compelled to address concussions in football. On February 3, 2013 President Obama also gave his opinion on the matter, saying that if he had a son, he is not sure he would let him play football. Furthermore, he stated he was 'glad the NFL is starting to take this (concussion) seriously'. To respond to President Obama, a Big Ten Football coach half-jokingly said, 'If I had a son, I am not sure I would let him go into politics!' Importantly though, the NFL has been taking this seriously at least since 1994, when the first Mild Traumatic Brain Injury Committee was formed.

Despite the fact that concussions can occur outside of sport, concussion management and awareness has taken center stage in professional American football. Media, money, and Monday nights have made professional football in the USA the epicenter of all things concussion related for over 100 years. Citing decades of scientific studies and media reports on the dangers of contact sports in 2013, thousands of former NFL players sued the NFL accusing the league of deliberately concealing information about life-altering brain injuries caused by playing football. The lawsuit was recently settled prior to verdict for USD 765,000,000, with the money going towards treatment and prevention of concussions. The NFL Player's Union also recently agreed to donate USD 100,000,000 over a period of 10 years to fund research on the etiology, prevention, and treatment of short- and long-term health problems associated with concussions. Although only involving several thousand professional athletes, the hope is the attention and money surrounding this agreement will 'trickle down' and lead to changes and advancements at all levels of football, from youth, high school, and college, and also other contact sports as well.

The incredible emphasis on concussions and head injuries in sports in all media outlets has had a significant effect in the participation of athletes in football and other sports. In 2013 the Pop Warner League experienced a 5–7% drop in participation due to parental concern and fears of long-term concussive effects on their children's brain. In Western Pennsylvania, a recent survey showed participation in football had declined by up to 20%. The same may be anticipated in hockey.

There have been approximately 25 football fatalities at all levels since 2004 according to the National Center for Sport Injury Research – or approximately 3 per year. When considering there are approximately 4 million athletes who play football annually, this is an extremely small incidence. There are many more deaths from skateboarding and bicycling in this age group. In terms of fatalities, it is more dangerous driving to and from the football field than participating. Yet despite these statistics and the tremendous improvements, the media continues to paint concussion management in sports in an extremely negative light.

The Treatment of Postconcussion Syndrome

In the 17th century, Moliere, the French playwright, parodied physicians when he wrote, 'the role of a physician is to amuse the patient until nature cures him'. Until recently, this facetious statement could describe the treatment of postconcussion syndrome. 'Treatment' essentially consisted of retreat from all physical or mental activity, avoiding stimulation of the mind or body, remaining in a darkened room if photophobia was present, and waiting for nature to cure the patient [9]. For many years, pharmacologic agents with their associated side effects were used liberally to manage symptoms. If one could not sleep, a hypnotic was given. If there were complaints of headache, an analgesic was prescribed. If there were mood or depressive symptoms, a selective serotonin reuptake inhibitor or other antidepressant was given [10]. It is not unusual for someone with a protracted postconcussion syndrome to be on 3–7 different psychoactive drugs.

Recently developed concussion centers have begun to reverse this trend and are beginning to address the underlying cause of these symptoms with specific treatment strategies. This includes balance, cognitive, and vestibular therapies designed to help retrain the brain to understand complex environments that include space, motion, and head/eye movements, which are often impaired in postconcussion syndrome.

Alternative Treatments

While many patients have benefitted from symptom management, in spite of the possible side effects, 10–20% of patients still experience prolonged postconcussion syndromes that respond insufficiently to symptom management. In these patients, alternative forms of treatment have been utilized with considerable anecdotal success. If the concept of neuroinflammation is truly an underlying part of the neuropathological substrate of these symptoms, then it seems sensible to use natural anti-inflammatory diets and dietary supplements to counter this process. Accordingly, in my practice, we have successfully used 2–3 g per day of omega-3 fatty acids (fish oil) for its anti-inflammatory effect in order to decrease the inflammatory prostaglandins and neuroinflammation. Many studies support this application [9, 11, 12]. In addition, we have described the use and their scientific basis of several other agents, such as resveratrol, a polyphenol found in various concentrations in plant sources; catechins, found in green tea; magnesium, which has neuroprotective features, yet is deficient in many athletes, and vitamin D_3, an anti-inflammatory agent which is also deficient in up to 75% of African-American athletes [11, 13, 14]. More recently, hyperbaric oxygen has been used by the military and also in our practice with, again anecdotal, very positive reports [15]. Importantly, randomized controlled studies are needed to substantiate these findings.

Conclusion

Over the past century, enormous progress has been made in terms of recognizing the gravity of concussions, diagnosis, implementing changes in sports regulation, and developing protective features and gear. Much research, however, remains to be done. Both sports medicine and athletic organizations are working together to further reduce concussion prevalence and severity. To that end, monitoring and adjusting game play regulations in high-risk contact sports, as well as improving protective gear, will be ongoing processes. The focus of future concussion research lies in the development of objective diagnostic tools, such as laboratory and imaging tests like high-definition fiber tracking, to provide additional objective data.

Perhaps the biggest challenge lies in the field of CTE research. While concussions are suspected to be a causal factor in the development of this neurodegenerative disease, the literature is plagued by ascertainment bias (i.e. whose brain is being selected to be studied), and we lack a clear understanding of associated risk factors, etiology, and prevalence.

In light of concussions and CTE, some have called for the abandonment of American football entirely; however, others continue to recognize the valuable benefits that accrue from team participation in contact sports. These include such character traits as perseverance in times of adversity, qualities of leadership, the benefits from team participation, and many more. Perhaps General Douglas MacArthur, superintendent of West Point said it best when he had the following quotation chiseled into the granite above the portals of the gymnasium at West Point that faced the athletic fields: 'On the fields of friendly strife are sown the seeds that on other days, on other fields will bear the fruits of victory'.

Acknowledgements

The authors would like to thank Robert Winkelman and Austin Amos, BA, for their valuable assistance in preparing this report.

References

1 Pellman EJ, Viano DC; National Football League's Committee on Mild Traumatic Brain Injury: Concussion in professional football: summary of research conducted by the National Football League's Committee on Mild Traumatic Brain Injury. Neurosurg Focus 2006;21:E12.

2 Omalu BI, DeKosky ST, Minster RL, Kamboh MI, Hamilton RL, Wecht CH: Chronic traumatic encephalopathy in a National Football League player. Neurosurgery 2005;57:128–134.

3 Gavett BE, Stern RA, McKee AC: Chronic traumatic encephalopathy: a potential late effect of sport-related concussive and subconcussive head trauma. Clin Sports Med 2011;30:179–188.

4 McKee AC, Stein TD, Nowinski CJ, Stern RA, Daneshvar DH, Alvarez VE, Lee HS, Hall G, Wojtowicz SM, Baugh CM, Riley DO, Kubilus CA, Cormier KA, Jacobs MA, Martin BR, Abraham CR, Ikezu T, Reichard RR, Wolozin BL, Budson AE, Goldstein LE, Kowall NW, Cantu RC: The spectrum of disease in chronic traumatic encephalopathy. Brain 2013;136:43–64.

5 Katayama Y, Becker DP, Tamura T, Hovda DA: Massive increases in extracellular potassium and the indiscriminate release of glutamate following concussive brain injury. J Neurosurg 1990;73:889–900.

6 Luo XG, Ding JQ, Chen SD: Microglia in the aging brain: relevance to neurodegeneration. Mol Neurodegener 2010;5:12.

7 Blaylock RL, Maroon JC: Immunoexcitotoxicity as a central mechanism in chronic traumatic encephalopathy – a unifying hypothesis. Surg Neurol Int 2011;2:107.

8 Bailes JE, Petraglia AL, Omalu BI, Nauman E, Talavage T: Role of subconcussion in repetitive mild traumatic brain injury. J Neurosurg 2013;119:1235–1245.

9 Maroon JC, LePere DB, Blaylock RL, Bost JW: Postconcussion syndrome: a review of pathophysiology and potential nonpharmacological approaches to treatment. Phys Sportsmed 2012;40:73–87.

10 McCrory P: Should we treat concussion pharmacologically? Br J Sports Med 2002;36:3–5.

11 Blaylock RL, Maroon JC: Natural plant products and extracts that reduce immunoexcitotoxicity-associated neurodegeneration and promote repair within the central nervous system. Surg Neurol Int 2012;3:19.

12 Hogyes E, Nyakas C, Kiliaan A, Farkas T, Penke B, Luiten PG: Neuroprotective effect of developmental docosahexaenoic acid supplement against excitotoxic brain damage in infant rats. Neuroscience 2003;119:999–1012.

13 Petraglia AL, Winkler EA, Bailes JE: Stuck at the bench: potential natural neuroprotective compounds for concussion. Surg Neurol Int 2011;2:146.

14 Ates O, Cayli S, Altinoz E, Gurses I, Yucel N, Sener M, Kocak A, Yologlu S: Neuroprotection by resveratrol against traumatic brain injury in rats. Mol Cell Biochem 2007;294:137–144.

15 Bennett MH, Trytko B, Jonker B: Hyperbaric oxygen therapy for the adjunctive treatment of traumatic brain injury. Cochrane Database Syst Rev 2012;12:1–42.

Additional Reading

Alsalaheen BA, Mucha A, Morris LO, Whitney SL, Furman JM, Camiolo-Reddy CE, Collins MW, Lovell MR, Sparto PJ: Vestibular rehabilitation for dizziness and balance disorders after concussion. J Neurol Phys Ther 2010;34:87–93.

Lau BC, Collins MW, Lovell MR: Sensitivity and specificity of subacute computerized neurocognitive testing and symptom evaluation in predicting outcomes after sports-related concussion. Am J Sports Med 2011;39:1209–1216.

Lovell M: The neurophysiology and assessment of sports-related head injuries. Phys Med Rehabil Clin N Am 2009;20:39–53.

Lovell M: The management of sports-related concussion: current status and future trends. Clin Sports Med 2009;28:95–111.

Jeffrey Bost, PA-C
Department of Neurosurgery, Presbyterian University Hospital
University of Pittsburgh Medical Center, Suite 5C
200 Lothrop Street, Pittsburgh, PA 15213 (USA)
E-Mail bostj@upmc.edu

Niranjan A, Lunsford LD (eds): Concussion. Prog Neurol Surg. Basel, Karger, 2014, vol 28, pp 14–27
DOI: 10.1159/000358748

Biomechanics of Concussion

Brian D. Stemper[a, b] · Frank A. Pintar[a, b]

[a]Medical College of Wisconsin and [b]VA Medical Center, Milwaukee, Wis., USA

Abstract

This report provides an overview of the biomechanics associated with mild traumatic brain injury (TBI), also known as concussion. Specifically, the role of angular acceleration in modulating concussion onset and severity is highlighted. Studies conducted and published from the 1960s to the 1980s provided initial estimates for TBI tolerance due to high rate head rotation. However, injury levels in those studies were more severe than what is considered to be concussion in the contemporary environment. Therefore, this issue deserves additional attention to provide quantitative estimates for concussive tolerance due to head rotational acceleration focusing on the types of clinical outcomes described today. Likewise, concussion in military personnel has notably increased in current conflicts due to the incorporation of improvised explosive devices and roadside bombs. Clinical evidence indicates that outcomes from concussion due to blast may be quite different from those due to head rotational acceleration. This report also provides an overview of blast concussion mechanisms and highlights some of the recent preclinical work in this area. As with head rotational acceleration, blast tolerance is necessary to understand the scope of this problem, better protect these personnel, and provide more informed return-to-duty guidelines for service members. © 2014 S. Karger AG, Basel

It has long been established that skull fractures and brain injuries result from physical inputs to the head. Skull fractures have been produced in laboratory experiments, and the fracture tolerance of the skull has been largely established through scientific studies that reproduced these injuries on human and animal cadaver models. Those studies concluded that the skull sustains fracture with local compressive displacements of the bone due to severe impact or crushing of the head. In some situations the skull may be impacted or accelerated, or may transmit blast overpressure, without sustaining fracture. In those cases, the brain is at risk of sustaining traumatic injury. The physics of what the skull experiences during traumatic brain injury (TBI) events is easier to establish than the mechanics of what the internal contents of the skull experience when the brain is injured. This field of study is referred to as biomechanics, or the study of the response of biological tissues to mechanical events. While the effects of vascular injury in the brain can more easily be correlated to imaging studies, concussion is not easily correlated to any imaging measure yet. Understanding the biomechanics of concussion or concussive events has also been a challenge due to the lack of establishing which particular tissues have been affected by such an event. From a biomechanics viewpoint, it is far easier to establish when a vessel is no longer intact than to establish when a concussion has occurred. This report provides a review of what is currently known about the biomechanics of concussion and will hopefully stir ongoing hypotheses as to where the answers may lie.

Basic Biomechanics

Beginning with a simple definition of motion, a rigid body may respond to an external force by translating or rotating. In three-dimensional space, the kinematics of a body are often referred to with six degrees of freedom: three dimensions of linear movement and three dimensions of angular movement. It is often convenient to characterize body kinematics by knowing where its center of gravity is. If one were to consider the human head a rigid body, its center of gravity would be approximately 2 cm anterior and 2 cm superior to the external auditory meatus in the midsagittal plane. Imagine then, a direction of impact force vector to the head. If the impact direction is in line with the center of gravity, the movement of the head will largely be translation in the direction of impact. If the impact direction is not in line with the center of gravity, the head will respond with some rotational movement and likely some translation as well. The ratio of translation to rotation depends on the distance of the force vector from the center of gravity. A vector more in line with the center of gravity will lead to primarily linear movement, whereas a vector further from the center of gravity induces a higher percentage or rotation. Thus, most head impacts will result in both translational and rotational movements. Once impacted, the rotational moment of inertia defines the resistance of the head to change in rotational velocity and is dependent upon the distribution of mass throughout its geometry. If an object's mass is concentrated near its center of gravity, it will rotate more easily than if the mass is distributed away from the center of gravity. The human head has somewhat evenly distributed mass and therefore has moderate rotational inertia.

Biomechanics of Traumatic Brain Injury

TBI results from a variety of mechanisms including impact, inertia, penetration, and blast overpressure. In civilian sporting and motor vehicle crash environments, injuries commonly result from impact to the head leading to a high rate of head acceleration or deceleration. Injuries develop within the tissues of the brain as strains are transferred from outer to inner regions, which results in pathologies distributed more diffusely than for other mechanisms such as blunt impact or penetration. The importance of head acceleration in the mechanism of concussive brain injury has been understood for decades [1]. It is generally accepted that mechanical measures modulate injury severity with greater loading conditions leading to more severe injuries [2], clinically diagnosed as concussion or diffuse axonal injuries. The effect of linear acceleration was investigated during the 1960s, wherein linear accelerations resulting from head impacts were correlated to intracranial pressure changes [3]. Further studies by the same group determined head acceleration levels required for concussion [4]. These data were later grouped to develop the Wayne State Tolerance Curve [2], which was used as the basis for the Head Injury Criterion (HIC) [5]. These relationships correlated the risk of injury with the magnitude of linear acceleration over a specific time duration.

Experimental studies, however, have identified that angular acceleration is more injurious to the brain than linear acceleration [6–8]. For example, a recent computational modeling study revealed that 90% of the total strain within the tissues of the brain during head acceleration due to blunt impact results from the rotational component, with only 10% attributed to the translational component [9]. Additionally, angular accelerations in the coronal plane were more injurious than in other planes due to the decreased inertial properties and anatomical structures that contribute to focal strain concentrations (i.e. falx cerebri) [10–13]. This point has been particularly well described using computational modeling [14–16]. In the case of rotationally induced injuries, kinematics such as angular acceleration, rotational velocity, and acceleration duration have been identified as primary determinants of diffuse brain injury severity [17–23]. Considerable experimental effort has been expended toward understanding the relationship between head rotational kinematics and injury severity. For example, a positive correlation was demonstrated between increasing rotational acceleration magnitude and injury severity [22–25]. In 2003, Gennarelli et al. [25] reported a theoretical relationship between increasing rotational acceleration magnitude and injury severity from mild concussion through severe diffuse axonal injury.

Other studies have identified lower tolerance at higher rotational velocities [22, 26, 27]. However, given its inherent limitations in the prediction of injury, i.e. high velocities resulting from very low acceleration with long duration, the focus of injury tolerance research may be better applied to the investigation of magnitude and duration as separate characteristics. Rotational velocity, being the integral of rotational acceleration versus time, inherently incorporates the effect of acceleration duration, but magnitude and duration of rotational acceleration are likely to have semi-independent effects [28]. As such, a complex relationship was identified between peak angular acceleration and pulse duration [20]. These theoretical and experimentally based observations have contributed to the development of rotationally based injury tolerance thresholds [18, 22, 26, 27, 29, 30]. Results of these studies, though, have not been conclusive and the independent effects of head angular acceleration pulse characteristics on injury thresholds remain ambiguous. Additionally, a majority of those

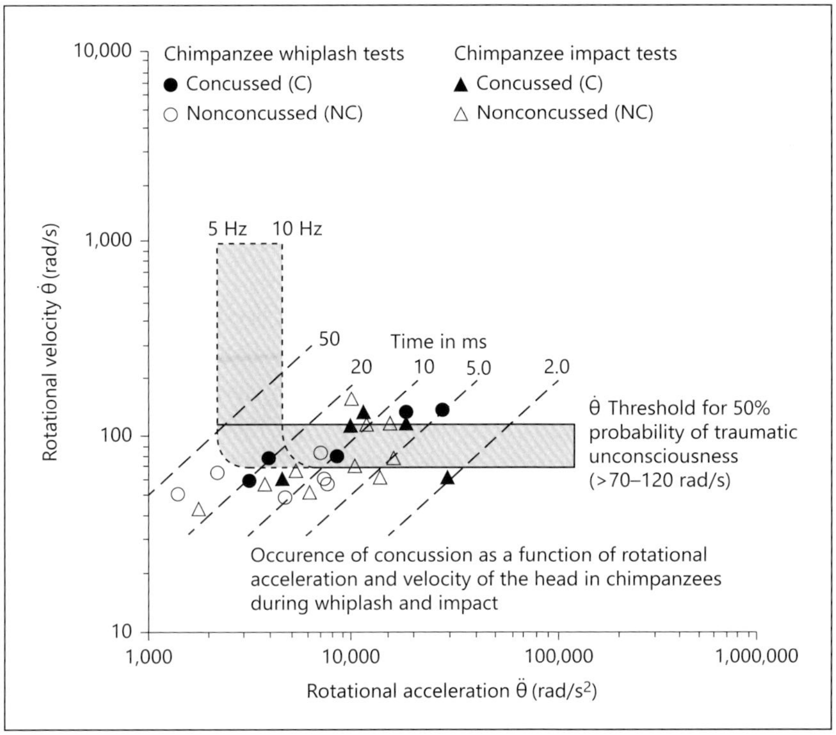

Fig. 1. Concussion tolerance curve relating rotational velocity to rotational acceleration of the head in chimpanzees. Rotational velocity inherently accounts for duration of head acceleration in its computation. From Ommaya et al. [23] with permission.

studies were generally focused on more severe injury levels, with outcome severity commonly exceeding what would be considered concussion in the contemporary clinical environment.

Rotational Acceleration Magnitude- and Duration-Based Injury Tolerance

The most comprehensive series of studies to focus on rotational acceleration as the mechanism of concussion was conducted by Ommaya et al. [8] in the 1960s using a primate injury model. Those studies recognized that peak rotational acceleration of the head significantly correlated with the production of concussion and also underlined the importance that rotational accelerations occur over a specific duration window (fig. 1). This eventually led to the formation of concussive injury tolerance curves that included head rotational acceleration and duration [22, 23, 31]. However, as indicated above, the determination of injury in those studies included outcomes that are likely of higher severity than what is considered to be concussion in the contemporary environment. Those outcomes included the loss of response to a piece of apple, loss of response to ear pinching, apnea greater than 3 s followed by irregular slow respirations, and bradycardia [32]. Some of those symptoms (e.g. apnea and bradycardia) are more commonly associated with severe head injury for contemporary diagnoses. Macroscopic pathological outcomes from those specimens included skull fractures, massive epidural and subdural hematomas, subarachnoid hemorrhage, intraventricular hemorrhage, and multiple brain contusions [23]. Other studies investigating head injury tolerance due to rotational acceleration have also focused on higher severities including diffuse axonal injury [18, 33].

Head injury tolerance to rotational acceleration deserves a second look, however, due to increasing concerns about behavioral and emotional disturbances resulting from single or repeated exposure to concussive events. This is particularly relevant in the setting of contact and collision sports, wherein participants may be exposed to hundreds of exposures over the course of a season [30, 34]. Another recent study indicated that a majority of concussions (>90%) resulting from participation in college football were graded as relatively minor according to multiple clinical assessments [35]. Recent reports have indicated that chronic cognitive deficiencies may occur even in the absence of frank neurologic dysfunction [34, 36]. These reports are particularly concerning given the long-term implications of repeated exposures to concussive injuries, including increased risk of neuropsychiatric disorders, cognitive dysfunction, and neurodegenerative disease [37–39].

Understanding the biomechanical tolerance for concussion in terms of measureable head kinematics is of critical importance now due to the increased clinical recognition of chronic cognitive and emotional disability from single or repeated concussive or subconcussive events. These tolerances can be directly applied in the field, given emerging technologies that allow for the measurement of head accelerations (linear and angular) in sporting and military helmets or directly on the head. However, as discussed above, relevant tolerance for concussion has not yet been developed, given the prior focus on higher severity injuries. Also of critical importance is the understanding of patient and biomechanical factors that can affect injury tolerance or outcomes that may include cumulative history of concussive or subconcussive accelerations, direction of head rotational acceleration, and gender, among others. This increased understanding of the importance of head rotational acceleration is evident in the recent focus on accurate injury mechanisms in preclinical models of concussion [40, 41]. Those types of preclinical models (fig. 2) combined with comprehensive behavioral and pathological assessments can help to define injury tolerance in the human.

Scaling Animals to Humans

As highlighted above, in vivo models are often necessary to study concussion tolerance and outcomes due to developing pathologies, secondary injuries, and subtle behavioral manifestations. However, relevance to the human condition is a major issue

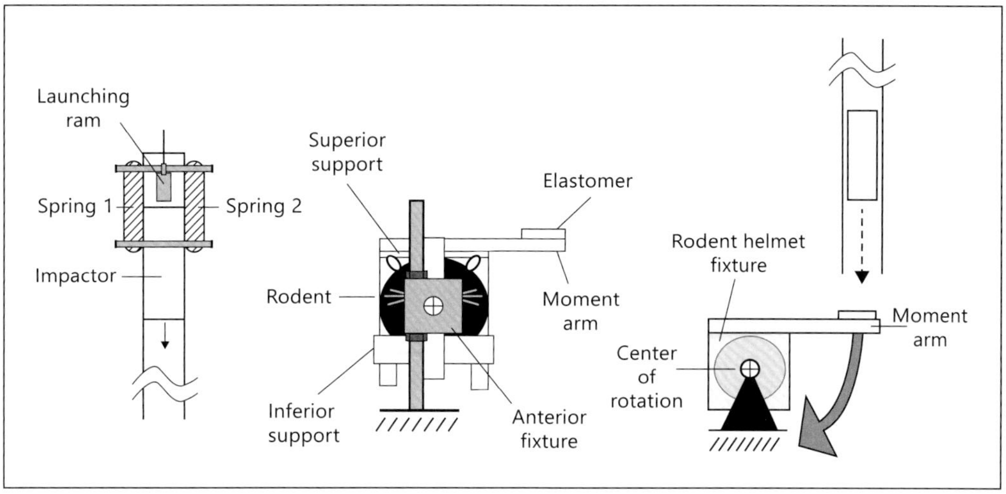

Fig. 2. Experimental rodent model that accurately reproduces the biomechanics of concussion. From Fijalkowski et al. [40].

for animal studies given different sizes and anatomical attributes of the head and cranial contents. Due to the effects of inertia, brain mass is known to influence the level of acceleration required for injury and, as such, is a logical first step in relating rodent and primate injury tolerance to humans. Because tissue strains are inertially induced during head rotations, greater accelerations are required in smaller brains for an equivalent injury level. Holbourn [11] theorized a scaling ratio that would enable rotational acceleration magnitudes to be scaled from one species to another based on the ratios of brain mass raised to the 2/3 power. To test this theory, Ommaya et al. [31] exposed different primate species with different brain masses to concussive brain injury. Theoretical tolerance curves were developed to describe cerebral concussion as a nonlinear function of angular acceleration magnitude and duration. The results validated Holbourn's theory as an inverse relationship was demonstrated between brain mass and rotational acceleration magnitude, wherein primates with decreased brain mass required increased rotational acceleration magnitude to induce an equivalent injury. These results are critical to the development of experimental models incorporating smaller species, and enable the scaling of biomechanics-based thresholds from rodent models to humans (fig. 3).

Biomechanics of Blast-Induced Concussion

While this report has focused primarily on the rotational acceleration injury mechanism to this point, military personnel are exposed to risks of sustaining concussion through blast mechanisms in the contemporary military environment due to the prevalence of improvised explosive devices. The incidence of blast-induced TBI of all severities for US

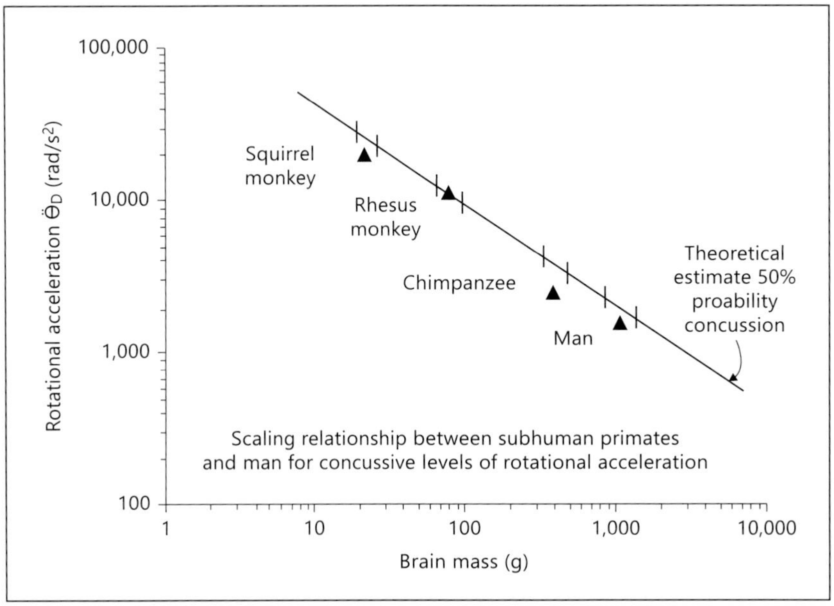

Fig. 3. Scaling relationships from primates to humans achieved using brain mass scaling ratios. Reprinted from [22] with permission from Elsevier.

veterans has risen considerably since the beginning of the conflicts in Iraq and Afghanistan. Injured veterans from previous military conflicts demonstrated primarily gunshot wounds that were focal in nature. However, a majority of head injuries sustained in the current conflicts are blast-induced [42], and are multifocal and polytraumatic in nature [43]. Multiple mechanisms of injury can result from a single blast event [44]. Three ways that TBI can occur during a blast are due to the initial overpressure wave, the blast wind accelerating the body and inducing contact with a fixed object (e.g. head impact with a wall), and/or blunt/penetrating injury from objects accelerated by the blast. The biomechanics of the last two mechanisms are more clearly understood as TBI results from more 'traditional' scenarios such as impact-induced head acceleration (discussed above) or penetration. However, the biomechanics of injury resulting from blast overpressure are less well understood. Blast produced by an explosive device includes a very fast-rising overpressure wave that has the potential to penetrate the skull and brain tissues [45]. As this pressure wave passes through the tissues, the mechanism of neural injury at the cellular level is poorly understood. The blast overpressure wave accelerates brain tissues of different densities at different relative rates, resulting in stretching and shearing forces [46]. Different brain tissues may be more susceptible to injury depending on density and material properties. Clinical presentation and chronic outcomes are affected by the severity and type of injured tissues. For example, injury to the hippocampus can lead to cognitive deficits, whereas injury to the cortex can result in motor deficits. Greater tissue distortion is generally associated with greater injury severity. Outcomes from blast exposure can be graded from concussion to severe TBI.

Injuries experienced as a consequence of blast exposure are categorized based upon the physical mechanisms resulting in biomechanical loads that exceed tolerance of the body. Primary blast injury is caused by the passage of blast overpressure waves, or shockwaves, through the tissues of the body. Secondary injury is associated with objects fragmented and propelled by the blast that can impact the body, resulting in blunt injuries. Tertiary injury is associated with the effects of the blast wind on the subject that may accelerate the body to strike a fixed object. Quaternary injuries are those not included in the other three classes. With respect to TBI, injuries can be associated with any of these injury classifications. Primary and tertiary mechanisms are responsible for closed-head TBI, which has become the most predominant injury in modern combat [47]. Penetrating injuries result from a completely different mechanism and involve skull fracture with passage of a projectile through the brain tissues. While the mechanisms of injury are better defined for tertiary injuries, involving head impact and rotational acceleration, through investigations described above, the mechanisms of injury resulting from blast overpressure are more ambiguous. This can be attributed, in part, to a general lack of consistency in experimental protocols for investigations of blast TBI that has resulted in inconsistent outcomes with regard to the timing and severity of behavioral deficits. Therefore, continued investigation is required to fully outline the influence of experimental factors, including magnitude and direction of overpressure exposure, on acute and chronic behavioral outcomes for a variety of changes relevant to the human condition, including neuromotor and cognitive deficits, elevated levels of anxiety, depression, and hedonistic behavior.

As stated above, contemporary military environments have brought the issue of blast TBI into clinical focus, which has moved the issue to the forefront of experimental research. However, experimental investigations have focused on mechanisms and outcomes using animal models since 2001 due to the high number of civilian and military war victims injured by explosive munitions during the 1990s [48–50]. With the recognition that blast TBI is a major outcome for military personnel in the wars in Iraq and Afghanistan due to the incorporation of improvised explosive devices, experimental research in this area has markedly increased in recent years. Those studies have focused on a variety of blast TBI-related issues, including effects of repeated blast exposures [51–53], biomarkers for determination of blast TBI prognosis [54, 55], imaging evidence of injury [56, 57], and behavioral changes following blast exposure [51, 57, 58].

A majority of those studies have incorporated rodent models (i.e. adult rats or mice) and shock tubes to simulate open-field blast exposure (fig. 4). Shock tubes are capable of generating a wide range of high-pressure shockwaves, with exposures simulating the primary component of open-field blast injury. Shock tubes are relatively simple experimental devices that generally consist of high- (driver) and low-pressure (driven) sections that are separated by a diaphragm. The high-pressure section is pressurized using compressed gas until it exceeds the bursting pressure of the diaphragm or until the desired pressure is attained and the diaphragm is ruptured using a mechanical device. Upon rupture of the diaphragm, an expanding pressure wave travels

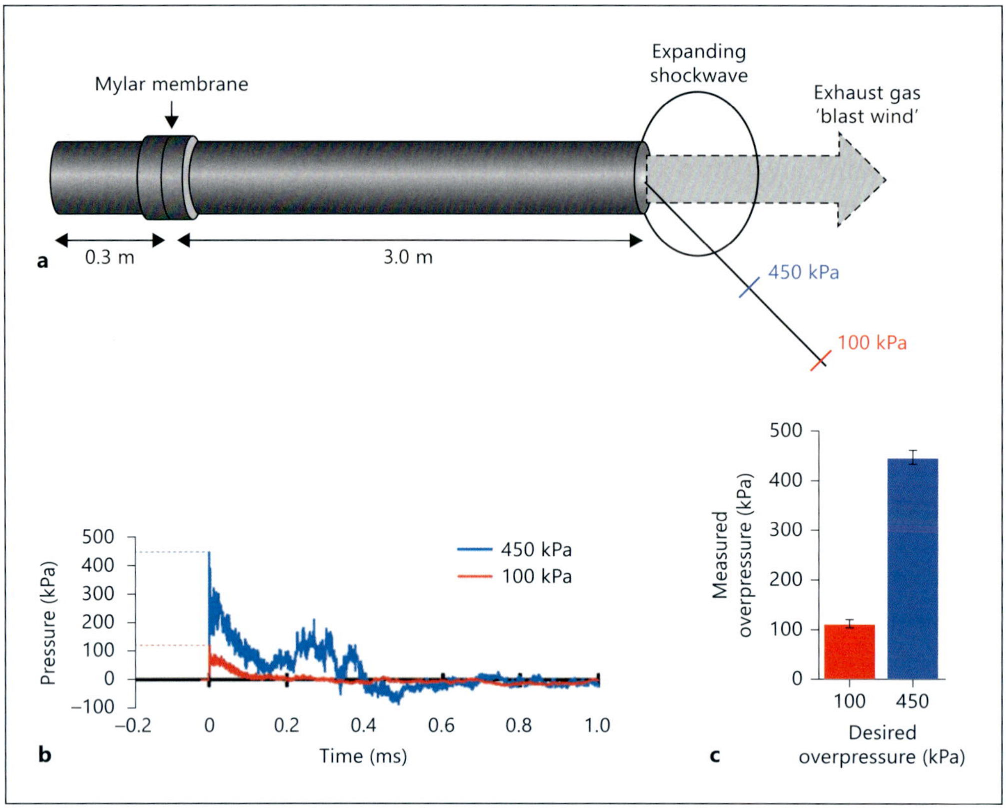

Fig. 4. a Diagram of a commonly used experimental shock tube setup for preclinical studies incorporating rodent models. **b** Experimentally recorded overpressure waves representing the Friedlander waveform with an extremely high rate of pressure onset followed by slower decay. **c** Maximum overpressure is commonly used to assess the severity of exposure, although other factors such as impulse are thought to play a role. From [57].

through the low-pressure section of the shock tube eventually forming a Friedlander-type waveform. Briefly, the characteristics of the waveform include an extremely short-duration rise (i.e. microseconds) in pressure to the peak overpressure level followed by an exponential decrease in pressure and eventual negative pressure (underpressure). Shockwave attributes are modifiable in a predictable manner using the shock tube by modulating the bursting pressure in the high-pressure section, type of pressurized gas, and controlling the ratio of driver-to-driven section lengths.

Long-Term Risks from Repetitive Concussion

Beyond the acute effects of a single mild TBI (mTBI), a growing body of evidence suggests that repetitive mTBI – either multiple injury events or cumulative subconcussive trauma – may be associated with an increased cumulative risk of chronic neurologic, neuropsychiatric, and neurobehavioral problems. Among the reported issues associated with repetitive concussion are increased risks of subsequent concussion, slower recovery time after an injury event, chronically elevated postconcussive symptoms, and long-term problems in memory and cognitive functioning [38, 39, 59]. The existing literature is based largely on results from studies of athletes with reported history of multiple mTBI events, with a smaller number of studies looking at the chronic effects of subconcussive contact through routine participation in contact or collision sports. Based on reports of multiple mTBI events and repetitive blast exposure, there are looming concerns about chronic effects of repetitive mTBI or subconcussive events in veterans.

The cumulative effect of repetitive concussive exposures under either blast or rotational mechanisms is dependent upon a number of exposure-related factors including the number of exposures, the relative severity of the exposures, and the frequency of the exposures. In general, a higher number of TBI, more severe TBI, and more frequent TBI are associated with higher levels of morbidity. These factors have been outlined to some degree in preclinical literature using rodent models of TBI. For example, three exposures to either weight drop, lateral fluid percussion, or impact acceleration injuries resulted in significant behavioral changes, including motor and cognitive deficits [60–62]. Likewise, more frequent exposures to multiple insults led to more deleterious behavioral outcomes [63]. However, a majority of those investigations were somewhat limited by incorporating rodent injury models that did not recreate accurate biomechanics and, therefore, the pathological cascade may be different, resulting in different behavioral manifestations, and biomechanical information is not directly scalable to the human.

Chronic Traumatic Encephalopathy

In addition to the concerns about chronic postconcussion symptoms and cognitive dysfunction, more recent reports are raising serious speculation that repetitive mTBI or cumulative subconcussive exposure may be associated with increased risk and earlier onset of neurodegenerative disease (i.e. dementia). While case studies of boxers affected by dementia go back several decades, more recent high-profile cases of retired football players and other nonboxing athletes affected by dementia have brought these concerns to the forefront of governing bodies in sports, the media, and the US Congress.

A growing number of postmortem examinations of the brains of athletes exposed to repetitive mTBI have provided case-series evidence of long-term effects from multiple mTBI events suffered earlier in life [64–67]. The distinctive neurodegenerative syndrome described in pathological studies of retired athletes is known as chronic traumatic encephalopathy (CTE), previously observed as 'punch drunk' syndrome or dementia pugilistica in boxers [66–68]. Recent reports cite the prevalence of CTE in nonboxers, including retired football players and other athletes [64, 69]. Less severe forms of CTE have also reportedly been identified in a small number of military veterans who are considerably younger than the athletes described in the literature [70].

CTE is a progressive brain disease that is pathologically and clinically distinctive from probable Alzheimer's disease and other common neurodegenerative diseases [64, 71]. Pathologically, CTE is characterized by extensive tau-immunoreactive neurofibrillary tangles and astrocytic tangles predominately distributed throughout the frontal and temporal cortices in a patchy, superficial distribution, with focal deposition at the depths of sulci and around small vessels. There are extensive tau neurofibrillary tangles in the limbic and paralimbic regions, diencephalon, basal ganglia, and brainstem. There is a relative paucity of β-amyloid deposits, although diffuse plaques are present in approximately 50% of cases. In advanced forms of CTE, there are also macroscopic abnormalities characterized by generalized cerebral atrophy and enlarged ventricles, atrophy of the medial temporal lobe structures and mammillary bodies, cavum septi pellucidi, and pallor of the substantia nigra [69]. To evaluate the hypothesis that chronic subconcussive exposures leads to CTE, the right combination of biomechanics will need to be determined from either well-controlled human studies or animal models. Existing animal models may yet help us understand the etiology of this disease.

Conclusion

Historically, concussion biomechanics were associated with head impact resulting in high rate head rotational acceleration. Experimental research has highlighted the effect of acceleration parameters, including magnitude, duration, and direction, on injury outcomes. However, significant efforts are still required to understand concussion tolerance to single and, perhaps more importantly, repetitive head impact scenarios. Unfortunately, a limited number of researchers are focused on concussion biomechanics, although an understanding of injury tolerance is likely to yield significant future benefits given the continued incorporation of head acceleration sensors in sporting and military environments. It is conceivable that these sensors could form the link between active sporting participation and head impact exposure limits that would be designed to limit participation prior to the onset of significant chronic illnesses. However, this information must be used responsibly and therefore significant validated data regarding concussion tolerance must be realized. Focusing research efforts on biomechanics tolerance to single and repetitive concussive and sub concussive exposures is the first step to realistic and validated exposure limits to protect athletes and military personnel.

References

1 Denny-Brown D, Russell WR: Experimental cerebral concussion. J Physiol 1940;99:153.
2 Gurdjian ES, Roberts VL, Thomas LM: Tolerance curves of acceleration and intracranial pressure and protective index in experimental head injury. J Trauma 1966;6:600–604.
3 Lissner HR, Lebow M, Evans FG: Experimental studies on the relation between acceleration and intracranial pressure changes in man. Surg Gynecol Obstet 1960;111:329–338.
4 Gurdjian ES, Lissner HR, Evans FG, Patrick LM, Hardy WG: Intracranial pressure and acceleration accompanying head impacts in human cadavers. Surg Gynecol Obstet 1961;113:185–190.
5 Versace J: A review of the severity index. 15th Stapp Car Crash Conference, San Diego, 1971.
6 Gennarelli TA, Thibault LE, Ommaya AK: Pathophysiological responses to rotational and translational accelerations of the head. 16th Stapp Car Crash Conference, Detroit, 1972.
7 Hirsch AE, Ommaya AK: Protection from brain injury: the relative significance of translational and rotational motions of the head after impact. 14th Stapp Car Crash Conference, Ann Arbor, 1970.
8 Ommaya AK, Hirsch AE, Martinez JL: The role of whiplash in cerebral concussion. 10th Stapp Car Crash Conference, New York, 1966.
9 Zhang J, Yoganandan N, Pintar FA, Gennarelli TA: Role of translational and rotational accelerations on brain strain in lateral head impact. Biomed Sci Instrum 2006;42:501–506.
10 Ommaya AK, Fisch FJ, Mahone RM, Caorrao P, Letcher F: Comparative Tolerances for Cerebral Concussion by Head Impact and Whiplash Injury in Primates. Warrendale, Society of Automotive Engineers, 1970.
11 Holbourn AHS: Mechanics of head injuries. Lancet 1943;2:438–441.
12 Gennarelli TA, Thibault LE, Ommaya AK: Comparison of translational and rotational acceleration in experimental cerebral concussion. 15th Stapp Car Crash Conference, San Diego, 1971.
13 Gennarelli TA, Adams JH, Graham DI: Acceleration induced head injury in the monkey. I. The model, its mechanical and physiological correlates. Acta Neuropathol Suppl 1981;7:23–25.
14 Lamy M, Baumgartner D, Willinger R, Yoganandan N, Stemper BD: Study of mild traumatic brain injuries using experiments and finite element modeling. Ann Adv Automot Med 2011;55:125–135.
15 Li J, Zhang J, Yoganandan N, Pintar F, Gennarelli T: Regional brain strains and role of falx in lateral impact-induced head rotational acceleration. Biomed Sci Instrum 2007;43:24–29.
16 Mao H, Zhang L, Jiang B, Genthikatti VV, Jin X, Zhu F, Makwana R, Gill A, Jandir G, Singh A, Yang KH: Development of a finite element human head model partially validated with thirty five experimental cases. J Biomech Eng 2013;135:111002–111015.
17 Gennarelli TA, Thibault LE, Tomei G, Wiser R, Graham DI, Adams JH: Directional dependence of axonal brain injury due to centroidal and non-centroidal acceleration. 31st Stapp Car Crash Conference, New Orleans, 1987.
18 Margulies SS, Thibault LE: A proposed tolerance criterion for diffuse axonal injury in man. J Biomech 1992;25:917–923.
19 Margulies SS, Thibault LE, Gennarelli TA: Physical model simulations of brain injury in the primate. J Biomech 1990;23:823–836.
20 Thibault LE, Gennarelli TA: Brain injury: an analysis of neural and neurovascular trauma in the nonhuman primate. 34th Annual Proceedings of the Association for the Advancement of Automotive Medicine, Scottsdale, 1990.
21 Gennarelli TA, Thibault LE, Adams JH, Graham DI, Thompson CJ, Marcincin RP: Diffuse axonal injury and traumatic coma in the primate. Ann Neurol 1982;12:564–574.
22 Ommaya AK, Hirsch AE: Tolerances for cerebral concussion from head impact and whiplash in primates. J Biomech 1971;4:13–21.
23 Ommaya AK, Corrao P, Letcher FS: Head injury in the chimpanzee. 1. Biodynamics of traumatic unconsciousness. J Neurosurg 1973;39:152–166.
24 Abel JM, Gennarelli TA, Segawa H: Incidence and severity of cerebral concussion in the rhesus monkey following sagittal plane angular acceleration. 22nd Stapp Car Crash Conference, Ann Arbor, 1978.
25 Gennarelli TA, Pintar FA, Yoganandan N: Biomechanical tolerances for diffuse brain injury and a hypothesis for genotypic variability in response to trauma. 47th Annual Proceedings of the Association for the Advancement of Automotive Medicine, Lisbon, 2003.
26 Bazarian JJ, Fisher SG, Flesher W, Lillis R, Knox KL, Pearson TA: Lateral automobile impacts and the risk of traumatic brain injury. Ann Emerg Med 2004;44: 142–152.
27 Higgins LS, Schmall RA: Device for investigation of head injury effected by non-deforming head accelerations. 11th Stapp Car Crash Conference, Anaheim, 1967.
28 Fijalkowski RJ, Stemper BD, Pintar FA, Yoganandan N, Gennarelli TA: Influence of insult duration on unconscious time following concussion. International IRCOBI Conference on the Biomechanics of Impact, Maastricht, 2007, pp 161–171.

29 Ono K, Kikuchi A, Nakamura M, Kobayashi H, Nakamura N: Human head tolerance to sagittal impact reliable estimation deduced from experimental head injury using subhuman primates and human cadaver skulls. 24th Stapp Car Crash Conference, Troy, 1980.
30 Rowson S, Duma SM, Beckwith JG, Chu JJ, Greenwald RM, Crisco JJ, Brolinson PG, Duhaime AC, McAllister TW, Maerlender AC: Rotational head kinematics in football impacts: an injury risk function for concussion. Ann Biomed Eng 2012;40:1–13.
31 Ommaya AK, Yarnell P, Hirsch AE: Scaling of experimental data on cerebral concussion in subhuman primates to concussion threshold for man. 11th Stapp Car Crash Conference, Anaheim, 1967.
32 Ommaya AK, Rockoff SD, Baldwin M: Experimental concussion; a first report. J Neurosurg 1964;21:249–265.
33 Higgens LS, Unterharnscheidt F: Pathomorphology of experimental head injury due to rotational acceleration. Acta Neuropathol 1969;12:200–204.
34 Breedlove EL, Robinson M, Talavage TM, Morigaki KE, Yoruk U, O'Keefe K, King J, Leverenz LJ, Gilger JW, Nauman EA: Biomechanical correlates of symptomatic and asymptomatic neurophysiological impairment in high school football. J Biomech 2012;45:1265–1272.
35 McCrea M, Guskiewicz KM, Marshall SW, Barr W, Randolph C, Cantu RC, Onate JA, Yang J, Kelly JP: Acute effects and recovery time following concussion in collegiate football players: the NCAA Concussion Study. JAMA 2003;290:2556–2563.
36 Talavage TM, Nauman EA, Breedlove EL, Yoruk U, Dye AE, Morigaki KE, Feuer H, Leverenz LJ: Functionally-detected cognitive impairment in high school football players without clinically-diagnosed concussion. J Neurotrauma 2013, Epub ahead of print.
37 Guskiewicz KM, Marshall SW, Bailes J, McCrea M, Cantu RC, Randolph C, Jordan BD: Association between recurrent concussion and late-life cognitive impairment in retired professional football players. Neurosurgery 2005;57:719–726.
38 Guskiewicz KM, Marshall SW, Bailes J, McCrea M, Harding HP Jr, Matthews A, Mihalik JR, Cantu RC: Recurrent concussion and risk of depression in retired professional football players. Med Sci Sports Exerc 2007;39:903–909.
39 Guskiewicz KM, McCrea M, Marshall SW, Cantu RC, Randolph C, Barr W, Onate JA, Kelly JP: Cumulative effects associated with recurrent concussion in collegiate football players: the NCAA Concussion Study. JAMA 2003;290:2549–2555.
40 Fijalkowski RJ, Stemper BD, Pintar FA, Yoganandan N, Crowe MJ, Gennarelli TA: New rat model for diffuse brain injury using coronal plane angular acceleration. J Neurotrauma 2007;24:1387–1398.
41 Davidsson J, Risling M: A new model to produce sagittal plane rotational induced diffuse axonal injuries. Front Neurol 2011;2:41.
42 Hoge CW, McGurk D, Thomas JL, Cox AL, Engel CC, Castro CA: Mild traumatic brain injury in U.S. soldiers returning from Iraq. N Engl J Med 2008;358:453–463.
43 Bauman RA, Ling G, Tong L, Januszkiewicz A, Agoston D, Delanerolle N, Kim Y, Ritzel D, Bell R, Ecklund J, Armonda R, Bandak F, Parks S: An introductory characterization of a combat-casualty-care relevant swine model of closed head injury resulting from exposure to explosive blast. J Neurotrauma 2009;26:841–860.
44 Ling G, Bandak F, Armonda R, Grant G, Ecklund J: Explosive blast neurotrauma. J Neurotrauma 2009;26:815–825.
45 Shah AS, Stemper BD, Yoganandan N, Pintar FA, Rangarajan N, Hallman JJ, Shender BS: Methodology to study attenuation of a blast wave through the cranium. ASME 2011 International Mechanical Engineering Congress and Exposition, Denver, 2011.
46 Taber KH, Warden DL, Hurley RA: Blast-related traumatic brain injury. J Neuropsychiatry Clin Neurosci 2006;18:141–145.
47 Warden D: Military TBI during the Iraq and Afghanistan wars. J Head Trauma Rehabil 2006;21:398–402.
48 Saljo A, Bao F, Haglid KG, Hansson HA: Blast exposure causes redistribution of phosphorylated neurofilament subunits in neurons of the adult rat brain. J Neurotrauma 2000;17:719–726.
49 Cernak I, Wang Z, Jiang J, Bian X, Savic J: Cognitive deficits following blast injury-induced neurotrauma: possible involvement of nitric oxide. Brain Inj 2001;15:593–612.
50 Cernak I, Wang Z, Jiang J, Bian X, Savic J: Ultrastructural and functional characteristics of blast injury-induced neurotrauma. J Trauma 2001;50:695–706.
51 Ahlers ST, Vasserman-Stokes E, Shaughness MC, Hall AA, Shear DA, Chavko M, McCarron RM, Stone JR: Assessment of the effects of acute and repeated exposure to blast overpressure in rodents: toward a greater understanding of blast and the potential ramifications for injury in humans exposed to blast. Front Neurol 2012;3:32.
52 Wang Y, Wei Y, Oguntayo S, Wilkins W, Arun P, Valiyaveettil M, Song J, Long JB, Nambiar MP: Tightly coupled repetitive blast-induced traumatic brain injury: development and characterization in mice. J Neurotrauma 2011;28:2171–2183.
53 Elsayed NM, Gorbunov NV: Pulmonary biochemical and histological alterations after repeated low-level blast overpressure exposures. Toxicol Sci 2007;95:289–296.

54 Balakathiresan N, Bhomia M, Chandran R, Chavko M, McCarron RM, Maheshwari RK: MicroRNA let-7i is a promising serum biomarker for blast-induced traumatic brain injury. J Neurotrauma 2012;29: 1379–1387.
55 Dalle Lucca JJ, Chavko M, Dubick MA, Adeeb S, Falabella MJ, Slack JL, McCarron R, Li Y: Blast-induced moderate neurotrauma (BINT) elicits early complement activation and tumor necrosis factor α (TNFα) release in a rat brain. J Neurol Sci 2012;318:146–154.
56 Bir C, Vandevord P, Shen Y, Raza W, Haacke EM: Effects of variable blast pressures on blood flow and oxygen saturation in rat brain as evidenced using MRI. Magn Reson Imaging 2012;30:527–534.
57 Budde MD, Shah A, McCrea M, Cullinan WE, Pintar FA, Stemper BD: Primary blast traumatic brain injury in the rat: relating diffusion tensor imaging and behavior. Front Neurol 2013;4:154.
58 Elder GA, Dorr NP, De Gasperi R, Gama Sosa MA, Shaughness MC, Maudlin-Jeronimo E, Hall AA, McCarron RM, Ahlers ST: Blast exposure induces post-traumatic stress disorder-related traits in a rat model of mild traumatic brain injury. J Neurotrauma 2012; 29:2564–2575.
59 Iverson GL, Gaetz M, Lovell MR, Collins MW: Cumulative effects of concussion in amateur athletes. Brain Inj 2004;18:433–443.
60 DeFord SM, Wilson MS, Rice AC, Clausen T, Rice LK, Barabnova A, Bullock R, Hamm RJ: Repeated mild brain injuries result in cognitive impairment in B6C3F1 mice. J Neurotrauma 2002;19:427–438.
61 Shultz SR, Bao F, Omana V, Chiu C, Brown A, Cain DP: Repeated mild lateral fluid percussion brain injury in the rat causes cumulative long-term behavioral impairments, neuroinflammation, and cortical loss in an animal model of repeated concussion. J Neurotrauma 2012;29:281–294.
62 Bolouri H, Säljö A, Viano DC, Hamberger A: Animal model for sport-related concussion; ICP and cognitive function. Acta Neurol Scand 2012;125:241–247.
63 Longhi L, Saatman KE, Fujimoto S, Raghupathi R, Meaney DF, Davis J, McMillan BSA, Conte V, Laurer HL, Stein S, Stocchetti N, McIntosh TK: Temporal window of vulnerability to repetitive experimental concussive brain injury. Neurosurgery 2005;56: 364–374.
64 McKee AC, Cantu RC, Nowinski CJ, Hedley-Whyte ET, Gavett BE, Budson AE, Santini VE, Lee HS, Kubilus CA, Stern RA: Chronic traumatic encephalopathy in athletes: progressive tauopathy after repetitive head injury. J Neuropathol Exp Neurol 2009;68:709–735.
65 Omalu BI, DeKosky ST, Minster RL, Kamboh MI, Hamilton RL, Wecht CH: Chronic traumatic encephalopathy in a National Football League player. Neurosurgery 2005;57:128–134.
66 Mortimer JA: Epidemiology of post-traumatic encephalopathy in boxers. Minn Med 1985;68:299–300.
67 Sabharwal RK, Sanchetee PC, Sethi PK, Dhamija RM: Chronic traumatic encephalopathy in boxers. J Assoc Physicians India 1987;35:571–573.
68 (Ex?) dementia pugilistica in ex-boxers. JAMA 1969; 210:2272.
69 Gavett BE, Stern RA, McKee AC: Chronic traumatic encephalopathy: a potential late effect of sport-related concussive and subconcussive head trauma. Clin Sports Med 2011;30:179–188, xi.
70 Omalu B, Hammers JL, Bailes J, Hamilton RL, Kamboh MI, Webster G, Fitzsimmons RP: Chronic traumatic encephalopathy in an Iraqi war veteran with posttraumatic stress disorder who committed suicide. Neurosurg Focus 2011;31:E3.
71 Gavett BE, Cantu RC, Shenton M, Lin AP, Nowinski CJ, McKee AC, Stern RA: Clinical appraisal of chronic traumatic encephalopathy: current perspectives and future directions. Curr Opin Neurol 2011; 24:525–531.

Brian D. Stemper, PhD
Department of Neurosurgery, Zablocki VA Medical Center
Neuroscience Research Labs-151
5000 W. National Ave., Milwaukee, WI 53295 (USA)
E-Mail bstemper@mcw.edu

Niranjan A, Lunsford LD (eds): Concussion. Prog Neurol Surg. Basel, Karger, 2014, vol 28, pp 28–37
DOI: 10.1159/000358749

The Neurophysiology of Concussion

David A. Hovda

Department of Neurosurgery, David Geffen School of Medicine at UCLA, Los Angeles, Calif., USA

Abstract

The following report reviews our current understanding of the neurobiological response to concussion which is often referred to as mild traumatic brain injury. The historical accomplishments to reveal the brain's response to this injury are discussed along with the neurochemical and metabolic cascade that results in an energy crisis. The massive ionic flux induced by cerebral concussion is discussed as it pertains to primarily potassium and calcium. The ensuing metabolic demands placed on cells exposed to this ionic flux is discussed as it relates to an injury-induced diaschisis. As this cascade produces neuronal dysfunction and corresponding deficits, it also results in a state of vulnerability to secondary insults and long-term neurological problems. While experimental studies are the primary focus of this report, relevant human observations are discussed and put into context. It is now clear that cerebral concussion is not a benign event. It carries with it neuroscientific consequences that result in symptoms and an increase in risk for many other challenges to the central nervous system.

© 2014 S. Karger AG, Basel

The concept of a dysfunctional brain following a concussion has been described for several centuries. Therefore, the concept that concussion is a mild traumatic brain injury (TBI) is well founded in the clinical and scientific literature. One of the more interesting concepts related to injuries to the human brain that produce temporary deficits was introduced by Constantin von Monakow in the early 1900s [1]. The key to understanding the mechanism(s) by which symptoms would appear and then over time subside eluded investigators for many years, and there was no hard scientific evidence why brain cells that were not biomechanically and irreversibly damaged were so vulnerable to secondary insults. Early studies in experimental TBI referred to intense excitation of the central nervous system at the moment of a blow to the head, which was thought to produce neurochemical changes given the interpretations of indirect measurements. Work by Walker and colleagues [2] studying cerebral concussion in various animals provided some of the first physiological recordings during the acute period after TBI. While many others had also conducted electroencephalographic (EEG) recordings early after TBI, the paper by Walker was one of the first to put forth the notion that trauma to the head produced a state of activation within the brain and not simply paralysis.

Much of this earlier work focused on measurement of cerebral electrical changes, the presence of acetylcholine in the cerebral spinal fluid, and cerebral circulation [3]. From electrical recordings, early investigators proposed that the electrical phenomena following concussion could be explained in terms of neuronal excitation as opposed to traumatic paralysis. This electrical discharge at the moment of injury was thought to be due to the depolarization of many cells and that this neuronal activation was the result of pressure waves induced by the blow. Consequently, the cell membrane would change its permeability allowing electrolytes to pass freely to and from the cell that most likely would be the basis for cerebral edema.

It was thought that the breakdown of the membrane would last for a short period of time. However, it was proposed that the acute breakdown would produce secondary factors such as anoxemia, hypoglycemia, edema, reduction in pH, loss of electrolytes, and accumulation of lactic acid. All of these secondary factors could impede the recovery of neurons that were not biomechanically and irreversibly damaged at the time of injury. Consequently, these proposed sequelae were thought to be the basis for neuronal dysfunction that would produce symptoms that could not otherwise be explained by cell death.

Such was the state of our understanding of the neurochemical pathomechanisms associated with mild TBI during the middle of the 20th century. It should be noted, however, that investigators at that time referred to the proposed neurochemical changes of TBI as the physiological response to TBI. It would later be referred to as the pathophysiology of TBI. New evidence suggesting that the former refers to physiology and not pathophysiology may be more accurate in describing the central nervous system's response to trauma.

As technology advanced over the years, it became possible to directly measure the neurotransmitters released by TBI-induced excitation as well as to detect the corresponding changes in neurochemistry. In terms of the conduction of these types of measurements during or after brain injury, most investigators focused on the responses to cerebral ischemia. Thought to be a 'cleaner' insult and getting around the inherent factors associated with the heterogeneity of TBI, many of the first insights into brain injury-induced changes in neurochemistry were done in models of cerebral ischemia/hypoxia. Nevertheless, investigators conducting work in both basic and clinical science have made great progress toward our understanding of the neurotransmitter, neurochemical, and neurometabolic response to TBI. These studies have demonstrated the unique aspect of trauma and the impact these postinjury changes have on cell death (or survival), cellular vulnerability, and/or dysfunction. The following brief review addresses the changes in neurotransmitters, the effects on ionic distribution, the implications for secondary cell death, edema, changes in cerebral metabolism, and the resulting impact on neuroplasticity and recovery of function.

Excitatory Neurotransmitters and Ionic Flux following Concussion

With the development of cerebral microdialysis it became possible to directly measure the concentration of the extracellular spaces after mild TBI in animals. Utilizing the fluid percussion (FPI) model of mild TBI in rodents [4], investigators began to determine that, in fact, the early electrophysiological studies were accurate in the conclusion that cerebral concussion resulted in an active response by the central nervous system. This active response consisted of the synaptic release of many neurotransmitters; however, the excitatory amino acid glutamate revealed itself as playing a fundamental role in the massive flux of ions and the resulting compromise of neuronal functioning which not only led to temporary deficits, but also to a state of energy crisis and vulnerability. In experimental animals it was determined that after FPI the dorsal hippocampus exhibited a very brief release of glutamate. In a series of elegant experiments, Katayama et al. [5] demonstrated that a mild FPI-induced release of glutamate was temporally related to the increase in extracellular potassium. In addition, these investigators conducted an injury severity study that illustrated a threshold for the concussion-induced massive increase in extracellular potassium. At levels of injury severity in which the hippocampus exhibited a small insignificant release of potassium for the first minute, it was determined that this was primarily due to concussion-induced synaptic activity. However, at a threshold described as 200 s for a righting response to return, a 'supra-physiological' level of potassium was reported. Furthermore, by using microdialysis as a delivery system pre-FPI, these investigators were able to determine that blocking synaptic activity had no effect on the more massive 'supra-physiological' levels, although it would stop the subthreshold release of potassium. These higher levels could, however, significantly reduce the preinjury administration of glutamatergic antagonists.

Given the history of calcium's role in the pathophysiology of cerebral ischemia, investigators studying TBI determined that calcium was involved in mild levels of injury. As described by others, calcium has always been known to have a fundamental role in central nervous system injury and corresponding cell death. At issue here in mild TBI was whether intracellular calcium would increase in cells that were not necessarily going to die, like what would be anticipated in cerebral concussion.

It was determined that even in mild TBI, using an FPI model in rats, calcium would accumulate in tissue that was not necessarily going on to die. Furthermore, following a lateral FPI, the regional and temporal characteristics of calcium accumulation were somewhat different than that reported for potassium and may be related to the well-described mitochondrial dysfunction. However, comparing calcium autoradiography to microdialysis results is not straightforward as the former provides regional information at a single time point, whereas the latter provides focal information in a within-subject design. Nevertheless, the consequences of the increase in extracellular potassium and the intracellular increase in calcium have particular significance in the metabolic demand of the tissue and its corresponding vulnerability after concussion.

In sum, the increase in extracellular potassium places an energy demand on cells to activate the sodium-potassium pump which is supported by adenosine triphosphate and the increase of intracellular calcium, which can be buffered by the mitochondria resulting in a reduction of this organelle's capacity to produce adenosine triphosphate via oxidative metabolism.

The Metabolic Cascade and Corresponding Vulnerability

As early as 1940, investigators were concerned that human cerebral concussion may be due to compression and displacement of the 'nutritive cerebrospinal fluid' that would deprive neurons of glucose, thereby resulting in a transient interruption of cerebral function [6]. With the FPI-induced increase in extracellular potassium it was hypothesized that there would be an increase in the use of glucose metabolism to activate the sodium potassium pump, which is the normal method by which cells equilibrate their ionic homeostasis. In cats using the arterial-venous difference, Andersen and Marmarou [7] reported a significant increase in the uptake of cerebral glucose acutely following FPI. It should be noted, however, that in an earlier study where investigators combined magnetic resonance spectroscopy and tissue pH measurements with periodic measurements following injury in cats, there was no evidence of metabolic changes seen later than 30 min after FPI [8].

With the development of [^{14}C] 2-deoxy-D-glucose autoradiography (2DG) came the ability to evaluate regional utilization of glucose for cerebral metabolism. Consequently, investigators began to use this technique following experimental mild TBI and found an acute increase in glucose uptake regionally. This uptake of glucose was determined to be on the order of minutes after FPI with different regions of the brain exhibiting various levels of metabolism. In fact, one group of scientists reported an increase in glucose metabolism within the brain stem of cats following FPI, suggesting that this may reflect the mechanism by which unconsciousness occurs following concussion.

In a series of experiments addressing the mechanism(s) by which the FPI would induce an increase of glucose metabolism, it was determined that this increase was due to the same mechanism(s) that caused the increase in extracellular potassium. Two experimental studies stand out in terms of directly addressing this issue. The first used a combination of microdialysis and 2DG where bilateral microdialysis probes were inserted into the cerebral cortex of rats and different types of excitatory amino acid antagonists were infused prior to injury followed by an acute 2DG study of each animal [9]. This study revealed that the preinfusion of kynurenic acid, 2-amino-5-phosphonovaleric acid, and 6-cyano-7-nitroquinoxaline-2,3-dione (CNQX) in a dose-dependent fashion revealed that although all subtypes of the glutamate receptor were involved in the post-FPI increase in glucose metabolism, the N-methyl-D-aspartate-activated channel (NMDA) played the most significant role. As is always the case in terms of evaluating 2DG autoradiography in pathological conditions, one is concerned regarding the 'steady state' assumptions required by the original equation to calculate the cerebral metabolic rate for glucose.

In terms of concern, the most likely problem would be that of a compromised blood-brain barrier or contamination of the tissue from microdialysis. In order to address some of these concerns, investigators designed an experiment that had been performed in models of cerebral ischemia addressing similar issues. In these experiments, investigators set out to determine if endogenous glutamate innervation of the CA_1 region of the hippocampus can provide an anatomical basis for a proposed mechanism behind the FPI-induced increase in glucose metabolism within the hippocampus. Five days prior to a lateral FPI, kainic acid (0.5 μg) was injected into the left ventricle, which resulted in unilateral severe cell loss within the CA_3 region, thereby eliminating the glutamatergic projection to CA_1. Immediately after lateral FPI, the 2DG study revealed that removal of the CA_3 projection to CA_1 protected these cells from the increase in glucose metabolism typically seen after FPI. More importantly, the contralateral hippocampus that remained intact as well as the overlying cerebral cortex bilaterally exhibited the post-FPI-induced increase in glucose metabolism. This strongly suggested that any compromise of the blood-brain barrier or a significant reduction in cerebral blood flow in interpreting the 2DG findings did not play a significant role.

In related studies it was determined that following FPI there is an increase in cerebral lactate, the byproduct of anaerobic glycolysis. Here again, investigators using microdialysis detected lactate acutely after FPI when the 2DG studies revealed an increase in glucose metabolism. In addition, using a similar approach for the experimental design for 2DG studies [9], kynurenic acid, ouabain, or barium were administered prior to injury [10]. The accumulation of lactate after FPI was attenuated by the preinjury administration of ouabain and kynurenic acid, and prolonged by barium. These results were interpreted as confirming that the lactate accumulation following FPI was the result of increased glycolysis to support ion-pumping mechanisms, thereby restoring the ionic balance which was disruption of stimulation of excitatory amino acid-coupled ion channels.

Given these acute neurochemical and metabolic findings, investigators began to look at the more long-term consequences of concussion of cerebral metabolism and any relationship to function. Two different studies addressed these issues systematically. Using 2DG or cytochrome oxidase histochemistry [11] to study rats at different times after lateral FPI, it was determined that the acute increase in glucose utilization was followed by a longer period of metabolic depression. This length of injury-induced metabolic depression lasted for up to 10 days and was not associated with levels of frank cerebral ischemia or with gross morphological cell death. Utilizing positron emission tomography (PET) modified for rodents, Moore et al. [12] were able to conduct a within-subject design comparing and contrasting the length of time of cerebral glucose depression and its spontaneous recovery with the recovery from injury-induced neurocognitive deficits. Although these animals did not exhibit frank ischemia, they did reveal a loss of coupling between neuronal activation and cerebral blood flow which could be reinstated with the administration of verapamil [13]. In addition, there is evidence for mitochondrial dysfunction and/or damage in experimental TBI.

These studies began to reveal that following concussion, cells in the brain were compromised in their ability to function, which resulted in deficits that spontaneously subsided with metabolic recovery. However, these studies also point to a period of time after concussion when the brain is not stable enough to absorb another energy demand which could be associated with a second injury or activation.

Evidence of a Postconcussive Vulnerable Brain

Investigators have been well aware that TBI places the brain in a vulnerable state. The literature is filled with efforts to protect the injured brain from seizures, cerebral hypertension, hyperthermia, and other types of secondary insults. Seminal papers by Becker, Jenkins, and colleagues [14, 15] demonstrated that following FPI, cells that were not biomechanically and irreversibly damaged were vulnerable to a sublethal level of reduction in cerebral blood flow. However, there have been studies indicating that FPI may produce a state of preconditioning for a second insult, but this may be restricted to time after injury, injury severity, or the age of the animal [16, 17].

There are most likely many different mechanisms by which cells become vulnerable after concussion. In terms of the neurochemical and neurometabolic cascade induced by injury, investigators have determined that a second concussion sustained during the period when rodents are recovering from the first injury produces a more prolonged period of cellular dysfunction and even cell death. Given the literature on post-TBI cellular vulnerability, it is not surprising that second insults that occur close in time would be extremely damaging to the brain. One only needs to explore the history of dementia pugilistica. However, following cerebral concussion, what may not be as clear is whether cells are too compromised to respond appropriately to physiological activation. For example, in human concussion, athletes who participate in high levels of activity shortly after injury exhibited worse neurocognitive performance than those who were more rested. There is evidence, however, that controlled exercise may be of benefit.

In addressing this question, there are experiments that have addressed electrical activation of the cerebral cortex after FPI as well as normal exercise. In terms of the former, following lateral FPI, rodents that received a direct cortical stimulation to the barrel field area of the concussed hemisphere not only exhibited an increase in cerebral glucose metabolism, but also significant cell death. Given that, as noted above, the concussed brain temporarily loses its cerebral blood flow to neuronal activation coupling [13], the combination of these studies points to the effect of an energy crisis after concussion which, if not recognized and managed properly, can result in permanent damage.

In an effort to enhance the upregulation of brain-derived neurotrophic factor after mild FPI, Griesbach et al. [18–20] proposed exposing injured rats to exercise. Although the review of this work is beyond the scope of this report, these investigators discovered that if animals were exposed to a voluntary running wheel soon after concussion, they would run spontaneously; however, when they were tested for spatial learning, their performance got worse and their brains did not respond in terms of upregulating brain-derived neurotrophic factor. However, if the investigators waited until the neurochemical and metabolic status normalized after concussion, voluntary exercise did result in neurocognitive improvement and an upregulation of brain-derived neurotrophic factor.

The concept of vulnerability may not necessarily be restricted to secondary cell death or a greater degree of neurological deficits. It may also be reflected in the compromising of the surviving cells to express plasticity. In a series of experiments in young developing rats, postnatal day 17–21 animals who sustained mild FPI were not capable of exhibiting the neuroanatomical and cognitive benefits of being raised in an enriched environment. However, just as in the voluntary exercise studies described above, if the exposure to an enriched environment is delayed until after the energy crisis subsides, then the capacity for plasticity in response to exposure to an enriched environment is reinstated [21]. This original finding was replicated in more detail and it was determined that the mechanism(s) behind this concussion-induced loss of capacity for plasticity may be related to alterations of the subunits of the same NMDA receptors that play such an important role in the neurochemical and metabolic cascade described above [22, 23]. It is interesting to note that following concussion in humans, there also appears to be changes in plasticity as studied using transcranial magnetic stimulation in the absence of magnetic resonance imaging (MRI), diffusion tensor imaging, or objective neuropsychological deficits.

Evidence of Neurochemical and Metabolic Cascade in Human Concussion

Most of the work associated with human concussion have been assessments of neuropsychological-neurological deficits, EEG recordings, and/or postmortem analysis of brain tissue. It was not until the development of sophisticated noninvasive imaging that acute studies for both cerebral metabolism and neurochemistry could be performed. The use of computed tomography (CT) did provide some insight into the damage caused in boxing; however, most patients who suffer from a concussion rarely exhibit abnormalities on a CT scan of the brain, although they may present with postconcussive symptoms. The introduction of PET revealed that acutely after TBI, even patients who have a diagnosis of a mild level of injury (as determined as having a Glasgow Coma Score of 14–15) produce a glucose uptake response similar to what is seen in animals [24].

In addressing the neurochemical signature of concussion, investigators have used magnetic resonance spectroscopy [25, 26]. Studying athletes from various sports in Europe, these investigators described a reduction in the N-acetylaspartate-creatine ratio after a single concussive event, which can last as long as 30 days. If these injured athletes sustain a second concussion while recovering from the first, the length of time for this ratio to recover to normal can exceed 45 days. Furthermore, others have described disruptions of connectivity within the concussed brain using MRI which would have gone undetected with CT.

In addition to these neurometabolic and neurochemical studies, researchers have used diffusion tensor imaging to explore the degree to which white matter disruption exists following cerebral concussion. In varsity level college athletes who had suffered a cerebral concussion without a loss of consciousness but who also exhibited symptoms for at least 1 month after injury, structural alterations were detected in several fiber tracts within the left hemisphere, including parts of the inferior/superior longitudinal and fronto-occipital fasciculi, the retrolenticular part of the internal capsule, and the posterior thalamic and acoustic radiations. Similar findings have been reported in experimental animal studies.

Investigators have also described how cells within the substantia nigra are very vulnerable and that this region exhibits extensive cell death when postinjury animals are exposed to a sublethal level of paraquat [27]. Additionally, changes in receptor subunits within the amygdala may be responsible for the increase in susceptibility in the acquisition of fear conditioning in mild FPI rats [28], which may be the basis behind the well-described comorbidity of mild TBI and posttraumatic stress disorder [29]. Finally, there is a rich literature on the relationship between TBI and Alzheimer's disease as well as other disorders.

Conclusion

The neurophysiology of concussion has a long and distinguished history. It is now clear that the neuroscience of this 'mild TBI' reveals that the symptoms and continuing problems suffered by individuals who have sustained a concussion are due to neurobiological responses. Therefore, the understanding of the basic cellular responses to this injury must be explored as they relate to age, type, and severity of concussion in order that appropriate management and/or treatment can be employed.

Acknowledgements

The author has no conflicts of interest. This work was supported by 5PO1NS058489 and RO1NS27544.

References

1 Feeney DM, Baron JC: Diaschisis. Stroke 1986;17:817–830.

2 Walker AE, Kolloros JJ, Case TJ: The physiological basis of concussion. J Neurosurg 1944;1:103–116.

3 Meyer JS, Denny-Brown D: Studies of cerebral circulation in brain injury. II. Cerebral concussion. Electroencephalogr Clin Neurophysiol 1955;7:529–544.

4 Dixon CE, Lyeth BG, Povlishock JT, Findling RL, Hamm RJ, Marmarou A, Young HF, Hayes RL: A fluid percussion model of experimental brain injury in the rat: neurological, physiological, and histopathological characterizations. J Neurosurg 1987;67:110–119.

5 Katayama Y, Becker DP, Tamura T, Hovda DA: Massive increases in extracellular potassium and the indiscriminate release of glutamate following concussive brain injury. J Neurosurg 1990;73:889–900.

6 Dixon KC: Mechanism of cerebral concussion. Lancet 1940;3:360.

7 Andersen BJ, Marmarou A: Post-traumatic selective stimulation of glycolysis. Brain Res 1992;585:184–189.

8 Unterberg AW, Andersen BJ, Clarke GD, Marmarou A: Cerebral energy metabolism following fluid-percussion brain injury in cats. J Neurosurg 1988;68:594–600.

9 Kawamata T, Katayama Y, Hovda DA, Yoshino A, Becker DP: Administration of excitatory amino acid antagonists via microdialysis attenuates the increase in glucose utilization seen following concussive brain injury. J Cereb Blood Flow Metab 1992;12:12–24.

10 Kawamata T, Katayama Y, Hovda DA, Yoshino A, Becker DP: Lactate accumulation following concussive brain injury: the role of ionic fluxes induced by excitatory amino acids. Brain Res 1995;674:196–204.

11 Hovda DA, Yoshino A, Kawamata T, Katayama Y, Becker DP: Diffuse prolonged depression of cerebral oxidative metabolism following concussive brain injury in the rat: a cytochrome oxidase histochemistry study. Brain Res 1991;567:1–10.

12 Moore AH, Osteen CL, Chatziioannou AF, Hovda DA, Cherry SR: Quantitative assessment of longitudinal metabolic changes in vivo following traumatic brain injury in the adult rat using FDG-microPET. J Cereb Blood Flow Metab 2000;20:1492–1501.

13 Maeda T, Lee SM, Hovda DA: Restoration of cerebral vasoreactivity by an L-type calcium channel blocker following fluid percussion brain injury. J Neurotrauma 2005;22:763–771.

14 Becker DP, Jenkins LW, Rabow L: The pathophysiology of head trauma; in Miller TA, Rowlands BJ (eds): The physiological basis of modern surgical care. St. Louis, Mosby, 1987, pp 763–788.

15 Jenkins LW, Moszynski K, Lyeth BG, Lewelt W, Dewitt DS, Allen A, Dixon CE, Povlishock JT, Majewski TJ, Clifton GL, Young HF, Becker DP, Hayes RL: Increased vulnerability of the mildly traumatized rat brain to cerebral ischemia: the use of controlled secondary ischemia as a research tool to identify common or different mechanisms contributing to mechanical and ischemic brain injury. Brain Res 1989;477:211–224.

16 Otori T, Friedland JC, Sinson G, McIntosh TK, Raghupathi R, Welsh FA: Traumatic brain injury elevates glycogen and induces tolerance to ischemia in rat brain. J Neurotrauma 2004;21:707–718.

17 Gurkoff GG, Giza CC, Shin D, Auvin S, Sankar R, Hovda DA: Acute neuroprotection to pilocarpine-induced seizures is not sustained after traumatic brain injury in the developing rat. Neuroscience 2009;164:862–876.

18 Griesbach GS, Hovda DA, Molteni R, Wu A, Gomez-Pinilla F: Voluntary exercise following traumatic brain injury: brain-derived neurotrophic factor upregulation and recovery of function. Neuroscience 2004;125:129–139.

19 Griesbach GS, Gomez-Pinilla F, Hovda DA: Time window for voluntary exercise-induced increases in hippocampal neuroplasticity molecules after traumatic brain injury is severity dependent. J Neurotrauma 2007;24:1161–1171.

20 Griesbach GS: Exercise after traumatic brain injury: is it a double-edged sword? PM R 2011;3:S64–S72.

21 Fineman I, Giza CC, Nahed BV, Lee SM, Hovda DA: Inhibition of neocortical plasticity during development by a moderate concussive brain injury. J Neurotrauma 2000;17:739–749.

22 Giza CC, Griesbach GS, Hovda DA: Experience-dependent behavioral plasticity is disturbed following traumatic injury to the immature brain. Behav Brain Res 2005;157:11–22.

23 Giza CC, Prins ML: Is being plastic fantastic? Mechanisms of altered plasticity after developmental traumatic brain injury. Dev Neurosci 2006;28:364–379.

24 Bergsneider M, Hovda DA, Lee SM, Kelly DF, McArthur DL, Vespa PM, Lee JH, Huang SC, Martin NA, Phelps ME, Becker DP: Dissociation of cerebral glucose metabolism and level of consciousness during the period of metabolic depression following human traumatic brain injury. J Neurotrauma 2000;17:389–401.

25 Slobounov S, Bazarian J, Bigler E, Cantu R, Hallett M, Harbaugh R, Hovda D, Mayer AR, Nuwer MR, Kou Z, Lazzarino G, Papa L, Vagnozzi R: Sports-related concussion: ongoing debate. Br J Sports Med 2014;48:75–76.

26 Vagnozzi R, Signoretti S, Cristofori L, Alessandrini F, Floris R, Isgro E, Ria A, Marziale S, Zoccatelli G, Tavazzi B, Del BF, Sorge R, Broglio SP, McIntosh TK, Lazzarino G: Assessment of metabolic brain damage and recovery following mild traumatic brain injury: a multicentre, proton magnetic resonance spectroscopic study in concussed patients. Brain 2010;133:3232–3242.
27 Hutson CB, Lazo CR, Mortazavi F, Giza CC, Hovda D, Chesselet MF: Traumatic brain injury in adult rats causes progressive nigrostriatal dopaminergic cell loss and enhanced vulnerability to the pesticide paraquat. J Neurotrauma 2011;28:1783–1801.
28 Reger ML, Poulos AM, Buen F, Giza CC, Hovda DA, Fanselow MS: Concussive brain injury enhances fear learning and excitatory processes in the amygdala. Biol Psychiatry 2012;71:335–343.
29 Stein MB, McAllister TW: Exploring the convergence of posttraumatic stress disorder and mild traumatic brain injury. Am J Psychiatry 2009;166:768–776.

Prof. David A. Hovda, PhD
Department of Neurosurgery, David Geffen School of Medicine at UCLA
10833 Le Conte Ave., 18-228 Semel, Box 957039
Los Angeles, CA 90095-7039 (USA)
E-Mail dhovda@mednet.ucla.edu

Niranjan A, Lunsford LD (eds): Concussion. Prog Neurol Surg. Basel, Karger, 2014, vol 28, pp 38–49
DOI: 10.1159/000358761

Chronic Traumatic Encephalopathy

Bennet Omalu

University of California, Davis, Medical Center, Sacramento, Calif., and San Joaquin General Hospital and San Joaquin County Coroner's Division, French Camp, Calif., USA

Abstract

Chronic traumatic encephalopathy (CTE) is a progressive neurodegenerative syndrome, which is caused by single, episodic, or repetitive blunt force impacts to the head and transfer of acceleration-deceleration forces to the brain. CTE presents clinically as a composite syndrome of mood disorders and behavioral and cognitive impairment, with or without sensorimotor impairment. Symptoms of CTE may begin with persistent symptoms of acute traumatic brain injury (TBI) following a documented episode of brain trauma or after a latent period that may range from days to weeks to months and years, up to 40 years following a documented episode of brain trauma or cessation of repetitive TBI. Posttraumatic encephalopathy is distinct from CTE, can be comorbid with CTE, and is a clinicopathologic syndrome induced by focal and/or diffuse, gross and/or microscopic destruction of brain tissue following brain trauma. The brain of a CTE sufferer may appear grossly unremarkable, but shows microscopic evidence of primary and secondary proteinopathies. The primary proteinopathy of CTE is tauopathy, while secondary proteinopathies may include, but are not limited to, amyloidopathy and TDP proteinopathy. Reported prevalence rates of CTE in cohorts exposed to TBI ranges from 3 to 80% across age groups.
© 2014 S. Karger AG, Basel

Definition of Chronic Traumatic Encephalopathy

Chronic traumatic encephalopathy (CTE) is defined as a progressive neurodegenerative syndrome, which is caused by single, episodic, or repetitive blunt force impacts to the head and transfer of acceleration-deceleration forces to the brain. CTE presents clinically after a prolonged latent period as a composite syndrome of mood disorders and behavioral and cognitive impairment, with or without sensorimotor impairment. Although CTE usually presents clinically after a prolonged latency period, some patients with CTE may not exhibit the classic prolonged latency period before clinical symptoms begin [1]. The final and definitive diagnosis of CTE remains microscopic tissue examination with histochemical and immunohistochemical tissue analysis of postmortem whole brains. However, in vivo premortem presumptive diagnosis of CTE has recently emerged using 2-(1-{6-[(2-[F-18]fluoroethyl)(methyl)amino]-2-naphthyl}ethylidene)malononitrile-positron emission tomography (FDDNP-PET) [2]. FDDNP-PET measures both tau tangle and amyloid plaque deposition in living brains. Premortem clinical diagnosis of CTE in living patients using radioligands like FDDNP remains a very promising trend in the near future for the management of CTE.

As part of the CTE spectrum, the spinal medulla may, in addition to the brain, exhibit distinctive neuropathologic changes of CTE. Since the spinal medulla is part of the central nervous system, and CTE is a disease of the central nervous system, CTE cases exhibiting spinal involvement should not be classified as a novel disease that is distinct from CTE. For such cases the myelopathic component may be emphasized by designating them as chronic traumatic myeloencephalopathy.

Like other neurodegenerative diseases, CTE exhibits cerebral and spinal proteinopathies comprising primary and secondary proteinopathies [3]. The primary proteinopathy of CTE is tauopathy, which may be accompanied by other secondary proteinopathies including, but not restricted to, amyloidopathy and/or TDP-43 proteinopathy [1, 4–9]. CTE is a distinct neurodegenerative disease with distinctive histomorphologic and proteinopathic phenotypes that are distinct from the phenotypes of the most prevalent neurodegenerative diseases including, but not limited to, Alzheimer's disease (AD), Lewy body disease (LBD), frontotemporal lobar degeneration, vascular brain injury, and cerebrovascular disease [10, 11]. However, similar to other neurodegenerative diseases, CTE can occur contemporaneously in the same individual with one or more other types of neurodegenerative diseases [1, 6–9]. CTE is a progressive disease that exhibits cumulative neuropathologic and proteinopathic changes with advancing age. Advanced or end-stage CTE in elderly patients can exhibit histomorphologic and proteinopathic phenotypes that resemble AD, and in such elderly patients it may not be feasible to differentiate CTE from AD with a reasonable degree of medical certainty [1, 8, 9].

Historically, a minority of doctors and authors, especially doctors and authors who may work or be associated with sporting organizations, have questioned or denied the existence of CTE [12–16]. In 1959 and 2006, the medical director of the New York State Athletic Commission [15, 16] and the Chairman of the Mild Traumatic Brain Injury Committee of the National Football League (NFL) [17, 18] both respectively published papers and opinions rejecting the notion or hypothesis that blows to the head can cause CTE in boxers and football players. However, CTE has remained a very well-established concept in the medical sciences across the centuries. It has become a generally accepted principle in the medical sciences that trauma to the brain can result in permanent brain damage that can manifest with a myriad of progressive symptoms. Over the centuries, CTE has been clearly recognized, described, and named with a variety of terminologies, which are enumerated in table 1 [19, 20]. The commonality of all these enumerated terminologies is the causal association of CTE with single,

Table 1. Syntactics and semantics of CTE across the centuries

1. Cerebral neurasthenia
2. Chronic postconcussion syndrome
3. Chronic TBI/chronic brain injury
4. Compensation hysteria
5. Concussion neurosis
6. Delayed traumatic apoplexy
7. Dementia pugilistica
8. Dementia traumatica
9. Encephalopathia traumatica
10. Litigation neurosis
11. Postconcussion neurosis
12. Postconcussion syndrome
13. Posttraumatic concussion state
14. Posttraumatic dementia
15. Posttraumatic head syndrome
16. Posttraumatic parkinsonism
17. Posttraumatic psychoneurosis
18. Posttraumatic stress disorder
19. Punch drunk/punch-drunk state
20. Terror neurosis
21. Traumatic constitution
22. Traumatic encephalitis
23. Traumatic encephalopathy
24. Traumatic encephalopathy of boxers
25. Traumatic hysterias
26. Traumatic insanity
27. Traumatic neurosis
28. Traumatic psychosis

episodic, or repetitive traumatic brain injury (TBI). It is pertinent to note that CTE can occur in a variety of human activities and circumstances in and out of sports, including in the military, whereby the human brain is exposed to biomechanical loading of kinetic energy and forces in one episode of trauma, in several (or just a few) episodes of trauma, and/or in numerous repetitive episodes of trauma over the years. For a single episode of trauma, like in motor vehicle crashes, brain trauma is more likely to involve severe TBI and posttraumatic encephalopathy (PTE) [21–23], while in repetitive episodes of trauma, brain trauma is more likely to involve subconcussions and concussions [24, 25].

Posttraumatic Encephalopathy versus Chronic Traumatic Encephalopathy

PTE and CTE are two distinct chronic disease entities, which are both sequelae of TBI. While both diseases are distinct, they can occur together as comorbidities in the same individual [1]. PTE can be defined as a clinicopathologic syndrome induced by focal and/or diffuse, gross and/or microscopic destruction of brain tissue following brain trauma [1, 23].

The spectrum of PTE changes comprises persistent sequelae of primary and secondary brain trauma, including, but not limited to, contusions and lacerations of the brain, secondary traumatic hypoxic-ischemic cerebral injury, secondary traumatic hypoxic-ischemic hippocampal necrosis, sclerosis and atrophy, traumatic intracranial hemorrhages, compression of the brain by traumatic epidural and subdural hemorrhages, and secondary traumatic cerebral herniations and necrosis. PTE injuries typically induce necrosis of brain tissue, cavitation and loss of brain tissue, anisomorphic astrogliosis, activation of microglia, and infiltration by histiocytes (foamy or pigment-laden histiocytes), resulting in gross scarring of the brain [21, 22, 26–28]. A widely recognized subtype of PTE is posttraumatic epilepsy [22, 29–33]. Posttraumatic epilepsy originates from a variety of pathogenetic mechanisms, including epileptogenic astroglial scars of the brain and mesial temporal lobe sclerosis [34, 35]. When posttraumatic changes similar to PTE occur in the spinal cord, a similar syndrome called posttraumatic myelopathy applies. PTE changes are more likely to present with focal lateralizing neurological symptoms and signs [36]. They are also more likely to be topographically focal and lobar in the brain [37], and focal and segmental in the spinal cord with attendant wallerian degeneration of nerve fibers [36].

PTE is not a neurodegenerative disease and is not progressive. CTE is a neurodegenerative disease and is progressive. Brains affected by PTE will show focal or diffuse gross destruction and disruption of brain tissue and brain anatomy caused by brain trauma, while brains affected by CTE will not show gross destruction and disruption of brain tissue and anatomy caused by brain trauma [5, 38, 39]. Historically, many of the cases which have been reported as CTE in boxers (dementia pugilistica) have been cases of combined PTE-CTE occurring together [4, 5, 8, 40]. In isolated CTE without PTE, the brain shows evidence of progressive neurodegeneration with proteinopathies (primary tauopathy with or without amyloidopathy, TDP-43 proteinopathy, or other secondary proteinopathies). There is no evidence of focal or diffuse structural destruction and necrosis of the brain. In isolated PTE without CTE, the brain shows evidence of focal or diffuse structural destruction and necrosis of the brain without evidence of neurodegeneration or progressive proteinopathy. In combined PTE-CTE, PTE changes are present in the brain, accompanied by the neurodegenerative proteinopathies of CTE [1]. Figure 1 illustrates an instance of combined PTE-CTE in a deceased retired 50-year-old boxer who had suffered a documented remote episode of a large right subdural hemorrhage following a fight, with compression and herniation of the right cerebral hemisphere. His brain showed diffuse right cerebral hemispheric multicystic necrosis and xanthochromia, accompanied by a diffuse tauopathy in the bilateral cerebral hemispheres and brainstem [1, 19]. In a postmortem TBI series [41], there was no association between posttraumatic epilepsy and tauopathy, further confirming that PTE and CTE are both distinct pathologies in the posttraumatic spectrum of brain diseases.

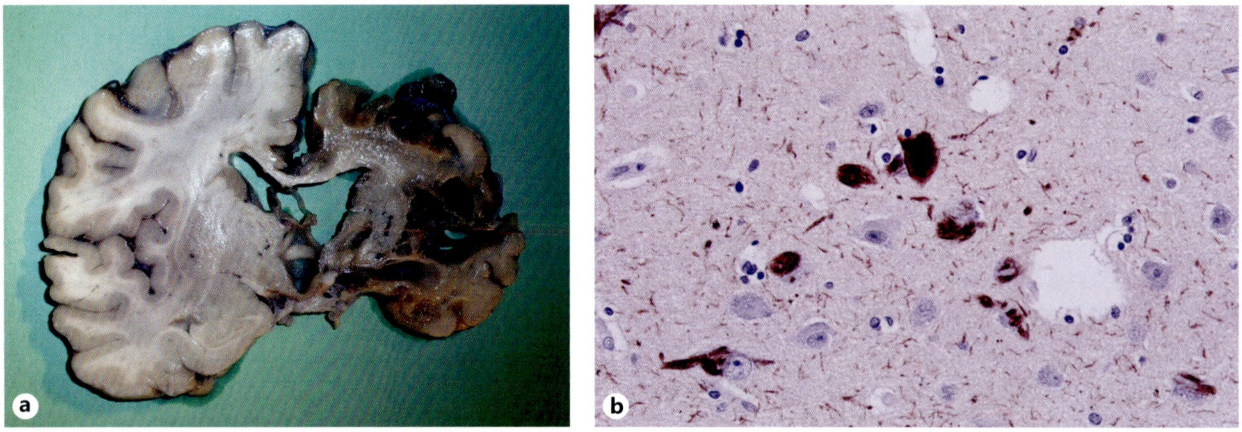

Fig. 1. a Gross photograph of a coronal section of the brain of a deceased retired boxer with combined PTE-CTE showing a global right cerebral multicystic necrosis. The left cerebral hemisphere looks grossly unremarkable. **b** Photomicrograph of a tau-immunostained section of the neocortex from the left cerebral hemisphere showing tauopathy (frequent NFTs and NTs). ×400 magnification.

Chronic Traumatic Encephalopathy Symptomatology and Clinimetrics

Symptoms of CTE may begin with persistent symptoms of acute TBI following a documented episode of brain trauma or after a latent period that may range from days to weeks to months and years, up to 40 years following a documented episode of brain trauma or cessation of repetitive TBI [1, 42, 43]. In 1969, The Royal College of Physicians of London reported that the prevalence of traumatic encephalopathy in ex-professional boxers was 47% in ex-boxers aged 50 years and over who boxed for more than 10 years. This prevalence rate dropped to 17% for older professional ex-boxers of the same age who boxed for 6–9 years, and 13% for those who boxed for less than 5 years. For younger retired professional boxers 30–49 years of age, the prevalence rates for the same durations of professional boxing were 25, 14, and 3% respectively [44, 45]. These reported prevalence rates across older and younger age groups of retired professional boxers suggest a positive correlation and association between duration of exposure to repetitive blows to the head and the risk of developing CTE. These rates also suggest that the prevalence rates of CTE increase with age, indicating that CTE progresses and advances with age.

In a magnetic resonance imaging (MRI)-based series of professional boxers and mixed martial arts fighters with a mean age of 27.3 years and a 5.1-year mean of participation in combat sports, 76% had at least one finding that will be associated with TBI [46]. In a postmortem series of contact sport athletes, 71% exhibited CTE neuropathologic changes [1]. In another postmortem series of individuals with a history of repetitive mild TBI, 80% showed CTE neuropathologic changes [8].

CTE symptoms are progressive and multidomain, primarily comprising mood disorders, behavioral impairment, and cognitive impairment, with or without incapacitating somatic and physical symptoms including motor dysfunction [1, 20]. The symptom severity and brain pathology burden of CTE progress and advance with increasing age, and the neuropathology of end-stage or advanced CTE, especially in the elderly, may resemble and be indistinct from high AD neuropathologic change [1, 8–10, 47].

Table 2 enumerates the symptoms and signs of CTE. There is no established and generally accepted threshold for CTE. Likewise, there are no established and generally accepted risk factors outside the fundamental risk factor and underlying causal factor, which is exposure to mild, moderate, and/or severe TBI. Apolipoprotein E-ε4 allele is a risk factor for AD and adverse outcomes following TBI, and has been suggested to be a risk factor for CTE; however, this risk quantification for CTE remains to be confirmed across populations [20, 47]. As expected for every disease model, the clinical presentation and symptoms of CTE exhibit broad variations across CTE sufferers. Several pathologic and clinical grading criteria and schemes have been proposed for CTE, but these classifications have not been widely accepted and applied [1, 8, 20].

Chronic Traumatic Encephalopathy Neuropathologic Changes

The brain of a CTE sufferer may appear grossly unremarkable without any focal or lobar necrosis, infarct, acute and chronic hemorrhage, or significant cortical atrophy (fig. 2). Conventional computerized tomography and MRI studies of the brain may appear within normal limits. Marked symmetrical dilatation of all ventricles (hydrocephalus ex vacuo) is typically absent as well as any marked atrophy of the subcortical ganglia. The centrum semiovale does not show any focal gross white matter necrosis or demyelination. However, typical CTE neuropathologic changes in elderly patients can be accompanied by the neuropathologic changes of normal aging and other neurodegenerative diseases including AD, frontotemporal lobar degeneration, Lewy body disease, vascular cognitive impairment, and cerebrovascular disease [1, 8].

Histologically, the neocortex may show minimal-to-mild neuronal loss and isomorphic astrogliosis. The centrum semiovale, subcortical white matter and spinal anterior, lateral and posterior funiculi may show mild patchy-to-diffuse rarefaction, with mild diffuse isomorphic fibrillary astrogliosis. There is mild diffuse activation of the white matter microglia with mildly increased numbers of neuropil histiocytes, which may be accentuated perivascularly. There are increased numbers of pigment-laden histiocytes in the Virchow-Robin spaces, which may be accompanied by sparse lymphocytic seeding. These neuropathologic changes are located in a diffuse manner involving all regions of the brain including the brainstem. The subcortical ganglia, midbrain, pontine and medullary nuclei, and spinal anterior and posterior horn neurons may also show minimal-to-mild neuronal loss. Hippocampal sclerosis or marked

Table 2. Reported symptoms and signs of CTE

A. Cognitive impairment
   1. Loss of memory and memory disturbances
   2. Deterioration in linguistic coherence and language impairment
   3. Deterioration in professional competence, work performance and socioeconomic status
      i. Poor attainment of set goals
   4. Impaired capacity to engage in complex intellectual reasoning and executive functioning
   5. Impaired attention and concentration
   6. Deterioration in capacity to manage money and personal bank accounts
   7. Visuospatial impairment and difficulties

B. Behavioral impairment and mood disorders
   1. Insomnia
      i. Deteriorating capacity to fall asleep and remain asleep for long
      ii. Waking up in the middle of the night and in the early morning, and not being able to fall back asleep
   2. Paranoid ideations and delusions
   3. Social phobias
   4. Breakdown of intimate and family relationships
      i. Spousal separation and divorces
   5. Disinhibition and loss of social etiquette
      i. Poor social judgment, social and sexual indiscretions and improprieties
      ii. Violent and criminal behaviors and tendencies
      iii. Socially disinhibited speech
      iv. Abuse of alcohol, prescription and illicit drugs
   6. Increasing impulsivity
   7. Increasing religiosity
   8. Mood disorders
      i. Rampant fluctuations in mood, and mood swings
         1. Sudden highs and lows; happy and sullen
         2. Intermittent periods of high-energy levels, drives and enthusiasm; low energy levels, no drive and no enthusiasm
      ii. Exaggerated responses to minor life stressors and issues of daily living
         1. Bouts of explosive anger, worry, and agitation
      iii. Increasing irritability and aggression
      iv. Anxiety and agitation
      v. Major depression, suicidal thoughts and ideations, parasuicides and suicides
         1. Apathy and feelings of hopelessness

C. Physical symptoms and motor dysfunction
   1. Headaches, generalized body aches and pain
   2. Motor speech impairment (dysarthria)
   3. Spasticity and parkinsonism including tremors
   4. Gait impairment and motor incoordination (ataxia)
   5. Muscle weakness, spasms, and pain, and other bulbar and spinal motor neuron symptoms

Posttraumatic epilepsy or seizure disorder is more a feature of PTE and not CTE.

loss of pyramidal neurons in the stratum pyramidalis of the hippocampus is typically absent. Essentially, routine hematoxylin and eosin-stained brain sections of the brain of a CTE sufferer may appear unremarkable with negligible pathologic changes. Immunohistochemical analysis of the brain with a battery of proteomic antibodies is required for the diagnosis of CTE [1, 8].

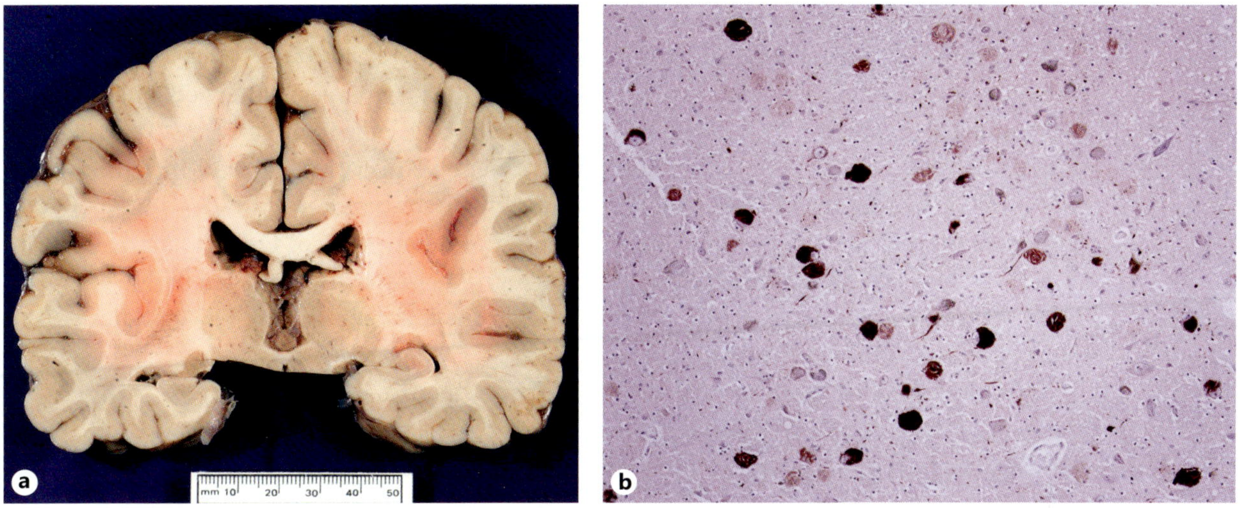

Fig. 2. a Gross photograph of a coronal section of the brain of a deceased football player with CTE. The brain appears grossly unremarkable without any significant cortical or subcortical atrophy. **b** Photomicrograph of a tau-immunostained section of a brainstem nucleus from the brain of a deceased NFL player with CTE showing frequent NFTs and NTs. ×100 magnification.

The primary proteinopathy of CTE is tauopathy manifested by the presence of neurofibrillary tangles (NFTs) and neuropil or neuritic threads (NTs) in all regions of the brain (fig. 2). Neuronal NFTs in CTE may be accompanied by astrocytic NFTs and plaques. The density of the neuronal NFTs may be sparse, moderate, or frequent in all regions of the brain, and may exhibit a distinctive skip phenomenon in the neocortex, whereby NFTs are haphazardly located, being present and absent in adjacent regions of the neocortex within the same lobe of the brain. Other topographic distributions of NFTs may include perivascular density accentuation and accentuation in the depths of the sulci. Subpial and periventricular tangles may also be present. The neocortical NFTs are more superficially located, found predominantly in laminae II and III. Topographic accentuation of tangle densities may also be observed in the amygdala, tegmental brainstem nuclei and hypothalamus [1, 8].

Secondary amyloidopathy may accompany the primary tauopathy of CTE in about 20–30% of cases, but is not a prerequisite or defining proteinopathy of CTE. Diffuse and neuritic amyloid plaques may be present, but diffuse amyloid plaques are more frequently encountered. Fully developed AD pathology with frequent neuritic amyloid plaques is more likely in older and elderly patients who suffer from CTE. With advancing age, advanced or end-stage CTE may progress and become fully developed AD neuropathologically, especially in elderly patients. Such a disease model is similar to that of cirrhosis of the liver, which is the end-stage outcome of many progressive chronic liver diseases. The underlying causes of end-stage cirrhosis of the liver may not be distinguishable histologically when cirrhosis is attained. Likewise, CTE-related end-stage AD neuropathology in a patient may not be distinguishable from non-CTE-related end-stage AD neuropathology [1, 8].

Cerebral amyloid angiopathy may also accompany CTE changes. Other secondary proteinopathies, which may accompany tauopathy in CTE may include TDP-43 proteinopathy and α-synucleinopathy. Secondary α-synucleinopathy is found in a minority of CTE sufferers (about 20%) and is more likely to be found in older and elderly patients, but is not a prerequisite or defining proteinopathy of CTE.

CTE is not Parkinson's disease. In CTE, the nigral neurons are damaged by NFTs and NTs (tauopathy), while in PD the nigral neurons are damaged by Lewy bodies (α-synucleinopathy) [1, 8].

Secondary TDP-43 proteinopathy, in the form of neuronal, glial, and neuritic inclusions, is not a prominent feature of CTE and is not a prerequisite proteinopathy for CTE diagnosis. However, in a minority of CTE sufferers, especially those with prominent clinical symptoms of motor neuron disease (muscle weakness, atrophy, fasciculations, and muscle pain), TDP-43 proteinopathy may become very widespread and prominent in the brain and spinal cord. In such cases, a primary diagnosis of frontotemporal lobar degeneration-TDP or motor neuron disease may be made, and CTE, if present, will be made as a secondary diagnosis [1, 8, 10, 48]. When CTE neuropathology occurs with those of other neurodegenerative diseases in the same brain, the standard of practice for diagnosis is to enumerate all neurodegenerative disease entities whose distinctive neuropathologies are present [10].

Chronic Traumatic Encephalopathy Pathogenesis and Neurobiology

The NFTs and NTs found in CTE are made of paired helical filamentous aggregates of abnormally hyperphosphorylated tau protein. All of the six isoforms of tau protein are present as well as 3-repeat and 4-repeat tau protein. Normal tau protein is a predominantly axonal microtubule-binding protein that promotes microtubule assembly and stability within the neuronal cytoskeletal system. Hyperphosphorylation of tau results in microtubule disassembly, impaired axonal transport, neuronal and synaptic dysfunction, and eventually neuronal death [49].

The impaired metabolism of tau, which results in abnormal tau hyperphosphorylation and accumulation, is seen in a variety of neurodegenerative and brain injury pathologies, including TBI. The neurochemical cascades are still not well elucidated; however, it is thought that TBI induces the activation and accumulation of kinases, which hyperphosphorylate tau. Accumulation of hyperphosphorylated tau in TBI is not thought to be a downstream consequence of amyloid-β (Aβ) accumulation and plaque formation. Amyloid precursor protein (APP) is upregulated by TBI and accumulates in neurons and axons within several hours following traumatic axonal injury. APP is cleaved by β- and γ-secretase enzymes to form Aβ peptides, which form amyloid plaques [49].

The specific cascade and threshold for the permanently impaired metabolism that results in chronic and progressive accumulation of hyperphosphorylated tau and Aβ peptide stemming from single, episodic, or repetitive TBI is still not clearly elucidated. Other epigenetic phenomena have been suggested; however, other accompanying cellular mechanisms of injury, which result in the cumulative outcome of CTE may also include chronic neuroinflammation, microglial activation, glutamate driven neuronal immunoexcitoxicity, mitochondrial dysfunction and oxidative stress, and calcium dysregulation [49–51]. The phenomenon of prion-like self-propagation has also been proposed as a possible mechanism of CTE pathogenesis, whereby hyperphosphorylated tau protein and Aβ peptide, like prion protein, form in a neuron and spread transynaptically to and recruit other unaffected neurons in other regions of the brain [52–54].

While the focus remains on primary and secondary proteinopathies of CTE (especially tauopathy), it is possible that these proteins and peptides that accumulate in CTE may be end-stage surrogate outcomes of other unelucidated cryptic and earlier subcellular and cellular processes. It is possible that by the time these proteins accumulate, the subcellular and cellular CTE cascades may have advanced remarkably. Future research, while exploring avenues of preventing protein accumulations, may also explore these possible cryptic subcellular and cellular processes in view of earlier intervention, prevention, and possibly treatment.

References

1 Omalu B, Bailes J, Hamilton RL, Kamboh MI, Hammers J, Case J, Fitzsimmons R: Emerging histomorphologic phenotypes of chronic traumatic encephalopathy in American athletes. Neurosurgery 2011;69:173–183, discussion 183.

2 Small GW, Kepe V, Siddarth P, Ercoli LM, Merrill DA, Donoghue N, Bookheimer SY, Martinez J, Omalu B, Bailes J, Barrio JR: PET scanning of brain tau in retired National Football League players: preliminary findings. Am J Geriatr Psychiatry 2013;21:138–144.

3 Chen-Plotkin AS, Lee VM, Trojanowski JQ: TAR DNA-binding protein 43 in neurodegenerative disease. Nat Rev Neurol 2010;6:211–220.

4 Geddes JF, Vowles GH, Nicoll JA, Revesz T: Neuronal cytoskeletal changes are an early consequence of repetitive head injury. Acta Neuropathol 1999;98:171–178.

5 Geddes JF, Vowles GH, Robinson SF, Sutcliffe JC: Neurofibrillary tangles, but not Alzheimer-type pathology, in a young boxer. Neuropathol Appl Neurobiol 1996;22:12–16.

6 McKee AC, Gavett BE, Stern RA, Nowinski CJ, Cantu RC, Kowall NW, Perl DP, Hedley-Whyte ET, Price B, Sullivan C, Morin P, Lee HS, Kubilus CA, Daneshvar DH, Wulff M, Budson AE: TDP-43 proteinopathy and motor neuron disease in chronic traumatic encephalopathy. J Neuropathol Exp Neurol 2010;69:918–929.

7 Hazrati LN, Tartaglia MC, Diamandis P, Davis KD, Green RE, Wennberg R, Wong JC, Ezerins L, Tator CH: Absence of chronic traumatic encephalopathy in retired football players with multiple concussions and neurological symptomatology. Front Hum Neurosci 2013;7:222.

8 McKee AC, Stein TD, Nowinski CJ, Stern RA, Daneshvar DH, Alvarez VE, Lee HS, Hall G, Wojtowicz SM, Baugh CM, Riley DO, Kubilus CA, Cormier KA, Jacobs MA, Martin BR, Abraham CR, Ikezu T, Reichard RR, Wolozin BL, Budson AE, Goldstein LE, Kowall NW, Cantu RC: The spectrum of disease in chronic traumatic encephalopathy. Brain 2013;136:43–64.

9 Omalu B, Hammers JL, Bailes J, Hamilton RL, Kamboh MI, Webster G, Fitzsimmons RP: Chronic traumatic encephalopathy in an Iraqi war veteran with posttraumatic stress disorder who committed suicide. Neurosurg Focus 2011;31:E3.
10 Hyman BT, Phelps CH, Beach TG, Bigio EH, Cairns NJ, Carrillo MC, Dickson DW, Duyckaerts C, Frosch MP, Masliah E, Mirra SS, Nelson PT, Schneider JA, Thal DR, Thies B, Trojanowski JQ, Vinters HV, Montine TJ: National Institute on Aging-Alzheimer's Association guidelines for the neuropathologic assessment of Alzheimer's disease. Alzheimers Dement 2012;8:1–13.
11 Montine TJ, Phelps CH, Beach TG, Bigio EH, Cairns NJ, Dickson DW, Duyckaerts C, Frosch MP, Masliah E, Mirra SS, Nelson PT, Schneider JA, Thal DR, Trojanowski JQ, Vinters HV, Hyman BT; National Institute on Aging; Alzheimer's Association: National Institute on Aging-Alzheimer's Association guidelines for the neuropathologic assessment of Alzheimer's disease: a practical approach. Acta Neuropathol 2012;123:1–11.
12 Randolph C, Karantzoulis S, Guskiewicz K: Prevalence and characterization of mild cognitive impairment in retired national football league players. J Int Neuropsychol Soc 2013;19:873–880.
13 McCrory P, Meeuwisse WH, Kutcher JS, Jordan BD, Gardner A: What is the evidence for chronic concussion-related changes in retired athletes: behavioural, pathological and clinical outcomes? Br J Sports Med 2013;47:327–330.
14 Kaplan HA, Browder J: Observations on the clinical and brain wave patterns of professional boxers. J Am Med Assoc 1954;156:1138–1144.
15 McCown IA: Protecting the boxer. J Am Med Assoc 1959;169:1409–1413.
16 McCown IA: Boxing injuries. Am J Surg 1959;98: 509–516.
17 Casson IR, Pellman EJ, Viano DC: Chronic traumatic encephalopathy in a National Football League player. Neurosurgery 2006;59:E1152.
18 Casson IR, Pellman EJ, Viano DC: Chronic traumatic encephalopathy in a National Football League player. Neurosurgery 2006;58:E1003, author reply E1003, discussion E1003.
19 Handbook of Neurological Sports Medicine. Champaign, Human Kinetic Publishing, 2014 (in press).
20 Jordan BD: The clinical spectrum of sport-related traumatic brain injury. Nat Rev Neurol 2013;9:222–230.
21 Cervos-Navarro J, Lafuente JV: Traumatic brain injuries: structural changes. J Neurol Sci 1991;103(Suppl): S3–S14.
22 Adams JH, Graham DI, Jennett B: The structural basis of moderate disability after traumatic brain damage. J Neurol Neurosurg Psychiatry 2001;71:521–524.
23 Proceedings of the Congress of Neurological Surgeons in 1964, Report of the Ad Hoc Committee to Study Head Injury Nomenclature. Clin Neurosurg 1966;12:386–394.
24 Bailes JE, Petraglia AL, Omalu BI, Nauman E, Talavage T: Role of subconcussion in repetitive mild traumatic brain injury. J Neurosurg 2013;119:1235–1245.
25 Talavage TM, Nauman EA, Breedlove EL, Yoruk U, Dye AE, Morigaki KE, Feuer H, Leverenz LJ: Functionally-detected cognitive impairment in high school football players without clinically-diagnosed concussion. J Neurotrauma 2014;31:327–338.
26 Bigler ED: Neuropathology of acquired cerebral trauma. J Learn Disabil 1987;20:458–473.
27 Valsamis MP: Pathology of trauma. Neurosurg Clin N Am 1994;5:175–183.
28 Patt S, Brodhun M: Neuropathological sequelae of traumatic injury in the brain. An overview. Exp Toxicol Pathol 1999;51:119–123.
29 Prince DA, Parada I, Scalise K, Graber K, Jin X, Shen F: Epilepsy following cortical injury: cellular and molecular mechanisms as targets for potential prophylaxis. Epilepsia 2009;50(Suppl 2):30–40.
30 Diaz-Arrastia R, Agostini MA, Madden CJ, Van Ness PC: Posttraumatic epilepsy: the endophenotypes of a human model of epileptogenesis. Epilepsia 2009;50(Suppl 2):14–20.
31 Dichter MA: Posttraumatic epilepsy: the challenge of translating discoveries in the laboratory to pathways to a cure. Epilepsia 2009;50(Suppl 2):41–45.
32 Pitkanen A, Immonen RJ, Grohn OH, Kharatishvili I: From traumatic brain injury to posttraumatic epilepsy: what animal models tell us about the process and treatment options. Epilepsia 2009;50(Suppl 2): 21–29.
33 Hunt RF, Scheff SW, Smith BN: Posttraumatic epilepsy after controlled cortical impact injury in mice. Exp Neurol 2009;215:243–252.
34 Swartz BE, Houser CR, Tomiyasu U, Walsh GO, DeSalles A, Rich JR, Delgado-Escueta A: Hippocampal cell loss in posttraumatic human epilepsy. Epilepsia 2006;47:1373–1382.
35 Statler KD: Pediatric posttraumatic seizures: epidemiology, putative mechanisms of epileptogenesis and promising investigational progress. Dev Neurosci 2006;28:354–363.
36 Povlishock JT, Katz DI: Update of neuropathology and neurological recovery after traumatic brain injury. J Head Trauma Rehabil 2005;20:76–94.
37 Graham DI, Adams JH, Nicoll JA, Maxwell WL, Gennarelli TA: The nature, distribution and causes of traumatic brain injury. Brain Pathol 1995;5:397–406.

38 Omalu BI, DeKosky ST, Hamilton RL, Minster RL, Kamboh MI, Shakir AM, Wecht CH: Chronic traumatic encephalopathy in a National Football League player: part II. Neurosurgery 2006;59:1086–1092, discussion 1092–1093.
39 Omalu BI, DeKosky ST, Minster RL, Kamboh MI, Hamilton RL, Wecht CH: Chronic traumatic encephalopathy in a National Football League player. Neurosurgery 2005;57:128–134; discussion 128–134.
40 McKee AC, Cantu RC, Nowinski CJ, Hedley-Whyte ET, Gavett BE, Budson AE, Santini VE, Lee HS, Kubilus CA, Stern RA: Chronic traumatic encephalopathy in athletes: progressive tauopathy after repetitive head injury. J Neuropathol Exp Neurol 2009;68:709–735.
41 Thom M, Liu JY, Thompson P, Phadke R, Narkiewicz M, Martinian L, Marsdon D, Koepp M, Caboclo L, Catarino CB, Sisodiya SM: Neurofibrillary tangle pathology and Braak staging in chronic epilepsy in relation to traumatic brain injury and hippocampal sclerosis: a post-mortem study. Brain 2011;134: 2969–2981.
42 Critchley M: Punch drunk syndromes: the chronic traumatic encephalopathy of boxers; in: Hommage à Clovis Vincent. Paris, Maloine, 1949, p 131.
43 Critchley M: Medical aspects of boxing, particularly from a neurological standpoint. Br Med J 1957;1: 357–362.
44 Royal College of Physicians of London. Committee on Boxing. Report on the Medical Aspects of Boxing. London, Royal College of Physicians of London, 1969, p 11.
45 Roberts AH: Brain Damage in Boxers. A Study of the Prevalence of Traumatic Encephalopathy among Ex-Professional Boxers. London, Pitman Medical and Scientific Publishing Co., 1969.
46 Orrison WW, Hanson EH, Alamo T, Watson D, Sharma M, Perkins TG, Tandy RD: Traumatic brain injury: a review and high-field MRI findings in 100 unarmed combatants using a literature-based checklist approach. J Neurotrauma 2009;26:689–701.
47 Stern RA, Daneshvar DH, Baugh CM, Seichepine DR, Montenigro PH, Riley DO, Fritts NG, Stamm JM, Robbins CA, McHale L, Simkin I, Stein TD, Alvarez VE, Goldstein LE, Budson AE, Kowall NW, Nowinski CJ, Cantu RC, McKee AC: Clinical presentation of chronic traumatic encephalopathy. Neurology 2013;81:1122–1129.
48 Mackenzie IR, Neumann M, Bigio EH, Cairns NJ, Alafuzoff I, Kril J, Kovacs GG, Ghetti B, Halliday G, Holm IE, Ince PG, Kamphorst W, Revesz T, Rozemuller AJ, Kumar-Singh S, Akiyama H, Baborie A, Spina S, Dickson DW, Trojanowski JQ, Mann DM: Nomenclature for neuropathologic subtypes of frontotemporal lobar degeneration: consensus recommendations. Acta Neuropathol 2009;117:15–18.
49 Blennow K, Hardy J, Zetterberg H: The neuropathology and neurobiology of traumatic brain injury. Neuron 2012;76:886–899.
50 Blaylock RL, Maroon J: Immunoexcitotoxicity as a central mechanism in chronic traumatic encephalopathy – a unifying hypothesis. Surg Neurol Int 2011;2:107.
51 Walker KR, Tesco G: Molecular mechanisms of cognitive dysfunction following traumatic brain injury. Front Aging Neurosci 2013;5:29.
52 Le MN, Kim W, Lee S, McKee AC, Hall GF: Multiple mechanisms of extracellular tau spreading in a non-transgenic tauopathy model. Am J Neurodegener Dis 2012;1:316–333.
53 Jucker M, Walker GF: Self-propagation of pathogenic protein aggregates in neurodegenerative diseases. Nature 2013;501:45–51.
54 Clavaguera F, Lavenir I, Falcon B, Frank S, Goedert M, Tolnay M: 'Prion-like' templated misfolding in tauopathies. Brain Pathol 2013;23:342–349.

Bennet Omalu, MD, MBA, MPH, CPE, DABP-AP, CP, FP, NP
San Joaquin County Coroner's Division
7000 Michael Canlis Boulevard
French Camp, CA 95231 (USA)
E-Mail bomalu@sjgov.org

Niranjan A, Lunsford LD (eds): Concussion. Prog Neurol Surg. Basel, Karger, 2014, vol 28, pp 50–62
DOI: 10.1159/000358765

Cumulative Effects of Repetitive Mild Traumatic Brain Injury

Julian E. Bailes[a] · Matthew L. Dashnaw[b] · Anthony L. Petraglia[b] · Ryan C. Turner[c, d]

[a]Department of Neurosurgery, NorthShore University HealthSystem, University of Chicago Pritzker School of Medicine, Evanston, Ill., [b]Department of Neurosurgery, University of Rochester Medical Center, Rochester, N.Y., and [c]Center for Neuroscience and [d]Department of Neurosurgery, West Virginia University, School of Medicine, Morgantown, W.Va., USA

Abstract

The majority of traumatic brain injuries (TBI) in the USA are mild in severity. Sports, particularly American football, and military experience are especially associated with repetitive, mild TBI (mTBI). The consequences of repetitive brain injury have garnered increasing scientific and public attention following reports of altered mood and behavior, as well as progressive neurological dysfunction many years after injury. This report provides an up-to-date review of the clinical, pathological, and pathophysiological changes associated with repetitive mTBI, and their potential for cumulative effects in certain individuals.

© 2014 S. Karger AG, Basel

While the understanding of mild traumatic brain injury (mTBI) pathophysiology has been greatly enhanced in recent years, the implications and clinical management of these injuries appears to have become more complex. It is estimated that several million concussions occur annually in the USA in sports and recreational activities [1]. In addition to sport-related prevalence, mTBI is of particular concern among military personnel. The prevalence of TBI has been projected to be 8–20% in those deployed to the recent conflicts in Iraq and Afghanistan, with mTBI accounting for the vast majority of cases [2]. The consequences of mTBI have garnered increasing scientific and public attention following reports of altered mood and behavior, as well as progressive neurological dysfunction in athletes and military personnel who have been exposed to repetitive concussions and subconcussive impacts. The mTBI research that has been produced over the previous decade supersedes the volume and content of all previous information [3]. Herein, we aim to review and highlight the pertinent clinical, histopathological, and pathophysiological research as it pertains to the cumulative effects of repetitive mTBI.

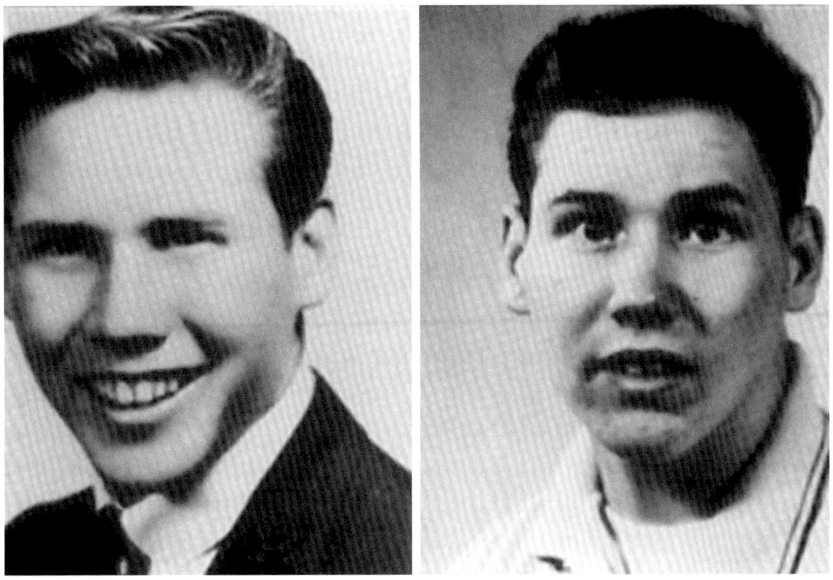

Fig. 1. Consecutive photographs of a high school football player 1 year apart, before and after concussive injury sustained in sport. His 4 concussions resulted in personality changes, diminished academic performance, and an inability to continue his sport. In addition, his appearance seems to reflect the brain injury, perhaps even at the brainstem level. From [55] with permission.

Clinical Effects of Repetitive Mild Traumatic Brain Injury

It is apparent that the spectrum of symptoms which may be expressed following mTBI is broader than originally thought. It has been established that only a small minority (approx. 10%) of athletic mTBI results in loss of consciousness, and that some concussions are not readily apparent until the next day. Disturbances of mood, balance, concentration, memory, school, athletic and work performance, anxiety, and other symptoms may be not obvious, occult, or passed over as not related to head trauma [4–6] (fig. 1).

Sleep disruption is another common consequence of TBI, and mTBI may be more strongly correlated with sleep disturbances than more severe TBI [7]. Until recently, there was a paucity of data on how cumulative TBIs affect sleep. Bryan [8] sought to investigate the incidence and severity of insomnia symptoms by lifetime TBIs in a clinical sample of deployed male personnel at a military TBI clinic in Iraq. Notably, 47.6% of patients with multiple TBIs exceeded the threshold for clinical insomnia, compared to 22.4% of those with a single TBI and only 5.6% of those with no history of TBI. It was also noted that sleep onset might be most vulnerable to disruption following an initial TBI and that disruption of sleep maintenance might intensify following additional TBI; however, further study would be needed to better understand how multiple TBIs might be related to different types of sleep disturbances.

There is a range of neurological sequelae that are likely related to concussive and subconcussive head injury. These include postconcussion syndrome (PCS), prolonged PCS (PPCS), posttraumatic stress disorder, mild cognitive impairment, chronic traumatic encephalopathy (CTE), and dementia pugilistica [3, 6]. Due to recent increased public awareness of the possible untoward effects of repetitive brain injury on athletes and soldiers, there has been a surge of data and interest in this field, particularly regarding CTE.

Most commonly, symptoms experienced after concussion usually resolve in 7–10 days [4, 5]. For patients with a prolongation of symptoms beyond this period, the terms PCS and PPCS are often used to define the constellation of symptoms and their duration [5]. Different analyses have defined the symptomatic period of PCS as ranging from 10 days to 3 months, and that of PPCS to range from 3 months to more than 6 months. In general, we consider the persistence of symptoms between 6 weeks and 3 months to be consistent with PCS, and symptoms lasting more than 3 months to be PPCS [6]. The symptoms which make up the aforementioned syndromes can be assigned to four general categories: somatic symptoms (headache, dizziness, fatigue, and nausea), sleep disturbances, emotional symptoms (depression and anxiety), and cognitive symptoms.

Studies of the effects of recurrent concussion in college football players have found (after observing 2,905 football players from 25 US colleges over 3 seasons) a 'dose-response' relationship between the number of previous concussions and risk of incident concussions. Players with a history of 3 or more previous concussions were 3 times more likely to have a concussion during the observed seasons than players with no concussion history. Those with more cumulative concussions were slower to recover from concussion symptoms than those with fewer concussions. Also, 30% of those with 3 or more previous concussions had symptoms lasting longer than 1 week compared with only 14.6% of those with 1 previous concussion. Of particular interest was that when repeat concussions occurred within the same season, 91.7% occurred within 10 days of the first injury, suggesting that there may be a period of particularly increased vulnerability to repeat concussion within the acute postinjury period [9]. Concerning long-term effects, research from the Center for Study of Retired Athletes showed that former professional football players with a history of 3 or more significant concussions had a fivefold greater risk of developing mild cognitive impairment, and a threefold greater incidence of being diagnosed and treated for depression during their retirement years [10, 11].

Pathophysiology of Repetitive Mild Traumatic Brain Injury

While the precise pathophysiologic mechanisms behind the clinical sequelae associated with repetitive brain injury are not entirely understood, diffuse axonal injury, microvascular changes, blood-brain barrier breakdown, and immunoexcitotoxicity

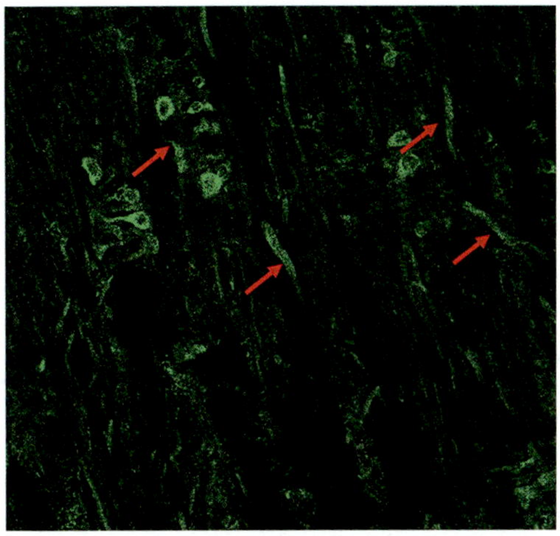

Fig. 2. Amyloid precursor protein staining following a standard, single impact rodent concussion model. Note the torn axons within the brainstem and corticospinal tract of the rat appearing as typical axon retraction bulbs.

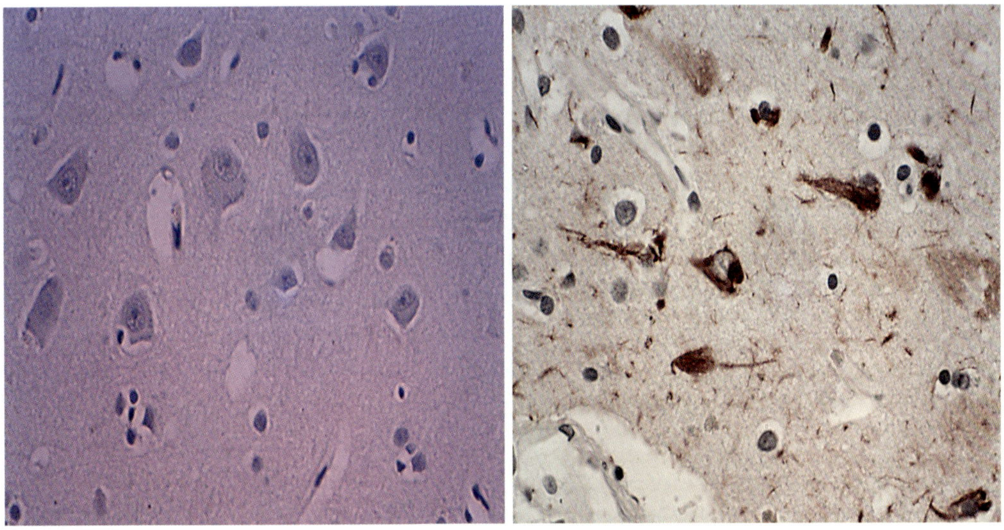

Fig. 3. Tau immunohistochemical staining showing a normal control (left) and CTE specimen (right), with characteristic tau protein deposits within the neurofibrillary tangles and neuritic threads.

have been implicated [3]. Much of our knowledge regarding the pathophysiology of repetitive concussion is gleaned from animal models of mTBI. The initial inciting event of mTBI results in diffuse axonal membrane disruption, with concomitant disruption of axonal transport and axonal swelling. This ultimately leads to axonal disconnection and wallerian degeneration [3, 12] (fig. 2). Providing further credence to the implication of axonal membrane disruption in CTE pathophysiology is the observation that abnormal tau protein accumulations, noted at autopsy on histopathological specimens of patients with CTE, are peptide derivatives of both membrane and cytoskeletal proteins which accumulate following brain injury (fig. 3).

As investigators have attempted to better understand the incidence, prevalence, and clinical course of CTE, Blaylock and Maroon [13] proposed *immunoexcitotoxicity* as the inciting mechanism. With this mechanism, the initial traumatic events serve to prime microglia, which undergo conversion to a destructive phenotype with repetitive sustained trauma and aging. The evoked proinflammatory state can be maintained for an extended period leading to a chronic neurodegenerative process (i.e. CTE), which may differ from the immediate sequelae of single-incident brain injury [13].

Because American football has a high incidence of concussion, and helmet telemetry devices can be used to measure biomechanical parameters and frequency of head impacts, it is the sport with the most available short-term biophysics data in the field of mTBI. In general, it has been felt that the greatest risk for concussion is with linear acceleration greater than 95 g, rotational acceleration greater than 5,500 rad/s^2, and with impacts occurring to the top, front, or back of the helmet [10, 14]. In addition to this, data have shown that linemen are subjected to the greatest number of impacts per season, followed by tight ends, running backs, and linebackers [14].

Evaluation of neuropsychiatric data in multiple head impacted athletes has yielded mixed results. Studies comparing preseason and postseason scores for the Automated Neuropsychological Assessment Metrics, Sensory Organization Test, Balance Error Scoring System, Graded Symptom Checklist, and ImPACT (Immediate Post-Concussion Assessment and Cognitive Testing) yielded no meaningful differences [15, 16]. On the contrary, Killam et al. [17] found that nonconcussed, collegiate athletes in contact sports scored lower than control subjects in two memory domains and lower overall scores on the Repeatable Battery for the Assessment of Neuropsychological Status (RBANS).

Furthermore, McAllister et al. [18] studied accelerometer data and neuropsychological outcomes in college football and ice hockey players compared with noncontact sport athletes and found that the contact-sport athletes had worse scores for new learning, even without having been diagnosed with a concussion. Also of note in this study was the finding that postseason cognitive impairment was correlated with greater subconcussive impact exposure. These findings were not consistent with those by Miller et al. [16] who found no preseason, midseason, or postseason difference with regard to Standardized Assessment of Concussion (SAC) and computerized neuropsychological testing in Division III football players. In summary, concerning neuropsychological testing in repeated head injury, there may be specific metrics that are more sensitive for detecting the effects of repetitive mTBI and there may be certain neuropsychiatric sequelae that require a greater length of time to develop than a single season [3]. Although no specific assessment can guide a determination of the cumulative effects, at present all of these factors can be incorporated, including the emerging concept of hit count or exposure, in arriving at a player's status regarding long-term exposure and advisability of continuing play versus retirement [3].

Recent findings now indicate that head impacts during contact sports may commonly occur, and these do not reach identification at the clinical level as no outward or visible sign of neurological dysfunction or symptomatology develops. These impacts, termed 'subconcussive impacts', have lasting effects as demonstrated by emerging evidence showing extensive tauopathy changes seen through autopsy analysis of brains of former professional football players and other athletes who did not have a diagnosis of concussion during their playing career, accelerometer data gathered in football players not known to have sustained a concussion or concussion-like symptoms during their competitive years, functional magnetic resonance (fMRI) studies, neuropsychological assessment, and in laboratory animals subjected to mTBI forces and later proven to have injury [3, 19]. Subconcussion is a cranial impact that does not result in known or diagnosed concussion on clinical grounds [3]. It may also occur with rapid acceleration-deceleration to the body or torso, particularly when the brain is free to move within the cranium, creating a 'slosh' phenomenon [20, 21]. Subconcussion has its greatest effect through repetitive occurrences whereby cumulative exposure becomes deleterious [3].

As defined by Omalu et al. [22] in 2005, CTE is a progressive neurodegenerative syndrome caused by episodic and repetitive blunt force impacts to the head and transfer of acceleration-deceleration forces to the brain. The clinical features of CTE generally involve a prolonged latency period prior to a composite syndrome of mood disorder, neuropsychiatric disturbance, and cognitive impairment [22–26]. Much of the clinical cognitive and behavioral changes and clinical status leading up to the death of patients determined to have CTE has been determined through postmortem interviews with next of kin. Insidious onset of loss recent memory, poor attention, frequent headaches, and bouts of disorientation and confusion are common early in the syndrome. While the rate of symptom development varies, there is often a progression of effects referable to poor prefrontal cortex executive function and limbic system dysfunction, including poor insight and judgment, worsening disorientation and confusion, onset of antisocial behaviors, failed business ventures and marriages, and substance and alcohol abuse [22–26].

In a review of clinical findings of football players with CTE, McKee et al. [24] reported that 80% suffered from mood disorder (mainly depression), memory loss, paranoia, and poor insight or judgment. While 60% had outbursts of anger, aggression, irritability, and apathy, 40% suffered from confusion, reduced concentration, and agitation. In more severe cases, both motor and brainstem-related deficits have been reported, including bradykinesia, staggering and propulsive gait, masked faces, tremor, dysarthria, dysphagia, and ocular abnormalities [26].

In a more recent study of 36 athlete subjects with a postmortem diagnosis of CTE, Stern et al. [25] reviewed the clinical presentation and course of symptoms obtained through postmortem telephone interviews with next of kin. They reported an overall triad of cognitive, behavioral, and mood impairments for nearly all subjects. However, upon further inspection, they reported two relatively distinct clinical presentations: those who had predominately behavior and/or mood disturbances (n = 22; symptoms including explosiveness, physical and verbal violence, depression, and inability to be controlled) which initially developed at a younger age, and a second group which appeared to involve predominately cognitive impairment (n = 11; symptoms including impairments in episodic memory and increased likelihood to progressive dementia) with noticeably less behavioral and mood disturbances. This second, older group had an initial presentation at an older age. Perhaps the most feared complications in those who have been subjected to repetitive TBI, and their loved ones, are the psychological sequelae, particularly depression and suicide.

TBI has been associated with several psychiatric disorders, impaired problem-solving, and aggression, which are established suicide risk factors. In a landmark study, Bryan and Clemans [2] tested the cumulative effect of mTBIs on the severity of psychiatric symptoms and suicide risk in a sample of deployed military personnel. They found that soldiers who had sustained more TBIs were more likely to report more severe psychological symptoms, namely posttraumatic stress, concussive symptoms, and depression, and were at an increased risk for suicide. When controlling for the effects of depression severity, posttraumatic stress disorder, and concussive symptoms, the number of TBIs was significantly associated with increased suicide risk. This study and others highlight the need for further study to help clarify the relationship between multiple mTBI occurrences, posttraumatic stress disorder, and related syndromes [27]. Currently, the diagnosis of CTE relies on autopsy and subsequent neuropathological examination [12, 28]. Both the gross and microscopic findings of brain specimens from those afflicted by repetitive brain injury will be described elsewhere. However, emerging positron emission tomography (PET) imaging with F^{18}DDNP shows promise for in vivo diagnosis of CTE or CTE-like changes (vide infra).

Our knowledge of CTE is still evolving. Many facets of the syndrome are incompletely understood, including the composition of tau protein, its isoforms, and predisposing cellular events, the prevalence and incidence amongst contact sport athletes and military combat veterans, and clinical course. Genetic predisposition certainly plays a major role, including the possibility of the influence of apolipoprotein E, but thus far has not been elucidated. The specifics of exposure, such as the number of diagnosed concussions, experience with subconcussive impacts and concept of the lifetime cranial hit count, interval between impacts, recovery time, age, and specific activity will likely all play roles in determining the risk of cumulative injury in select individuals [3].

Advancing Recognition of Repetitive Mild Traumatic Brain Injury and Development of Chronic Traumatic Encephalopathy: Potential Role for Imaging in Diagnosis

The continued reliance on neuropathological examination for diagnosis of CTE diminishes the ability to not only understand disease pathophysiology, but also prevents identification of neuropathologic changes prior to symptom onset [24]. Furthermore, without early identification of disease, there is little hope for treatment development and implementation. The prevalence of the disease, its clinical course, the relationship of tau protein accumulation to symptoms, and many other aspects of CTE are currently incompletely understood due to an inability for a premorbid diagnosis. Consequently, increasing focus has been placed on the development of imaging modalities for diagnosing concussive and subconcussive injury [23, 25]. While the short-term deficits associated with concussive injury have been historically difficult to quantify using traditional imaging modalities such as computed tomography (CT) and magnetic resonance imaging (MRI), the development of new imaging modalities and techniques have allowed for increased investigation and understanding of the neuropathological changes associated with neurotrauma [26–28]. Some of the most promising techniques and modalities are briefly summarized in the following sections.

Perhaps the most well-investigated technique for detecting axonal injury associated with neurotrauma is diffusion tensor imaging (DTI). Both preclinical and clinical studies have indicated a significant correlation between the occurrence of TBI and abnormalities detected using DTI. In addition, changes observed using DTI in a rodent model of TBI correlate with long-term outcome [29]. Similarly, preliminary studies in retired athletes have shown a relationship between concussive history and measures of injury using DTI, particularly in the callosal white matter [24]. How these measures change with age [30–33] and the development of CTE remains unclear, but DTI appears promising for the detection and tracking of structural correlates of repetitive brain injury [34–38].

Functional MRI (fMRI) has been identified as a promising diagnostic tool based on its use in recognizing subconcussive injury [39–41]. fMRI is unique amongst imaging modalities since it is the only modality that pairs functional with anatomic and structural assessment. As such, brain-behavior relationships can be observed. Equally important, prior studies have shown the ability of fMRI to distinguish between injuries of varying severity [42, 43].

In terms of gaining insight into neurotrauma pathophysiology, few techniques have been as instrumental as magnetic resonance spectroscopy, which is advantageous in that it is noninvasive and capable of measuring biochemical markers altered by TBI [44, 45]. Specific metabolites or metabolite ratios, such as N-acetylaspartate and ATP, can be measured and provide insight into reversible neuronal or mitochondrial dysfunction. Similarly, an increase in the N-acetylaspartate:creatinine ratio indicates persistent damage following neurotrauma. Other advantages of magnetic resonance spectroscopy include the ability to track metabolites, and therefore recovery, longitudinally over the course of a season or career – both before and after injury or trauma exposure [46–48]. Prior work by Lin et al. [49, 50] demonstrated persistent changes in some metabolites in professional athletes in relation to control subjects. Consequently, these metabolite measurements may represent a unique means for not only understanding neurotrauma, but also for following such patients temporally, both of which are likely to be important in understanding the development of chronic symptoms, CTE-like effects, or a CTE clinical syndrome, as well as identifying safe return-to-play guidelines.

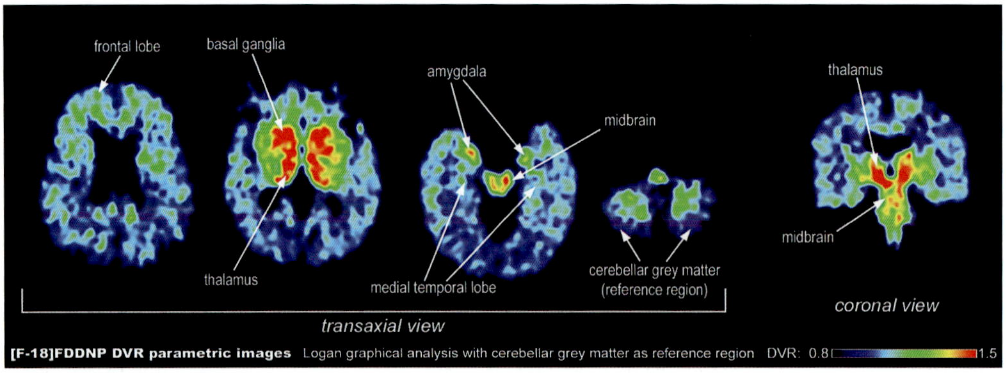

Fig. 4. [F-18]FDDNP distribution volume ratio (DVR) parametric images showing the brain of a retired NFL player with decline in normal brain function. Transaxial images show typical distribution pattern of increased [F-18]FDDNP signal in the frontal lobe, basal ganglia and thalamus, amygdala and the rest of medial temporal lobe, and midbrain. Cerebellar gray matter is used as reference and is shown for visual comparison with the affected areas.

A final imaging modality poised to contribute to the identification and understanding of neurotrauma and the progression to neurodegenerative disease such as CTE, is PET. While traditional PET studies are unlikely to play a role, limited primarily to observation of regions of hypometabolism after injury, the development of tau-binding radiolabeled ligands has drastically increased the likelihood PET will play a role in future work, as has been suggested in former boxers [51, 52]. Specifically, Small et al. [53] have shown in a limited series of cases the ability to identify an increased tau burden within the brains of retired professional football players subjected to repetitive neurotrauma. This work in particular represents the first effort clearly showing the potential of premortem CTE diagnosis. Using F^{18}DDNP, which labels amyloid but most importantly is the only definitive in vivo marker of tau protein deposits, characteristic findings in preliminary studies demonstrate accumulation of tau in the amygdala, subcortical regions, and areas of the mesencephalon (fig. 4). This specific pattern has not been seen in other forms of brain maladies including Alzheimer's disease and other dementias, depression, and mild cognitive impairment. Current clinical research should elucidate the ultimate potential for F^{18}DDNP to provide an in vivo diagnosis of a CTE pattern of injury.

Return to Play

The decision-making process regarding return to play in sports is often difficult and involves many complex factors. The practice of neurological sports medicine is fraught with innumerable potential factors and circumstances, which results in each decision needing to be individualized [6]. The circumstances that are involved in the various sports, which entail both regular purposeful head contact as well as those that have the potential for frequent collisions, are all considered prior to formulating a final course of action.

Table 1. Retirement decision factors[a]

Season-ending factors
Prolonged PCS
≥2 major concussions[b] in a single season
Abnormality on neurologic examination
Diminished academic performance
Diminished athletic performance
CT or MRI brain scan showing traumatic abnormality
Career-ending factors
Chiari malformation[c]
Intracranial hemorrhage
Diminished academic performance or cognitive abilities
Persistent prolonged PCS
Lowering of threshold for concussion (as judged by physicians, athletes, coaches, certified athletic trainers)
≥3 major concussions
CT or MRI scan documentation of structural brain injury
Nonresolving fMRI scan deficits
CTE symptoms

[a] All return-to-play and retirement decisions are individualized; some features are relative contraindications for return to play. [b] Major concussion: symptomatic for >1 week or loss of playing time. [c] If symptomatic or associated with sports concussions.

The care of the athlete involved in contact or collision sports has traditionally been based upon clinical factors meshed with concussion grading scales. In recent years, the grading of concussions has fallen into disfavor for several reasons. In the past, it was customary that for each grade of concussion, a predetermined and standardized approach to the length of time off and the safe return strategy. However, with more accrued experience and clinical experience, we now know that return to play must be approached in a flexible, graded, and individualized system of care [3, 5]. The full spectrum of postconcussion symptomatology should be considered in every case in order to arrive at an optimal plan for continuation of the respective sport, or for retirement in some instances. If, however, it appears that the cumulative result of repetitive mTBI places the athlete's future participation at risk, there are accepted factors which help guide retirement decision-making (table 1).

Conclusion

There has been tremendous progress in the understanding of the potential for cumulative effects for those having sustained mTBI, especially if repetitive concussions or subconcussive impacts have occurred [54]. Not only do we have a better appreciation of the acute symptomatology of mTBI, but we also know more about the potential for chronic effects. In addition to the clinical course, emerging technologies including neuroimaging studies and biomarkers provide hope that improved outcomes are on the horizon [12, 53].

References

1 Daneshvar DH, Nowinski CJ, McKee AC, Cantu RC: The epidemiology of sport-related concussion. Clin Sports Med 2011;30:1–17.

2 Bryan CJ, Clemans TA: Repetitive traumatic brain injury, psychological symptoms, and suicide risk in a clinical sample of deployed military personnel. JAMA Psychiatry 2013;70:686–691.

3 Bailes JE, Petraglia AL, Omalu BI, Nauman E, Talavage T: Role of subconcussion in repetitive mild traumatic brain injury. J Neurosurg 2013;119:1235–1245.

4 McCrory P, Meeuwisse W, Aubry M, Cantu B, Dvorak J, Echemendia R, Engebretsen L, Johnston K, Kutcher J, Raftery M, Sills A, Benson B, Davis G, Ellenbogen R, Guskiewicz K, Herring SA, Iverson G, Jordan B, Kissick J, McCrea M, McIntosh A, Maddocks D, Makdissi M, Purcell L, Putukian M, et al: Consensus statement on concussion in sport – the 4th International Conference on Concussion in Sport held in Zurich, November 2012. Phys Ther Sport 2013;14:e1–e13.

5 Petraglia AL, Maroon JC, Bailes JE: From the field of play to the field of combat: a review of the pharmacological management of concussion. Neurosurgery 2012;70:1520–1533.

6 Sedney CL, Orphanos J, Bailes JE: When to consider retiring an athlete after sports-related concussion. Clin Sports Med 2011;30:189–200, xi.

7 Ouellet MC, Beaulieu-Bonneau S, Morin CM: Insomnia in patients with traumatic brain injury: frequency, characteristics, and risk factors. J Head Trauma Rehabil 2006;21:199–212.

8 Bryan CJ: Repetitive traumatic brain injury (or concussion) increases severity of sleep disturbance among deployed military personnel. Sleep 2013;36:941–946.

9 Guskiewicz KM, McCrea M, Marshall SW, Cantu RC, Randolph C, Barr W, Onate JA, Kelly JP: Cumulative effects associated with recurrent concussion in collegiate football players: the NCAA Concussion Study. JAMA 2003;290:2549–2555.

10 Guskiewicz KM, Marshall SW, Bailes J, McCrea M, Cantu RC, Randolph C, Jordan BD: Association between recurrent concussion and late-life cognitive impairment in retired professional football players. Neurosurgery 2005;57:719–726.

11 Guskiewicz KM, Marshall SW, Bailes J, McCrea M, Harding HP Jr, Matthews A, Mihalik JR, Cantu RC: Recurrent concussion and risk of depression in retired professional football players. Med Sci Sports Exerc 2007;39:903–909.

12 Turner RC, Lucke-Wold BP, Robson MJ, Omalu BI, Petraglia AL, Bailes JE: Repetitive traumatic brain injury and development of chronic traumatic encephalopathy: a potential role for biomarkers in diagnosis, prognosis, and treatment? Front Neurol 2012;3:186.

13 Blaylock RL, Maroon J: Immunoexcitotoxicity as a central mechanism in chronic traumatic encephalopathy – a unifying hypothesis. Surg Neurol Int 2011;2:107.

14 Broglio SP, Eckner JT, Martini D, Sosnoff JJ, Kutcher JS, Randolph C: Cumulative head impact burden in high school football. J Neurotrauma 2011;28:2069–2078.

15 Gysland SM, Mihalik JP, Register-Mihalik JK, Trulock SC, Shields EW, Guskiewicz KM: The relationship between subconcussive impacts and concussion history on clinical measures of neurologic function in collegiate football players. Ann Biomed Eng 2012; 40:14–22.

16 Miller JR, Adamson GJ, Pink MM, Sweet JC: Comparison of preseason, midseason, and postseason neurocognitive scores in uninjured collegiate football players. Am J Sports Med 2007;35:1284–1288.

17 Killam C, Cautin RL, Santucci AC: Assessing the enduring residual neuropsychological effects of head trauma in college athletes who participate in contact sports. Arch Clin Neuropsychol 2005;20:599–611.

18 McAllister TW, Flashman LA, Maerlender A, Greenwald RM, Beckwith JG, Tosteson TD, Crisco JJ, Brolinson PG, Duma SM, Duhaime AC, Grove MR, Turco JH: Cognitive effects of one season of head impacts in a cohort of collegiate contact sport athletes. Neurology 2012;78:1777–1784.

19 Pardini J, Bailes J, Maroon J: Mild traumatic brain injury in adults and concussion in sports; in Winn HR (ed): Youmans Neurological Surgery, ed 6. Saunders, Philadelphia, 2011, pp 3380–3389.

20 Smith DW, Bailes JE, Fisher JA, Robles J, Turner RC, Mills JD: Internal jugular vein compression mitigates traumatic axonal injury in a rat model by reducing the intracranial slosh effect. Neurosurgery 2012;70:740–746.

21 Turner RC, Naser ZJ, Bailes JE, Smith DW, Fisher JA, Rosen CL: Effect of slosh mitigation on histologic markers of traumatic brain injury: laboratory investigation. J Neurosurg 2012;117:1110–1118.
22 Omalu BI, DeKosky ST, Minster RL, Kamboh MI, Hamilton RL, Wecht CH: Chronic traumatic encephalopathy in a National Football League player. Neurosurgery 2005;57:128–134.
23 Randolph C, Karantzoulis S, Guskiewicz K: Prevalence and characterization of mild cognitive impairment in retired National Football League players. J Int Neuropsychol Soc 2013;19:873–880.
24 McKee AC, Stein TD, Nowinski CJ, Stern RA, Daneshvar DH, Alvarez VE, Lee HS, Hall G, Wojtowicz SM, Baugh CM, Riley DO, Kubilus CA, Cormier KA, Jacobs MA, Martin BR, Abraham CR, Ikezu T, Reichard RR, Wolozin BL, Budson AE, Goldstein LE, Kowall NW, Cantu RC: The spectrum of disease in chronic traumatic encephalopathy. Brain 2013; 136:43–64.
25 Stern RA, Daneshvar DH, Baugh CM, Seichepine DR, Montenigro PH, Riley DO, Fritts NG, Stamm JM, Robbins CA, McHale L, Simkin I, Stein TD, Alvarez VE, Goldstein LE, Budson AE, Kowall NW, Nowinski CJ, Cantu RC, McKee AC: Clinical presentation of chronic traumatic encephalopathy. Neurology 2013;81:1122–1129.
26 McKee AC, Cantu RC, Nowinski CJ, Hedley-Whyte ET, Gavett BE, Budson AE, Santini VE, Lee HS, Kubilus CA, Stern RA: Chronic traumatic encephalopathy in athletes: progressive tauopathy after repetitive head injury. J Neuropathol Exp Neurol 2009;68:709–735.
27 Omalu B, Hammers JL, Bailes J, Hamilton RL, Kamboh MI, Webster G, Fitzsimmons RP: Chronic traumatic encephalopathy in an Iraqi war veteran with posttraumatic stress disorder who committed suicide. Neurosurg Focus 2011;31:E3.
28 Saulle M, Greenwald BD: Chronic traumatic encephalopathy: a review. Rehabil Res Pract 2012;2012: 816069.
29 Baugh CM, Stamm JM, Riley DO, Gavett BE, Shenton ME, Lin A, Nowinski CJ, Cantu RC, McKee AC, Stern RA: Chronic traumatic encephalopathy: neurodegeneration following repetitive concussive and subconcussive brain trauma. Brain Imaging Behav 2012;6:244–254.
30 McCrory P: Sports concussion and the risk of chronic neurological impairment. Clin J Sport Med 2011; 21:6–12.
31 Prichep LS, McCrea M, Barr W, Powell M, Chabot RJ: Time course of clinical and electrophysiological recovery after sport-related concussion. J Head Trauma Rehabil 2013;28:266–273.
32 Signoretti S, Lazzarino G, Tavazzi B, Vagnozzi R: The pathophysiology of concussion. PM R 2011; 3(10 Suppl 2):S359–S368.
33 Lakhan SE, Kirchgessner A: Chronic traumatic encephalopathy: the dangers of getting 'dinged'. Springerplus 2012;1:2.
34 MacDonald CL, Dikranian K, Song SK, Bayly PV, Holtzman DM, Brody DL: Detection of traumatic axonal injury with diffusion tensor imaging in a mouse model of traumatic brain injury. Exp Neurol 2007;205:116–131.
35 Shah S, Yallampalli R, Merkley TL, McCauley SR, Bigler ED, Macleod M, Chu Z, Li X, Troyanskaya M, Hunter JV, Levin HS, Wilde EA: Diffusion tensor imaging and volumetric analysis of the ventral striatum in adults with traumatic brain injury. Brain Inj 2012;26:201–210.
36 Shenton ME, Hamoda HM, Schneiderman JS, Bouix S, Pasternak O, Rathi Y, Vu MA, Purohit MP, Helmer K, Koerte I, Lin AP, Westin CF, Kikinis R, Kubicki M, Stern RA, Zafonte R: A review of magnetic resonance imaging and diffusion tensor imaging findings in mild traumatic brain injury. Brain Imaging Behav 2012;6:137–192.
37 Smits M, Houston GC, Dippel DW, Wielopolski PA, Vernooij MW, Koudstaal PJ, Hunink MG, van der Lugt A: Microstructural brain injury in post-concussion syndrome after minor head injury. Neuroradiology 2011;53:553–563.
38 Maller JJ, Thomson RH, Lewis PM, Rose SE, Pannek K, Fitzgerald PB: Traumatic brain injury, major depression, and diffusion tensor imaging: making connections. Brain Res Rev 2010;64:213–240.
39 Gavett BE, Cantu RC, Shenton M, Lin AP, Nowinski CJ, McKee AC, Stern RA: Clinical appraisal of chronic traumatic encephalopathy: current perspectives and future directions. Curr Opin Neurol 2011; 24:525–531.
40 Tremblay S, De BL, Henry LC, Boulanger Y, Evans AC, Bourgouin P, Poirier J, Theoret H, Lassonde M: Sports concussions and aging: a neuroimaging investigation. Cereb Cortex 2013;23:1159–1166.
41 McDonald BC, Saykin AJ, McAllister TW: Functional MRI of mild traumatic brain injury (mTBI): progress and perspectives from the first decade of studies. Brain Imaging Behav 2012;6:193–207.
42 Talavage TM, Nauman EA, Breedlove EL, Yoruk U, Dye AE, Morigaki KE, Feuer H, Leverenz LJ: Functionally-detected cognitive impairment in high school football players without clinically-diagnosed concussion. J Neurotrauma 2013, Epub ahead of print.
43 Breedlove EL, Robinson M, Talavage TM, Morigaki KE, Yoruk U, O'Keefe K, King J, Leverenz LJ, Gilger JW, Nauman EA: Biomechanical correlates of symptomatic and asymptomatic neurophysiological impairment in high school football. J Biomech 2012;45: 1265–1272.

44 Tshibanda L, Vanhaudenhuyse A, Galanaud D, Boly M, Laureys S, Puybasset L: Magnetic resonance spectroscopy and diffusion tensor imaging in coma survivors: promises and pitfalls. Prog Brain Res 2009; 177:215–229.
45 Henry LC, Tremblay S, Leclerc S, Khiat A, Boulanger Y, Ellemberg D, Lassonde M: Metabolic changes in concussed American football players during the acute and chronic post-injury phases. BMC Neurol 2011;11:105.
46 Bigler ED, Maxwell WL: Neuropathology of mild traumatic brain injury: relationship to neuroimaging findings. Brain Imaging Behav 2012;6:108–136.
47 Henry LC, Tremblay S, Boulanger Y, Ellemberg D, Lassonde M: Neurometabolic changes in the acute phase after sports concussions correlate with symptom severity. J Neurotrauma 2010;27:65–76.
48 Kleindienst A, Tolias CM, Corwin FD, Muller C, Marmarou A, Fatouros P, Bullock MR: Assessment of cerebral S100B levels by proton magnetic resonance spectroscopy after lateral fluid-percussion injury in the rat. J Neurosurg 2005;102:1115–1121.
49 Lin A, Ramadan S, Box H, Stanwell P, Stern R: Neurochemical changes in athletes with chronic traumatic encephalopathy. Radiological Society of North America, Chicago, 2010.
50 Lin AP, Liao HJ, Merugumala SK, Prabhu SP, Meehan WP III, Ross BD: Metabolic imaging of mild traumatic brain injury. Brain Imaging Behav 2012;6: 208–223.
51 Venneti S, Wagner AK, Wang G, Slagel SL, Chen X, Lopresti BJ, Mathis CA, Wiley CA: The high affinity peripheral benzodiazepine receptor ligand DAA1106 binds specifically to microglia in a rat model of traumatic brain injury: implications for PET imaging. Exp Neurol 2007;207:118–127.
52 Provenzano FA, Jordan B, Tikofsky RS, Saxena C, Van Heertum RL, Ichise M: F-18 FDG PET imaging of chronic traumatic brain injury in boxers: a statistical parametric analysis. Nucl Med Commun 2010; 31:952–957.
53 Small GW, Kepe V, Siddarth P, Ercoli LM, Merrill DA, Donoghue N, Bookheimer SY, Martinez J, Omalu B, Bailes J, Barrio JR: PET scanning of brain tau in retired National Football League players: preliminary findings. Am J Geriatr Psychiatry 2013;21:138–144.
54 Dashnaw ML, Petraglia AL, Bailes JE: An overview of the basic science of concussion and subconcussion: where we are and where we are going. Neurosurg Focus 2012;33:E5–E9.
55 Schieder R: Head and Neck Injuries in Football, ed 1. Baltimore, Williams and Wilkins, 1973.

Julian E. Bailes, MD
Department of Neurosurgery, NorthShore University HealthSystem
University of Chicago Pritzker School of Medicine
2650 Ridge Avenue, Kellogg-3rd Floor
Evanston, IL 60201 (USA)
E-Mail jbailes@northshore.org

Niranjan A, Lunsford LD (eds): Concussion. Prog Neurol Surg. Basel, Karger, 2014, vol 28, pp 63–74
DOI: 10.1159/000358763

Understanding Concussive Injuries Using Investigational Imaging Methods

Luke C. Henry
University of Pittsburgh, UPMC Sports Concussion Program, Pittsburgh, Pa., USA

Abstract
Concussions have long been understood to be an invisible injury. Indeed, conventional imaging techniques [computed tomography and magnetic resonance imaging (MRI)] are largely ineffective in elucidating concussive injuries. More advanced techniques are being used experimentally to help delineate the underlying pathophysiology of concussive injuries on metabolic as well as ultrastructural levels. The current report reviews the data from several of these techniques including functional MRI, single-photon emission computed tomography, positron emission tomography, diffusion tensor imaging, and magnetic resonance spectroscopy. Each technique is briefly described, followed by a summary of the findings specific to concussive injuries. Overall, there is mounting evidence to suggest that each technique has utility in describing and explaining postinjury changes in the brain. Overall, concussive injuries are evident using the various aforementioned neuroimaging modalities and suggest at a minimum the concussed brain is different in the acute and subacute postinjury phases with several other studies suggesting that changes are persistent well beyond, especially in those patients with persistent symptoms. © 2014 S. Karger AG, Basel

Understanding the physical consequences of a concussive injury has proven to be an arduous if not elusive task. Symptoms varying anywhere from minutes to months or even years can be present in concussed patients despite any apparent physical injury. Reconciling the neural effects of concussion with the apparent absence of visible damage has continued to be rather puzzling even with the advent and widespread clinical use of imaging techniques such as computed tomography (CT) and magnetic resonance imaging (MRI). In a large-scale study investigating the utility of CT scans [1] only 16% of scans were read as positive. However, it is worth noting that within this 16%, the criteria fitting 'mild' traumatic brain injury (mTBI) were only loosely defined and those patients with a positive scan shared several characteristics in common, including intracranial abnormalities, loss of consciousness, skull fractures, and lower Glasgow Coma Scale and Galveston Orientation and Amnesia Test scores. Though still used in emergency settings because of their relative cost-effectiveness and wide availability [2], CT scans have very limited utility in research due to their inability to detect finite lesions and contusions, especially relative to even basic structural MRI [3–5].

MRI has much higher resolution, capacity to image different planes, and provides better distinction between tissue types, i.e. gray matter, white matter, and cerebrospinal fluid. Typical injuries detected by MRI resulting from sport concussion include small cortical contusions or subdural hematomas. Additionally, MRI is also sensitive to small white matter hemorrhages [2] thought to be reflective of diffuse axonal injury [6]. Though more effective at detecting abnormalities than CT [3, 4], MRI has proven inconsistent with only moderate predictive validity in sports concussion [3, 4], and concussion in general [1, 6, 7]. MRI, though clearly superior to CT, is still unable to detect lesions in the vast majority of concussed athletes [3, 8], which limits its use from not only a clinical standpoint, but also from a research standpoint. However, there are several emerging investigational neuroimaging techniques that are capable of detecting functional, metabolic, and more finite structural changes resulting from concussive injuries. Even as the research using these techniques is in many ways still in its infancy with respect to concussive injuries, much of what is presently known about the pathophysiological processes in the concussed brain is based on findings using these technologies. This report will focus on functional MRI (fMRI), single-photon emission computed tomography (SPECT), positron emission tomography (PET), diffusion tensor imaging (DTI), and magnetic resonance spectroscopy (MRS).

Functional Magnetic Resonance Imaging

fMRI is based on the same basic concept as MRI, though instead of capitalizing on hydrogen protons to create an image, it takes advantage of the magnetic properties of hemoglobin. The most common paradigm used in fMRI research tracks blood oxygenation changes by detecting the blood oxygenation level-dependent (BOLD) signal [2]. The underlying assumption is that blood flow is increased in areas related to the cognitive process inherent to the task and the subsequent increased metabolic demand. Changes in blood flow as a result of an injury are therefore thought to represent impaired or altered functional capacity.

Though the body of literature on fMRI is limited, the results in the few studies that have used fMRI consistently find differences between concussed individuals and control subjects, though the nature of those changes is not always the same. Chen et al. [9, 10] found reduced activation localized to the dorsolateral prefrontal cortex using a working memory paradigm. Furthermore, this work demonstrated that atypical BOLD signals correlated with self-reported symptoms in concussed athletes regardless of how remote the injuries were, ranging from 1 to 14 months after injury. Likewise, Mayer et al. [11] also reported hypoactivation in concussed patients within several cortical and subcortical areas in correlation with poor performance on tasks of auditory orientation and attention inhibition relative to noninjured controls.

In contrast, other studies have found the BOLD signal in the concussed brain to be characterized by hyperactivation. Using a series of different working memory tasks, McAllister et al. [12–14] showed enhanced and more widespread BOLD signals in the dorsolateral prefrontal cortex of concussed subjects relative to age-matched controls within 1 month after injury where the increased activation was noted to be disproportionately high for moderate-to-difficult tasks [14]. Using a motor-sequencing task, Jantzen et al. [15] noted an atypically increased BOLD response in parietal and lateral frontal cortical areas. This preliminary finding was confirmed by Jantzen [16], who demonstrated increased activation in the parietal, lateral frontal, and cerebellar regions in concussed subjects relative to preinjury scans even when cognitive performance was equivalent. Similarly, Lovell et al. [17] scanned concussed athletes in the acute postconcussion phase (1 week after concussion) and approximately 1 month after injury. Briefly, athletes who displayed hyperactivation on a cognitive task in the acute phase had prolonged recovery times relative to those athletes who demonstrated typical activation in the acute phase.

The disparity in the fMRI findings may be due to several factors, with differences in techniques, tasks, and research questions among them. What seems ubiquitous is that there are changes in activation patterns. These changes may be reflective of brain reorganization which would imply more permanent changes in the neural substrate. The changes may also represent neural compensation to buttress performance where the brain is recruiting more area without permanent alterations to the existing neural pathways. Such a notion implies transience to the observed alterations. Finally, changes in brain activation may be reflective of what Hillary et al. [18, 19] termed the 'latent support hypothesis', which essentially posits that the concussed brain is less functionally able and therefore needs to recruit other brain areas to complete a given task in a manner similar to the nonconcussed brain – only this is done with increasingly easier tasks that would normally not require neural recruitment. That is to say, in the concussed brain, a task normally requiring moderate brain activation would require more widespread activation that would otherwise be reserved for more difficult tasks.

While it seems there is ample evidence to support changes in the concussed brain under cognitive demand, there is also evidence to suggest that even at rest, the injured brain behaves differently. Studies investigating functional connectivity of the brain at rest have found acute postinjury changes in the strength, but not the number, of connections [20, 21] and overall reduced interhemispheric connectivity [22]. Further research looking at the default mode network shows a similar reduction in connection strength and in number, as well as a moderating effect of the number of injuries sustained [22]. Similar findings in more chronic patients have shown functional connectivity changes between frontal lobe circuits and the hippocampus at resting states in patients with diffuse axonal injury [23]. Again, the extant literature shows the concussed brain to behave differently than the noninjured brain. The differences in activation may in fact be showing reorganization; however, a more conservative interpretation of the data suggests that these changes are more likely a reflection of the concussed brain's use of existing support resources early after neural disruption to help mitigate demand and improve efficiency during recovery.

Single-Photon Emission Tomography and Positron Emission Tomography

Similar to resting state fMRI, and available at a fraction of the cost, SPECT also provides information about changes in cerebral blood perfusion, but does so through an intravenously injected radioactive ligand that accumulates in different brain areas in proportion to the delivery of nutrients to provide an overall picture of regional cerebral blood flow [2]. There have been several studies using SPECT to investigate mTBI, the majority of which have focused on chronic postinjury patient samples. The few studies that have examined concussive injuries in the acute/subacute phase have shown consistent findings. The acute postinjury phase is characterized by hypoperfusion in a similar pattern to more severely brain-injured patients [24, 25]. Hypoperfusion is most evident in temporal and frontal regions, though these differences are moderated by age, with children showing more hypoperfusion in the former and adults in the latter [26]. Subacutely, hypoperfusion remains evident in the frontal and temporal regions [27, 28], though there does not seem to be a relationship to hypoperfused areas and neurocognitive performance [28].

Chronic postinjury studies have shown similar findings to those conducted more immediately after injury and moderately correlate with clinical outcome [29–31]. Several studies comparing SPECT with CT and MRI have consistently shown SPECT to be far superior to its conventional counterparts at detecting abnormalities in the concussed brain [31–35]. Although there is variability in the findings, the vast majority of studies have shown hypoperfusion in the frontal and temporal areas [27, 29, 30, 32, 36, 37] in addition to other brain regions such as the basal ganglia [35] and cerebellum [38, 39]. Further, these abnormalities anatomically correlate to abnormalities in the blood-brain barrier and cortical rhythm generators [40]. However, the strength of SPECT findings in relation to neurocognitive function varies greatly: one study showed no relationship at all [32], another suggested a moderate relationship [29], and others found the relationship to be quite strong [30, 34, 38, 39, 41].

PET offers an advantage that neither SPECT nor fMRI can offer. PET constructs a highly sensitive functional three-dimensional image of the brain from the emissions of a radio isotope and can directly detect blood flow, much like SPECT and fMRI, as well as track glucose and oxygen metabolism in the brain. The majority of PET studies have focused on nonsport-related mTBI patients with persistent symptomatology and found that the frontotemporal regions are the most consistently impaired regions [36, 42–45]. Only one study using PET was conducted on a single patient within the acute phase where hypoperfusion in the frontal and temporal areas was evident [46].

However, given the paltry sample size, making any suppositions with respect to PET in the acute/subacute phase is speculative at best. PET appears to offer reasonable correlation with neuropsychological deficit [36, 45, 47], which is consistent with fMRI and SPECT findings.

Diffusion Tensor Imaging

Regardless of the directionality and the duration of the functional and hemodynamic changes, what is apparent is that changes are indeed present in the concussed brain. Importantly, there also seems to be some degree of correlation between those functional changes and self-reported symptoms; however, what functional imaging is able to demonstrate with respect to alterations in neural networks and cerebral blood flow, it still cannot account for an underlying anatomical substrate. DTI provides information about brain microstructure by quantifying isotropic (typical of gray matter) and anisotropic (typical of white matter) water diffusion. DTI measurements are based on the fact that the network of fibers within the brain is composed of a distinct microstructure that inherently constrains the flow of water molecules. Diffusion tensors numerically model the direction of fastest diffusion in a pattern aligned with fiber orientation. DTI's main utility in neurology is detecting the presence of axonal injury [2].

There are several ways to analyze DTI data depending on the research or clinical question. Fractional anisotropy (FA) and mean diffusivity (MD) are the most often used measures of diffusivity [2]. FA is derived from three eigenvalues, the longest (λ_1), middle (λ_2), and shortest (λ_3) distances around a given tensor which correspond to linear (cigar-shaped) and planar (plate-shaped) anisotropic diffusion, and isotropic (spherical) diffusion, respectively, which define the shape of the tensor as an ellipse. Diffusion anisotropy can be modeled more completely using a set of three matrices where each plane is parameterized in a barycentric space with the three extremes at each corner [2], making it possible to separate the eigenvalues in order to obtain values of axial diffusivity taken from the linear plane and radial diffusivity derived by averaging the planar and spherical planes. MD is simply the average diffusivity along all three eigenvectors divided by three which gives the overall diffusion of water regardless of direction.

There is mounting evidence suggesting that DTI is a useful imaging modality in the investigation of mTBI/concussion. Stemming back just over a decade, researchers have found decreases in FA along the corpus callosum as well as the internal capsule [48] where others have found a strong correlation between the extent of the changes in FA and the severity of the brain injury [49]. Several studies focusing on the acute postinjury phase have successfully detected changes in FA/MD in concussed patients.

Postinjury alterations can be detected within the first week. Though not unanimous across studies, vulnerable brain areas include the corpus callosum (both genu and splenium), the internal capsule, and the cortical spinal tracts as has been illustrated in both case [49, 50] and group studies [51–53]. Furthermore, the observed axonal shearing in people with mTBI has functional consequences. Lee et al. [50] noted that brain areas affected by axonal injury corresponded to the types of neuropsychological dysfunctions that patients exhibited. Similarly, Miles et al. [53] observed neuropsychological correlations between FA/MD changes and neurocognitive performance.

Diffusion alterations are not limited to the acute postconcussion phase. Changes are also evident in the chronic postinjury phase for months to even years after injury. Several studies investigating mTBI in adult trauma samples have found diffuse white matter differences spanning the corpus callosum [52] as well as cortical white matter in frontotemporal [52] and midbrain regions [54] manifest as changes in FA, MD, radial diffusivity, and/or axial diffusion. Further, diffusivity changes are present in asymptomatic and symptomatic patients alike, though symptomatic patients have demonstrated overall higher MD values than both controls and asymptomatic patients in the corpus callosum, thalamic radiations, and frontotemporal brain areas [55]. A study investigating concussed college athletes who had been symptomatic for at least 1 month found no changes in FA, but did find that concussed athletes showed significantly increased MD in the left hemisphere (specifically parts of the inferior/superior longitudinal and frontooccipital fasciculi, the retrolenticular part of the internal capsule, and posterior thalamic and acoustic radiations) [56].

Converging evidence points to DTI's utility in detecting diffusivity changes in acute and chronic postinjury time points; however, questions remain about its clinical utility. Perhaps the single largest factor in the trepidation about DTI as a clinical tool lies in the disparity of the findings. Indeed, while there appear to be a few brain areas that are more vulnerable to diffuse axonal injury, findings often indicate polarizing results with some studies showing decreased FA/increased MD [48, 53, 57–60] while others demonstrate increased FA/decreased MD [51, 52, 61, 62].

These differences may be due to the use of different patient populations (i.e. trauma vs. sport-related, age, gender), different imaging techniques, and different time intervals. The reasons for the differences are multifactorial, ranging from the postprocessing analysis techniques to the study target population. It may very well be that there are different, still unknown factors that cause an individual's brain to respond differently than another's. Such differences are unlikely to be detected in group-based studies and thus postinjury differences specific to individual participants may be washed out. Irrespective of the directionality of the changes in diffusivity, there are likely vast differences in the underlying pathophysiology of those brains that exhibit decreased FA/increased MD and those showing the opposite. It has been intimated that decreased FA/increased MD indicates vasogenic edema, which will likely resolve over time [63]. Conversely, increased FA/reduced MD may indicate cytotoxic edema, characterized by axonal swelling and more restricted diffusion of water, thereby explaining the increase in FA and decrease in MD [63]. As yet, it is difficult to make a case for one or the other being more severe than the other, though it is speculated that increased FA/decreased MD may result in a poorer prognosis [64].

Magnetic Resonance Spectroscopy

Concussions are well understood to be primarily a neurometabolic injury [65]. Certainly the findings in other imaging modalities reviewed in the current report would support such a notion. With that in mind, there is perhaps no better imaging tool available to provide in vivo analysis of the metabolic processes of the concussed brain than MRS. Using standard clinical MR scanners, MRS is ideal for repeated measurements and tracking therapeutic outcomes. MRS can be quantified using two different methods: absolute quantitation and relative quantitation (RQ). Absolute quantitation is a simple and straightforward method where the concentration of a given metabolite is reported. It is generally considered to be the more precise method as it makes no assumptions about the stability of a given neurometabolite, an assumption that is inherent in RQ. However, absolute quantitation is much more difficult to process than RQ, and introduces more individual variance [66]. RQ, on the other hand has been successfully applied in the diagnosis of several pathologies including epilepsy, cancer, dementia, and multiple sclerosis, to name a few. RQ also normalizes the neurometabolic concentrations to an extent as they are expressed as ratios. As mentioned, a key assumption in RQ is the stability of certain metabolites, namely creatine (Cr) and choline, which are used as reference metabolites. This can complicate the interpretation of spectra as any detectable changes may in fact be due to a change in either the metabolite being measured, a change in the reference metabolite, or both. There are several neurometabolites that can be imaged using MRS, but only a few of the more often used/reported are discussed in the current review, including Cr, myo-inositol (m-I), glutamate (Glu) and N-acetylaspartate (NAA).

Cr is synthesized endogenously in the liver and kidneys and is also available exogenously in fish and meats [67]. It is essential for maintaining the supply of ATP inter- and intracellularly through Cr kinase and the phosphocreatine system which bridge sites of ATP consumption and production. Because the brain accounts for roughly 20% of the body's energy consumption, an extremely high rate of ATP turnover is necessary to maintain electrical membrane potentials as well as signaling activities [67]. Studies investigating the role of Cr in brain trauma have not revealed any changes in its concentration, but have demonstrated its neuroprotective role. That is to say, higher levels of Cr minimize cell damage [67].

m-I is synthesized throughout the body, but mostly within the brain where its concentration is also the greatest [68]. It serves as a precursor molecule for inositol lipid synthesis, and is also an osmolyte. The concentration of m-I is maintained via three mechanisms responsible for (1) the transport of inositol across the plasma membrane mediated by specific carrier molecules, (2) the synthesis of an isomer, and (3) the efflux of inositol mediated by a volume-sensitive osmolyte channel. In functioning cells the osmotic pressure is in a constant state of flux which must be tightly regulated so that the cell does not sustain damage due to changes in cell volume. Acutely, this is done by the movement of NA^+, K^+, H^+, and Cl^- across the membrane, and chronically by the transport of osmolytes, namely m-I. Physical trauma to the brain can compromise the blood-brain barrier resulting in leakage of ions and macromolecules into the cerebral extracellular space which in turn translates into an upregulation of an m-I transporter (sodium m-I transporter) and cellular uptake of m-I.

Glu, a member of the family of biogenic amines, is the most frequently occurring neurotransmitter in the central nervous system [7, 69]. It is produced from α-ketoglutarate, and once released after catabolism, Glu is taken up from the synaptic cleft by neurons and glia. Within glia, specifically astrocytes, it is converted to glutamine, a nonneuroexcitatory amino acid, by glutamine synthase which occurs almost exclusively in neuroglia [70]. The role of Glu differs depending on the type of receptor that it binds with: Glu is excitatory at ionotropic receptors, but modulatory at metabotropic receptors [69]. However, Glu has a role beyond that of neurotransmitter. It is also an important neurometabolite used in the production of nitrogen, which is key in the synthesis of proteins and nucleic acid, and essential to the production of other important molecules, including GABA.

NAA is present at exceptionally high concentrations in the brain second only to Glu, and is the largest peak in spectra of healthy brain tissue [71]. NAA is synthesized in neuronal mitochondria by Asp-NAT using acetyl-CoA and L-aspartate. Aspartoacylase hydrolyzes NAA, localized primarily in oligodendrocytes, producing acetate and aspartate. It is synthesized and exported from neuronal mitochondria [72] where it is exported to oligodendrocytes as a key contributor in the formation of myelin lipid formation. NAA is also thought to be an osmoregulator [73]. It had been hypothesized that upon sustaining brain trauma, a loss of NAA was equal to traumatic axonal injury in white matter and neuronal loss in gray matter [74, 75].

Within the acute/subacute postinjury phase there are nearly ubiquitous biochemical changes in the concussed brain. Neuronal injury is hallmarked by reduced NAA [76–79] as well as energetic and neurotransmitter disruption as highlighted by alterations in Cr and Glu (increase in white matter, decrease in gray matter), respectively. It is worth noting that these findings are not present in all studies in adults [80] or in the lone pediatric study [81]. The role that development may play in concussion is a complex issue and neurometabolism is likely quite different between adult and pediatric populations at baseline, let alone after injury [82].

In the chronic postinjury phase, studies have also demonstrated abnormalities from individuals with mTBI with otherwise normal-appearing MR scans [83–88]. Significantly depressed concentrations of NAA have been measured in mTBI despite normal findings on conventional MRI [79, 89, 90], with the greatest reductions seen in injury-prone brain tissues which typically include frontal areas and gray-white matter junctions. In contrast, levels of m-I have been shown to be augmented in mTBI [79, 91], although they have also shown the opposite [92]. There are methodological differences between studies. While not all MRS research findings are identical, the prevailing findings strongly support the notion that mTBI results in metabolic disturbance that in many cases resolves, but changes persist. The looming question in this regard is what differentiates those that do recover from those that do not? Though the MRS research is burgeoning and encouraging, more studies further delineating the injury are necessary and require particular attention to gender differences, age-related differences, and predictive factors of recovery.

Conclusion

Concussions represent a significant challenge to the clinical community where they have long been thought of as an invisible injury; however, fMRI, SPECT, PET, DTI, and MRS have all been shown to have utility in characterizing mTBI in acute/subacute and chronic populations. Though there are differences between studies that are at times difficult to account for, the converging evidence flies in the face of the long-held belief that concussions are an invisible injury. Even across modalities as disparate as those reviewed here, the consistency of the metabolic dysfunction, be it imaged using fMRI, SPECT, PET, or more precisely with MRS, point to some common brain regions, namely frontal and temporal cortices and their underlying structures. These changes are further substantiated when the more recent and burgeoning DTI findings are considered. Thus, we can now begin to conceptualize concussions as much more than a mere bump on the head with only transient symptoms. Indeed, the more we are able to see by way of metabolic and structural changes, the more we are able to see concussions for what they really are. Even as research continues to make leaps and bounds in understanding concussive injuries, there are still far more questions than answers, which only underscores the substantial gap between what we can understand empirically and what patients experience subjectively. This lacuna will likely never be entirely closed, though sound research employing the imaging techniques reviewed here as well as electrophysiological and neurocognitive assessment will help advance the clinical treatment and management of concussive injuries.

References

1 Iverson GL, Lovell MR, Smith S, Franzen MD: Prevalence of abnormal CT-scans following mild head injury. Brain Inj 2000;14:1057–1061.

2 Toga AW, Mazziotta JC: Brain Mapping: The Methods, ed 2. San Diego, Academic Press, 2002.

3 Jordan BD, Zimmerman RD: Computed tomography and magnetic resonance imaging comparisons in boxers. JAMA 1990;263:1670–1674.

4 Newton MR, et al: A study comparing SPECT with CT and MRI after closed head injury. J Neurol Neurosurg Psychiatry 1992;55:92–94.

5 Snow RB, Zimmerman RD, Gandy SE, Deck MD: Comparison of magnetic resonance imaging and computed tomography in the evaluation of head injury. Neurosurgery 1986;18:45–52.
6 Bazarian JJ, Blyth B, Cimpello L: Bench to bedside: evidence for brain injury after concussion – looking beyond the computed tomography scan. Acad Emerg Med 2006;13:199–214.
7 Barr M: The Human Nervous System: An Anatomical Viewpoint, ed 8. Baltimore, Lipincott Williams & Wilkins, 2005, p 470.
8 Jordan BD, et al: CT of 338 active professional boxers. Radiology 1992;185:509–512.
9 Chen JK, et al: Functional abnormalities in symptomatic concussed athletes: an fMRI study. Neuroimage 2004;22:68–82.
10 Chen JK, et al: Neural substrates of symptoms of depression following concussion in male athletes with persisting postconcussion symptoms. Arch Gen Psychiatry 2008;65:81–89.
11 Mayer AR, et al: Auditory orienting and inhibition of return in mild traumatic brain injury: a fMRI study. Hum Brain Mapp 2009;30:4152–4166.
12 McAllister TW: Mixed neurologic and psychiatric disorders: pharmacological issues. Compr Psychiatry 1992;33:296–304.
13 McAllister TW, et al: Mechanisms of working memory dysfunction after mild and moderate TBI: evidence from functional MRI and neurogenetics. J Neurotrauma 2006;23:1450–1467.
14 McAllister TW, et al: Differential working memory load effects after mild traumatic brain injury. Neuroimage 2001;14:1004–1012.
15 Jantzen KJ, et al: A prospective functional MR imaging study of mild traumatic brain injury in college football players. AJNR Am J Neuroradiol 2004;25: 738–745.
16 Jantzen KJ: Functional magnetic resonance imaging of mild traumatic brain injury. J Head Trauma Rehabil 2010;25:256–266.
17 Lovell MR, et al: Functional brain abnormalities are related to clinical recovery and time to return-to-play in athletes. Neurosurgery 2007;61:352–359, discussion 359–360.
18 Hillary FG: Neuroimaging of working memory dysfunction and the dilemma with brain reorganization hypotheses. J Int Neuropsychol Soc 2008;14:526–534.
19 Hillary FG, et al: The nature of processing speed deficits in traumatic brain injury: is less brain more? Brain Imaging Behav 2010;4:141–154.
20 Nakamura T, Hillary FG, Biswal BB: Resting network plasticity following brain injury. PLoS One 2009;4:e8220.
21 Slobounov SM, et al: Alteration of brain functional network at rest and in response to YMCA physical stress test in concussed athletes: RsFMRI study. Neuroimage 2011;55:1716–1727.
22 Johnson B, et al: Alteration of brain default network in subacute phase of injury in concussed individuals: resting-state fMRI study. Neuroimage 2012;59:511–518.
23 Marquez de la Plata CD, et al: Deficits in functional connectivity of hippocampal and frontal lobe circuits after traumatic axonal injury. Arch Neurol 2011;68:74–84.
24 Abu-Judeh HH, et al: SPECT brain perfusion findings in mild or moderate traumatic brain injury. Nucl Med Rev Cent East Eur 2000;3:5–11.
25 Abu-Judeh HH, et al: SPET brain perfusion imaging in mild traumatic brain injury without loss of consciousness and normal computed tomography. Nucl Med Commun 1999;20:505–510.
26 Gowda NK, et al: Technetium Tc-99m ethyl cysteinate dimer brain single-photon emission CT in mild traumatic brain injury: a prospective study. AJNR Am J Neuroradiol 2006;27:447–451.
27 Audenaert K, et al: Imaging of mild traumatic brain injury using 57Co and 99mTc HMPAO SPECT as compared to other diagnostic procedures. Med Sci Monit 2003;9:MT112–MT117.
28 Hofman PA, et al: MR imaging, single-photon emission CT, and neurocognitive performance after mild traumatic brain injury. AJNR Am J Neuroradiol 2001;22:441–449.
29 Umile EM, Plotkin RC, Sandel ME: Functional assessment of mild traumatic brain injury using SPECT and neuropsychological testing. Brain Inj 1998;12:577–594.
30 Bonne O, et al: Cerebral blood flow in chronic symptomatic mild traumatic brain injury. Psychiatry Res 2003;124:141–152.
31 Jacobs A, et al: One-year follow-up of technetium-99m-HMPAO SPECT in mild head injury. J Nucl Med 1996;37:1605–1609.
32 Kant R, et al: Tc-HMPAO SPECT in persistent post-concussion syndrome after mild head injury: comparison with MRI/CT. Brain Inj 1997;11:115–124.
33 Gray BG, et al: Technetium-99m-HMPAO SPECT in the evaluation of patients with a remote history of traumatic brain injury: a comparison with X-ray computed tomography. J Nucl Med 1992;33:52–58.
34 Ichise M, et al: Technetium-99m-HMPAO SPECT, CT and MRI in the evaluation of patients with chronic traumatic brain injury: a correlation with neuropsychological performance. J Nucl Med 1994; 35:217–226.
35 Lewine JD, et al: Objective documentation of traumatic brain injury subsequent to mild head trauma: multimodal brain imaging with MEG, SPECT, and MRI. J Head Trauma Rehabil 2007;22:141–155.
36 Umile EM, et al: Dynamic imaging in mild traumatic brain injury: support for the theory of medial temporal vulnerability. Arch Phys Med Rehabil 2002;83: 1506–1513.

37 Hashimoto K, Abo M: Abnormal regional benzodiazepine receptor uptake in the prefrontal cortex in patients with mild traumatic brain injury. J Rehabil Med 2009;41:661–665.

38 Amen DG, et al: Impact of playing American professional football on long-term brain function. J Neuropsychiatry Clin Neurosci 2011;23:98–106.

39 Hattori N, et al: Differential SPECT activation patterns associated with PASAT performance may indicate frontocerebellar functional dissociation in chronic mild traumatic brain injury. J Nucl Med 2009;50:1054–1061.

40 Korn A, et al: Focal cortical dysfunction and blood-brain barrier disruption in patients with postconcussion syndrome. J Clin Neurophysiol 2005;22:1–9.

41 Amen DG, et al: Reversing brain damage in former NFL players: implications for traumatic brain injury and substance abuse rehabilitation. J Psychoactive Drugs 2011;43:1–5.

42 Varney NR, Pinkston JB, Wu JC: Quantitative PET findings in patients with posttraumatic anosmia. J Head Trauma Rehabil 2001;16:253–259.

43 Chen SH, et al: A study of persistent post-concussion symptoms in mild head trauma using positron emission tomography. J Neurol Neurosurg Psychiatry 2003;74:326–332.

44 Ruff RM, et al: Selected cases of poor outcome following a minor brain trauma: comparing neuropsychological and positron emission tomography assessment. Brain Inj 1994;8:297–308.

45 Gross H, et al: Local cerebral glucose metabolism in patients with long-term behavioral and cognitive deficits following mild traumatic brain injury. J Neuropsychiatry Clin Neurosci 1996;8:324–334.

46 Abu-Judeh HH, et al: Discordance between FDG uptake and technetium-99m-HMPAO brain perfusion in acute traumatic brain injury. J Nucl Med 1998;39:1357–1359.

47 Humayun MS, et al: Local cerebral glucose abnormalities in mild closed head injured patients with cognitive impairments. Nucl Med Commun 1989;10:335–344.

48 Arfanakis K, et al: Diffusion tensor MR imaging in diffuse axonal injury. AJNR Am J Neuroradiol 2002;23:794–802.

49 Huisman TA, et al: Diffusion tensor imaging as potential biomarker of white matter injury in diffuse axonal injury. AJNR Am J Neuroradiol 2004;25:370–376.

50 Lee JW, Choi CG, Chun MH: Usefulness of diffusion tensor imaging for evaluation of motor function in patients with traumatic brain injury: three case studies. J Head Trauma Rehabil 2006;21:272–278.

51 Wilde EA, et al: Diffusion tensor imaging of acute mild traumatic brain injury in adolescents. Neurology 2008;70:948–955.

52 Henry LC, et al: Acute and chronic changes in diffusivity measures after sports concussion. J Neurotrauma 2011;28:2049–2059.

53 Miles L, et al: Short-term DTI predictors of cognitive dysfunction in mild traumatic brain injury. Brain Inj 2008;22:115–122.

54 Hartikainen KM, et al: Persistent symptoms in mild to moderate traumatic brain injury associated with executive dysfunction. J Clin Exp Neuropsychol 2010;32:767–774.

55 Messe A, et al: Diffusion tensor imaging and white matter lesions at the subacute stage in mild traumatic brain injury with persistent neurobehavioral impairment. Hum Brain Mapp 2011;32:999–1011.

56 Cubon VA, et al: A diffusion tensor imaging study on the white matter skeleton in individuals with sports-related concussion. J Neurotrauma 2011;28:189–201.

57 Kumar R, et al: Serial changes in the white matter diffusion tensor imaging metrics in moderate traumatic brain injury and correlation with neuro-cognitive function. J Neurotrauma 2009;26:481–495.

58 Newcombe VF, et al: Concordant biology underlies discordant imaging findings: diffusivity behaves differently in grey and white matter post acute neurotrauma. Acta Neurochir Suppl 2008;102:247–251.

59 Newcombe VF, et al: Analysis of acute traumatic axonal injury using diffusion tensor imaging. Br J Neurosurg 2007;21:340–348.

60 Wilde EA, et al: Diffusion tensor imaging of the cingulum bundle in children after traumatic brain injury. Dev Neuropsychol 2010;35:333–351.

61 Mayer AR, et al: A prospective diffusion tensor imaging study in mild traumatic brain injury. Neurology 2010;74:643–650.

62 Chu Z, et al: Voxel-based analysis of diffusion tensor imaging in mild traumatic brain injury in adolescents. AJNR Am J Neuroradiol 2010;31:340–346.

63 Kou Z, et al: The role of advanced MR imaging findings as biomarkers of traumatic brain injury. J Head Trauma Rehabil 2010;25:267–282.

64 Bazarian JJ, et al: Diffusion tensor imaging detects clinically important axonal damage after mild traumatic brain injury: a pilot study. J Neurotrauma 2007;24:1447–1459.

65 Giza CC, Hovda DA: The neurometabolic cascade of concussion. J Athl Train 2001;36:228–235.

66 Jansen JF, et al: 1H MR spectroscopy of the brain: absolute quantification of metabolites. Radiology 2006;240:318–332.

67 Andres RH, et al: Functions and effects of creatine in the central nervous system. Brain Res Bull 2008;76:329–343.

68 Fisher SK, Novak JE, Agranoff BW: Inositol and higher inositol phosphates in neural tissues: homeostasis, metabolism and functional significance. J Neurochem 2002;82:736–754.

69 Kandel E, Schwartz J, Jessell T: Principles of Neuroscience, ed 4, New York, McGraw-Hill, 2000, p 1414.
70 Broer S, Brookes N: Transfer of glutamine between astrocytes and neurons. J Neurochem 2001;77:705–719.
71 Moffett JR, et al: N-acetylaspartate in the CNS: from neurodiagnostics to neurobiology. Prog Neurobiol 2007;81:89–131.
72 Patel TB, Clark JB: Synthesis of N-acetyl-L-aspartate by rat brain mitochondria and its involvement in mitochondrial/cytosolic carbon transport. Biochem J 1979;184:539–546.
73 Taylor DL, et al: Extracellular N-acetylaspartate in the rat brain: in vivo determination of basal levels and changes evoked by high K+. J Neurochem 1994; 62:2349–2355.
74 Urazaev AK, et al: Synthesis and release of N-acetylaspartylglutamate (NAAG) by crayfish nerve fibers: implications for axon-glia signaling. Neuroscience 2001;106:237–247.
75 Gehl LM, et al: Biosynthesis of NAAG by an enzyme-mediated process in rat central nervous system neurons and glia. J Neurochem 2004;90:989–997.
76 Vagnozzi R, et al: Assessment of metabolic brain damage and recovery following mild traumatic brain injury: a multicentre, proton magnetic resonance spectroscopic study in concussed patients. Brain 2010;133:3232–3242.
77 Vagnozzi R, et al: Temporal window of metabolic brain vulnerability to concussion: a pilot 1H-magnetic resonance spectroscopic study in concussed athletes – part III. Neurosurgery 2008;62:1286–1295, discussion 1295–1296.
78 Henry LC, et al: Neurometabolic changes in the acute phase after sports concussions correlate with symptom severity. J Neurotrauma 2010;27:65–76.
79 Henry LC, et al: Metabolic changes in concussed American football players during the acute and chronic post-injury phases. BMC Neurol 2011;11: 105.
80 Chamard E, et al: A prospective study of physician-observed concussion during a varsity university hockey season: metabolic changes in ice hockey players. Part 4 of 4. Neurosurg Focus 2012;33:E4:1–7.
81 Maugans TA, et al: Pediatric sports-related concussion produces cerebral blood flow alterations. Pediatrics 2012;129:28–37.
82 Hädel S, et al: Effects of age and sex on the concentrations of glutamate and glutamine in the human brain. J Magn Reson Imaging 2013;38:1480–1487.
83 Babikian T, et al: MR spectroscopy: Predicting long-term neuropsychological outcome following pediatric TBI. J Magn Reson Imaging 2006;24:801–811.
84 Govindaraju V, et al: Volumetric proton spectroscopic imaging of mild traumatic brain injury. AJNR Am J Neuroradiol 2004;25:730–737.
85 Holshouser BA, et al: Prospective longitudinal proton magnetic resonance spectroscopic imaging in adult traumatic brain injury. J Magn Reson Imaging 2006;24:33–40.
86 Kirov I, et al: Characterizing 'mild' in traumatic brain injury with proton MR spectroscopy in the thalamus: initial findings. Brain Inj 2007;21:1147–1154.
87 Shutter L, et al: Prognostic role of proton magnetic resonance spectroscopy in acute traumatic brain injury. J Head Trauma Rehabil 2006;21:334–349.
88 Tremblay S, et al: Sports concussions and aging: a neuroimaging investigation. Cereb Cortex 2013;23: 1159–1166.
89 Cecil KM, et al: High-field proton magnetic resonance spectroscopy of a swine model for axonal injury. J Neurochem 1998;70:2038–2044.
90 Garnett MR, et al: Evidence for cellular damage in normal-appearing white matter correlates with injury severity in patients following traumatic brain injury: a magnetic resonance spectroscopy study. Brain 2000;123:1403–1409.
91 Garnett MR, et al: Early proton magnetic resonance spectroscopy in normal-appearing brain correlates with outcome in patients following traumatic brain injury. Brain 2000;123:2046–2054.
92 Chamard E, et al: Neurometabolic and microstructural alterations following a sports-related concussion in female athletes. Brain Inj 2013;27:1038–1046.

Luke C. Henry, PhD
University of Pittsburgh, UPMC Sports Concussion Program
3200 S. Water Street
Pittsburgh, PA 15203 (USA)
E-Mail henryl@upmc.edu

Niranjan A, Lunsford LD (eds): Concussion. Prog Neurol Surg. Basel, Karger, 2014, vol 28, pp 75–85
DOI: 10.1159/000358766

Neurometabolic, Electrophysiological, and Imaging Abnormalities

Emilie Chamard[a] · Maryse Lassonde[a, b] · Hugo Théoret[a, b]

[a]Centre de Recherche en Neuropsychologie et Cognition, Department of Psychology, University of Montreal, and [b]Centre de Recherche du CHU Sainte Justine, Montreal, Que., Canada

Abstract

Sport-related concussions affect millions of athletes every year, but they generally present no anatomic alterations when examined using conventional magnetic resonance imaging or a computed tomography scan. Because the damage occurring after a head injury seems to be more functional than structural, these techniques are unable to detect subtle alterations. The absence of detectable structural alterations using traditional neuroimaging methods, the presence of persistent symptoms in some athletes, and the risk of developing neurodegenerative diseases emphasize the importance of assessing the impacts of a head injury with alternative neuroimaging techniques. Electrophysiological methods, magnetic resonance spectroscopy, and diffusion tensor imaging are useful techniques that are sensitive to the effects of a brain trauma, which provide complementary information to allow a more complete understanding of the multiple pathophysiological processes involved in concussive events. This report summarizes recent data using neurophysiological and neuroimaging techniques to better understand the acute and chronic effects of sport-related concussions.

© 2014 S. Karger AG, Basel

Sport-related concussions affect millions of athletes every year, but only a limited proportion of cases result in visible anatomic alterations using conventional structural neuroimaging techniques such as magnetic resonance imaging (MRI) or a computed tomography scan. While these methods should be used for suspected intracerebral lesions or skull fractures, they contribute little to the evaluation and management of a sport-related concussion since the damages occurring after injury seem to be more functional than structural [1]. However, the presence of persistent postconcussion symptoms and the recent association between a history of multiple concussions in former retired athletes and a higher risk of developing neurodegenerative disease [2] suggest the importance of understanding the pathophysiology of concussion with the use of alternative techniques.

In the last decade, many studies have assessed the functional and anatomical impacts of a concussion using magnetic resonance spectroscopy (MRS), diffusion tensor imaging (DTI), and electrophysiology [electroencephalography (EEG) and transcranial magnetic stimulation (TMS)]. These methods provide complementary information on the neurochemical (MRS) and microstructural (DTI) alterations that follow a concussion and offer important clues to the electrical activity of neurons (EEG) following injury. In this report, recent findings obtained with these tools in the acute and long-term phases of brain trauma in athletes are reviewed.

Neurometabolism

MRS allows the detection and quantification of various metabolites in the brain, and, consequently, the detection of neuronal damage and change in neurochemistry following brain trauma. MRS is particularly useful for corroborating evidence of diffuse axonal injury following head trauma since damage appears to affect the physical structure of neurons as well as their composition. The principal metabolites of interest are N-acetylaspartate (NAA), a marker of neuronal integrity; myo-inositol (m-I), a marker of glial cells and an important osmolyte; choline-containing compounds (Cho), markers of neuronal damage and membrane turnover, and glutamate/glutamine (Glx), a marker of excitatory neurotransmission.

The first study to demonstrate neurochemical changes in the acute phase of a concussion was by Cimatti [3], who found a decrease in NAA in 6 concussed athletes (a soccer player, a biker, and 4 boxers) by comparing their baseline data to posttrauma scans on whole-brain analysis. Based on analysis of regions of interest, a decrease in NAA has also been reported in the prefrontal and motor areas, as well as a decrease in Glx in the motor area of American football players in the days following head trauma [4]. These changes in primary motor cortex neurochemistry were correlated with the severity of self-reported symptoms in concussed athletes [4].

In another study assessing the time course of metabolic recovery in the frontal lobe, a decrease in NAA was found in the acute phase of male and female concussed athletes [5]. This study showed that concussions open a temporal window of brain vulnerability due to a metabolic imbalance that does not coincide with the resolution of clinical symptoms, which occurs between 3 and 15 days. The impairments in cellular metabolism mostly returned to the levels of control athletes within 30 days, but can last up to 45 days if the athlete suffers a subsequent injury during this period [5]. This suggests that the impairments in cellular metabolism occurring after a brain trauma are transient, and return to normal levels after approximately 1 month.

However, pathological decreases in NAA in the prefrontal and motor areas 6 months after injury [6], and in the corpus callosum (CC) in the subacute phase [7], have been shown in asymptomatic athletes. The recovery time of NAA seems to be longer than initially postulated, suggesting that the brain is still vulnerable months after a concussion. This last study by Johnson et al. [7] also demonstrated the usefulness of a multiparametric approach that combines MRS with functional MRI (fMRI).

Immediately after the resolution of postconcussion symptoms, athletes demonstrated reduced NAA in the genu and splenium of the CC that were not correlated with fMRI measures of functional interhemispheric connectivity as was the case in control athletes. The authors attributed these differences in concussed athletes to persistent membrane damage in the CC [7].

Cerebral metabolic recovery cannot be monitored solely by the quantification of NAA changes in the brain since persistent alterations in neurochemistry are not limited to NAA and affect other metabolites. Lower levels of Glx in the primary motor cortex that return to normal levels within 6 months after the injury have been reported in the acute phase in American football players [6]. These results are in contradiction to the study of Lin et al. [8], who showed higher levels of Glx and Cho in the chronic phase. However, the latter study recruited 5 professional athletes, aged between 31 and 54 years, with a history of multiple concussions and subconcussive trauma who were evaluated in the chronic phase of their injuries to investigate the posterior cingulate gyrus. These discrepancies suggest different neurometabolic profiles which are dependent on the cerebral region and the time elapsed since injury. With regards to m-I, changes are present months to years after concussion [6, 9, 10]. However, the direction of m-I changes are not entirely clear, as a study found a decrease in female athletes in the hippocampus and primary motor cortex [9] while other studies found an increase in male athletes in the primary motor cortex [6] and hippocampus [10]. Finally, persistent alterations have recently been reported in healthy former athletes who sustained their last concussion more than three decades prior to testing [10]. Chronic neurometabolic alterations, characterized by a decrease of Cho and an elevation of m-I in the medial temporal lobes, may indicate that disrupted cellular mechanisms are related to long-term detrimental effects [10].

In summary, recent studies have demonstrated neurometabolic impairments in the acute, subacute, and chronic phases following concussion in young asymptomatic athletes of both sexes, as well as in healthy former athletes (table 1). However, the persistence and direction of these changes still have to be confirmed. Also, the effects of gender, time elapsed since the last concussive event, and the impact of multiple concussions or repeated subconcussive blows have to be clarified, as they could explain some discrepancies between published data. Nevertheless, MRS studies have demonstrated the persistent vulnerability of cellular metabolism following brain trauma that could be one of the factors contributing to a higher risk of sustaining additional concussions.

Electrophysiology

EEG and quantitative EEG measure the electrical activity of the brain by recording ongoing brain function through the summation of action potentials. In sports traumatology, a study by Thompson et al. [11] demonstrated an overall decrease in am-

Table 1. Summary of MRS studies on sport-related concussions

Study	Subjects	Delay after concussion	Results
Cimatti [3]	6 concussed athletes	36–48 h	decreased NAA in some but not all cases
Henry et al. [4]	12 control athletes 12 concussed athletes	1–6 days	decreased NAA in DLPC and M1; decreased Glx in M1
Vagnozzi et al. [5]	5 control volunteers 13 concussed athletes	3, 15, 30, and 45 days	decreased NAA in frontal lobes that resolve within 30 days but can be further exacerbated to 45 days by subsequent injury within the restorative time frame
Henry et al. [6]	10 control athletes 10 concussed athletes	1–6 days and 6 months	persistent decrease of NAA in DLPC and M1; recovery of Glx in the chronic phase while concentration was lower in the acute phase; increase of m-I in M1 only in the chronic phase
Johnson et al. [7]	20 control volunteers 28 concussed athletes	within 30 days (within 24 h after symptom resolution)	decreased NAA in the genu of the CC; concussed athletes recovering from their first concussion showed the greatest alteration in NAA ratios; trend of increasing NAA ratios that coincided with increasing number of concussions
Chamard et al. [9]	10 control athletes 10 concussed athletes	≥7 months (mean 18 months)	lower levels of m-I in the hippocampus and M1
Tremblay et al. [10]	15 retired control athletes 15 retired concussed athletes	30 years	higher levels of m-I and lower level of Cho in the left hippocampus; higher levels of Cho in the right prefrontal cortex

DLPC = Dorsolateral prefrontal cortex; M1 = primary motor cortex.

plitude in all frequency bands across the spectrum, i.e. delta, theta, alpha, alpha-2, beta, and beta-2 amplitudes approximately 3 months after concussion. These lower amplitudes were associated with greater postural instability, which the authors attributed to insufficient brain resource allocation, and abnormal balance of excitatory and inhibitory drives in standing posture [11]. The resolution of symptoms and cognitive alterations following brain trauma does not appear to follow the resolution of electrophysiological markers. In a prospective study using quantitative EEG, concussed athletes presented significantly more symptoms in the first 3 days following the injury, which resolved by days 5–8. The resolution of cognitive alterations was faster, and concussed athletes exhibited poorer performance than controls only on the day of the injury. However, abnormalities in electrical brain activity were still present 8 days after injury and returned to the level of controls on day 45, which suggests a discrepancy between the recovery of symptoms, cognitive dysfunction, and physiological recovery [12]. These two studies suggest subtle changes following a head trauma in concussed athletes that appear to be independent of functional recovery. However, none of these studies recorded brain activity when the athletes were performing a cognitive task.

EEG recordings while athletes carry out a cognitive task or during sensory stimulation [event-related potentials (ERPs)] have also been studied to assess brain function in concussed athletes. ERPs consist of various waves labelled after their polarity (P for positive and N for negative) and latency that are the direct result of a specific sensory, cognitive, or motor process. Many studies in sports traumatology have used an oddball task, which consists of the presentation of two types of stimuli having different probabilities of occurrence (frequent or rare). Athletes must give a motor response when the rare stimulus appears (target stimulus). The appearance of the target stimuli elicits a positive wave called P3b (also known as P3 or P300), a marker of the amount of attentional resources allocated to a task, and stimulus classification speed, following stimulus presentation. Other important ERP components, the P3a waves, represent an involuntary attention switch to changes in the environment. Using this task in the auditory modality, a study by Gosselin et al. [13] showed a reduction in the amplitude of the P3b wave in symptomatic and asymptomatic athletes having suffered a concussion compared to controls athletes. Since the latency of the P3b is associated with stimulus classification speed, the reduced latency of ERP signals in concussed athletes and the absence of a difference between the control and concussed group in neuropsychological tests point to a higher sensitivity of electrophysiological testing in the auditory modality than neuropsychological assessment [13].

Reduction in the amplitude of P3a and P3b waves using an auditory oddball task were also found in asymptomatic athletes having suffered multiple concussions and who were less than 1 year from their last injury, as opposed to a control group and a group of athletes that had suffered multiple concussions but for whom more than 2 years had passed since the last event [14]. These results suggest that sport-related concussions can cause brain function abnormalities months following the injury, but these dysfunctions seem to resolve in the long-term phase. However, a subsequent study using a modified visual oddball task demonstrated long-term electrophysiological changes in athletes with multiple concussions compared to athletes having experienced one concussion and control athletes independently of the time elapsed since injury [15]. The long-lasting P3b amplitude suppression was found despite equivalent neuropsychological performance and the absence of postconcussion symptoms, suggesting a cumulative effect of concussions on brain electrophysiology that persists in the chronic phase.

The long-term sequelae were also investigated in a study conducted with former retired athletes that had suffered their last concussion more than three decades prior to testing [16]. Nineteen healthy former athletes who sustained their last concussion in early adulthood were compared to 21 healthy former athletes who never had a concussion. Significantly delayed and attenuated P3a and P3b components were found in the concussed athletes in an auditory oddball task, in conjunction with poorer performance on neuropsychological tests of episodic memory, bradykinesia, and significantly prolonged intracortical inhibition evaluated with TMS [16]. In general, these studies demonstrated acute and chronic dysfunctions, which can be observed by changes in latency and amplitude of waves involved in cognitive processes. For a more detailed review of ERP abnormalities in concussed athletes, readers may refer to Gosselin et al. [17].

Neurophysiological studies in sports traumatology have also used TMS to better understand the complexity of cerebral perturbations following concussion. This method uses electromagnetic induction to allow the study of the inhibitory and excitatory mechanisms of the motor system following brain trauma. A technique frequently used is the cortical silent period (CSP), for which a greater duration is thought to reflect dysfunctional intracortical inhibitory systems. The presence of long-lasting alterations in the motor system of athletes with multiple concussions was first demonstrated by De Beaumont et al. [18]. This study also showed that additional concussions further increased the duration of the CSP, which point to a cumulative effect of concussions on intracortical inhibitory systems. A prolonged CSP was also present in a study with concussed athletes having experienced a brain trauma more than 1 year prior to testing [19]. However, no differences were found between concussed and control groups relative to other TMS parameters measuring sensorimotor integration (short latency afferent inhibition and long latency afferent inhibition). In addition, somatosensory-evoked potentials were found to be normal, pointing to intact somatosensory processing and sensorimotor integration following a concussion, while the long-term neurophysiological dysfunctions seem to be specific to intracortical inhibitory mechanisms of the primary motor cortex [19]. The specificity of the alterations is thought to reflect specific and stable alterations of GABAb receptor activity in the primary motor cortex [16, 19]. Furthermore, these neurophysiological dysfunctions appear to persist many years after the last concussion [16]. Indeed, retired athletes presented a significantly prolonged CSP while no differences were found using other TMS paradigms (resting motor threshold, paired-pulse intracortical inhibition and intracortical facilitation, and input/output curve) [16].

Taken together, electrophysiological studies in concussed athletes suggest persistent, long-term effects that seem to be independent of the time elapsed since the last concussion (table 2). However, the persistent effects on brain electrophysiology appear to increase with a history of multiple concussions, suggesting a cumulative effect of concussions.

Microstructural Alterations

DTI is a magnetic resonance technique allowing the mapping of diffusion processes in the brain, and subsequently allowing the analysis of microstructure and the organization and integrity of white matter (WM) tissue. Traumatic axonal injury follow-

Table 2. Summary of electrophysiological studies on sport-related concussions

Study	Subjects	Delay after concussion	Results
Thompson et al. [11]	12 control athletes 12 concussed athletes	70–131 days	decrease in EEG power in all bandwidths associated with postural instability
McCrea et al. [12]	28 control athletes 27 concussed athletes	1, 8, and 45 days	abnormalities in electrical brain activity in concussed athletes on day 1 and 8 after injury, but not on day 45
Gosselin et al. [13]	10 control athletes 10 symptomatic concussed athletes 10 asymptomatic concussed athletes	2–32 weeks	reduction in P3b wave in asymptomatic and symptomatic concussed athletes
Theriault et al. [14]	10 control athletes 10 multiple concussed athletes (<1 year after concussion) 10 multiple concussed athletes (>2 years after concussion)	5–12 months or 22–60 months	reduction in the amplitude of P3a and P3b waves in asymptomatic athletes having suffered concussion <1 year prior to testing
De Beaumont et al. [15]	15 control athletes 15 athletes with 1 concussion 15 athletes with multiple concussions	≥9 months	reduction in the amplitude of P3b wave in multiple concussed athletes
De Beaumont et al. [16]	21 former control athletes 19 former concussed athletes	30 years	ERP: delayed and attenuated P3a and P3b waves TMS: prolonged CSP
De Beaumont et al. [18]	15 control athletes 15 athletes with 1 concussion 15 athletes with multiple concussions	≥9 months	prolonged CSP in multiple concussed athletes
Tremblay et al. [19]	14 control athletes 12 concussed athletes	>1 year	prolonged CSP and enhancement of long-interval intracortical inhibition

ing a concussion can be assessed by the main DTI indices: fractional anisotropy (FA) and mean diffusivity (MD). In concordance with studies using MRS and electrophysiology, acute and chronic effects have been reported in concussed athletes using DTI. WM alterations affecting the corticospinal tract and the CC in the acute phase (1–6 days after injury) that persist in the chronic phase (6 months after injury) have been found in concussed American football players [20]. Moreover, differences in diffusion and anisotropy have been found in boxers, characterized by an increase in the average diffusion constant (a measure similar to MD) and a decrease in FA in the CC and the posterior limb of the internal capsule [21]. A similar pattern of results (MD increase) has been reported by Cubon et al. [22], who showed alterations in diffusivity in several large tracts of the left hemisphere, notably the inferior/superior longitudinal and frontooccipital fasciculi, the internal capsule, and acoustic radiations. Moreover, alterations in diffusion measures seem to correlate with functional alterations on a working memory task in concussed athletes using fMRI, suggesting an association between microstructural and functional deficits following a sport-related concussion [23].

Most studies to date have been conducted with male athletes or with groups composed of both male and female athletes, while gender differences have previously been demonstrated with regards to the risk of sustaining a concussion, the recovery period, and postconcussion impacts [1]. Recently, a study conducted exclusively with female athletes months to years after a concussion found no differences in FA, but an increase in MD in large WM tracts including the forceps minors, inferior/superior longitudinal fasciculi, inferior frontooccipital fasciculus, cingulum, uncinate fasciculus, anterior thalamic radiations, and corticospinal tract [9]. Moreover, a region-of-interest approach for the CC revealed a significant reduction in FA levels in the segment containing fibers projecting to the primary motor cortex in female concussed athletes [9]. The absence of difference with respect to FA in whole-brain analysis is in agreement with the study by Cubon et al. [22], which points to a higher sensitivity of MD to detect subtle microstructural damage following a sport-related concussion. The chronic alteration in WM integrity also appears to be related to depressive symptoms, as reported in a study with retired National Football League (NFL) athletes [24]. In that study, depressive symptoms assessed with BDI-II correlated negatively with FA, notably in the right frontal aslant tract, in the right uncinate fasciculus, in the left superior fasciculus, and in the forceps minor. This last tract differentiated depressed from nondepressed athletes with 100% sensitivity and 95% specificity, which opens the possibility to use DTI as a biomarker for depression in concussed athletes [24].

Finally, while the microstructural effects of brain trauma have been well studied, the effect of subconcussive impacts in contact sports as an additional mechanism of brain injury has yet to be fully defined. In one study, professional soccer players without a symptomatic concussion were compared to swimmers [25]. No differences relative to FA and MD were found between the groups, but soccer players demonstrated increased axial and radial diffusivity (associated respectively with axon and myelin integrity) in several WM tracts of the brain, suggesting possible demyelination [25]. Furthermore, the association between soccer heading and subclinical evidence of WM alterations following subconcussive blows to the head was studied in soccer players [26]. Results showed that heading was associated with lower FA in temporooccipital WM that was also associated with poorer memory. The authors concluded that heading in soccer is associated with microstructural alterations and reduced neurocognitive performance [26].

Taken together, these studies suggest the presence of alterations in WM integrity in the acute, subacute, and long-term stages of a concussion (table 3). While these alterations seem to affect multiple large WM tracts in the brain, the CC and the corticospinal tracts seem to be particularly vulnerable to the effects of head injuries.

Table 3. Summary of DTI studies on sport-related concussions

Study	Subjects	Delay after concussion	Results
Chamard et al. [9]	10 control athletes 10 concussed athletes	≥7 months (mean 18 months)	higher level of MD in forceps minors, inferior/superior longitudinal fasciculus, cingulum, uncinate fasciculus, anterior thalamic radiations, corticospinal tract, and CC
Henry et al. [20]	10 control athletes 18 concussed athletes	1–6 days and 6 months	persistent increased of FA in dorsal regions of corticospinal tracts and the CC; persistent increased AD in the right corticospinal tract; persistent decreased MD in the corticospinal tract and CC
Zhang et al. [21]	19 control volunteers 49 concussed athletes	not specified	decreased FA and increased ADC in the CC and the posterior limb of the internal capsule
Cubon et al. [22]	10 control athletes 10 concussed athletes	≥1 month	increased MD in left hemisphere: inferior/superior longitudinal and frontooccipital fasciculi, retrolenticular part of the internal capsule, and posterior thalamic and acoustic radiations
Zhang et al. [23]	15 control athletes 15 concussed athletes	30 days	decreased ADC in left DLPC that correlated with functional changes (fMRI) in a working memory task
Strain et al. [24]	26 retired professional football players	not applicable	negative correlation between forceps minor, right frontal aslant tract, right uncinate fasciculus, and left superior longitudinal fasciculus and total BDI-II; FA of the forceps minor differentiated depressed from nondepressed athletes with 100% sensitivity and 95% specificity
Koerte et al. [25]	12 soccer players 11 swimmers	not applicable	increased AD and RD in several WM tracts
Lipton et al. [26]	37 soccer players	not applicable	association between heading and lower FA at three locations in temporooccipital WM; association between lower levels of FA and poorer memory scores with a threshold of 1,800 headings per year

AD = Axial diffusivity; ADC = average diffusion constant; DLPC = dorsolateral prefrontal cortex; RD = radial diffusivity.

Conclusion

The present report reviewed recent studies in sports traumatology investigating the effects of sport-related concussions on neurophysiology, cellular metabolism, and WM integrity. Even if postconcussion symptoms and neurocognitive deficits generally appear to return to baseline after a period of 7–10 days [1], there is evidence of subclinical brain alterations in the acute, subacute, and long-term phases of injury. These alterations, which are detectable by EEG, quantitative EEG, TMS, MRS, and DTI, suggest that the brain remains vulnerable to the effects of the concussion, and they could play a role in the higher susceptibility of concussed athletes to suffer further head injury. Also, they could play a role in the higher severity of postconcussion symptoms and the longer rehabilitation time needed by concussed athletes to recover from a subsequent injury to the head. However, many factors still have to be confirmed. For example, future studies should assess the potential cumulative impact of previous concussions or the effects of repetitive subconcussive blows to the head since this is an important issue in many contact sports. Also, the impact of age at the time of the injury, gender, potential genetic influence, and time elapsed since the last concussion have to be assessed to better understand the complex pathophysiology of a sport-related concussion.

References

1 McCrory P, Meeuwisse W, Aubry M, Cantu B, Dvorak J, Echemendia R, Engebretsen L, Johnston K, Kutcher J, Raftery M, Sills A, Benson B, Davis G, Ellenbogen R, Guskiewicz K, Herring SA, Iverson G, Jordan B, Kissick J, McCrea M, McIntosh A, Maddocks D, Makdissi M, Purcello L, Putukian M, Schneider K, Tatoru C, Turner M: Consensus statement on Concussion in Sport – the 4th International Conference on Concussion in Sport held in Zurich, November 2012. Phys Ther Sport 2013;14:1–13.

2 Guskiewicz K, Marshall S, Bailes J: Association between recurrent concussion and late-life cognitive impairment in retired professional football players. Neurosurgery 2005;57:719–726.

3 Cimatti M: Assessment of metabolic cerebral damage using proton magnetic resonance spectroscopy in mild traumatic brain injury. J Neurosurgical Sci 2006;50:83–88.

4 Henry LC, Tremblay S, Boulanger Y, Ellemberg D, Lassonde M: Neurometabolic changes in the acute phase after sports concussions correlate with symptom severity. J Neurotrauma 2010;27:65–76.

5 Vagnozzi R, Signoretti S, Tavazzi B, Floris R, Ludovici A, Marizali S, Tarascio G, Amorini AM, Di Pietro V, Delfini R, Lazzarino G: Temporal window of metabolic brain vulnerability to concussion: a pilot 1H-magnetic resonance spectroscopic study in concussed athletes – part III. Neurosurgery 2008;62:1286–1295.

6 Henry LC, Tremblay S, Leclerc S, Khiat A, Boulanger Y, Ellemberg D, Lassonde M: Metabolic changes in concussed American football players during the acute and chronic post-injury phases. BMC Neurol 2011;11:105–114.

7 Johnson B, Gay M, Zhang K, Neuberger T, Horovitz SG, Hallett M, Sebastianelli W, Slobounov S: The use of magnetic resonance spectroscopy in the subacute evaluation of athletes recovering from single and multiple mild traumatic brain injury. J Neurotrauma 2012;29:2297–2304.

8 Lin AP, Ramadan S, Box H, Stanwell P, Stern R: Neurochemical changes in athletes with chronic traumatic encephalopathy. 96th Scientific Assembly and Annual Meeting of the Radiological Society of North America, Chicago, 2010.

9 Chamard E, Lassonde M, Henry L, Tremblay J, Boulanger Y, De Beaumont L, Theoret H: Neurometabolic and microstructural alterations following a sports-related concussion in female athletes. Brain Inj 2013;27:1038–1046.

10 Tremblay S, De Beaumont L, Henry LC, Boulanger Y, Evans AC, Bourgouin P, Poirier J, Théoret H, Lassonde M: Sports concussions and aging: a neuroimaging investigation. Cereb Cortex 2012;23:1159–1166.

11 Thompson J, Sebastianelli W, Slobounov S: EEG and postural correlates of mild traumatic brain injury in athletes. Neurosci Lett 2005;377:158–163.

12 McCrea M, Prichep L, Powell MR, Chabot R, Barr WB: Acute effects and recovery after sport-related concussion: a neurocognitive and quantitative brain electrical activity study. J Head Trauma Rehabil 2010;25:283–292.

13 Gosselin N, Thériault M, Leclerc S, Montplaisir J, Lassonde M: Neurophysiological anomalies in symptomatic and asymptomatic concussed athletes. Neurosurgery 2006;58:1151–1161.

14 Theriault M, De Beaumont L, Gosselin N, Filipinni M, Lassonde M: Electrophysiological abnormalities in well functioning multiple concussed athletes. Brain Inj 2009;23:899–906.

15 De Beaumont L, Brisson B, Lassonde M, Jolicoeur P: Long-term electrophysiological changes in athletes with a history of multiple concussions. Brain Inj 2007;21:631–644.

16 De Beaumont L, Théoret H, Mongeon D, Messier J, Leclerc S, Tremblay S, Ellemberg D, Lassonde M: Brain function decline in healthy retired athletes who sustained their last sports concussion in early adulthood. Brain 2009;132:695–708.

17 Gosselin N, Saluja RS, Chen JK, Bottari C, Johnston K, Ptito A: Brain functions after sports-related concussion: insights from event-related potentials and functional MRI. Phys Sports Med 2010;38:27–37.
18 De Beaumont L, Lassonde M, Leclerc S, Theoret H: Long-term and cumulative effects of sports concussion on motor cortex inhibition. Neurosurgery 2007; 61:329–336, discussion 336–337.
19 Tremblay S, De Beaumont L, Lassonde M, Theoret H: Evidence for the specificity of intracortical inhibitory dysfunction in asymptomatic concussed athletes. J Neurotrauma 2011;28:493–502.
20 Henry LC, Tremblay J, Tremblay S, Lee A, Brun C, Lepore N, Theoret H, Ellemberg D, Lassonde M: Acute and chronic changes in diffusivity measures after sports concussion. J Neurotrauma 2011;28: 2049–2059.
21 Zhang L, Heier LA, Zimmerman RD, Jordan B, Ulug AM: Diffusion anisotropy changes in the brains of professional boxers. AJNR Am J Neuroradiol 2006; 27:2000–2004.
22 Cubon VA, Putukian M, Boyer C, Dettwiler A: A diffusion tensor imaging study on the white matter skeleton in individuals with sports-related concussion. J Neurotrauma 2011;28:189–201.
23 Zhang K, Johnson B, Pennell D, Ray W, Sebastianelli W, Slobounov S: Are functional deficits in concussed individuals consistent with white matter structural alterations: combined fMRI and DTI study. Exp Brain Res 2010;204:57–70.
24 Strain J, Didehbani N, Cullum CM, Mansinghani S, Conover H, Kraut MA, Hart J, Womack KB: Depressive symptoms and white matter dysfunction in retired NFL players with concussion history. Neurology 2013;81:25–32.
25 Koerte IK, Ertl-Wagner B, Reiser M, Zafonte R, Shenton ME: White matter integrity in the brains of professional soccer players without a symptomatic concussion. JAMA 2012;308:1859–1861.
26 Lipton ML, Kim N, Zimmerman ME, Kim M, Stewart WF, Branch CA, Lipton RB: Soccer heading is associated with white matter microstructural and cognitive abnormalities. Radiology 2013;268:850–857.

Prof. Hugo Théoret
Department of Psychology, University of Montreal
CP 6128, Succ. Centre-Ville
Montreal, QC H3C 3J7 (Canada)
E-Mail hugo.theoret@umontreal.ca

Niranjan A, Lunsford LD (eds): Concussion. Prog Neurol Surg. Basel, Karger, 2014, vol 28, pp 86–93
DOI: 10.1159/000358767

Detection of White Matter Injury in Concussion Using High-Definition Fiber Tractography

Samuel S. Shin[a] · Sudhir Pathak[b] · Nora Presson[b] · William Bird[b] · Lauren Wagener[b] · Walter Schneider[b] · David O. Okonkwo[a] · Juan C. Fernandez-Miranda[a]

[a]Department of Neurological Surgery and [b]Learning Research and Development Center, University of Pittsburgh, Pittsburgh, Pa., USA

Abstract

Over the last few decades, structural imaging techniques of the human brain have undergone significant strides. High resolution provided by recent developments in magnetic resonance imaging (MRI) allows improved detection of injured regions in patients with moderate-to-severe traumatic brain injury (TBI). In addition, diffusion imaging techniques such as diffusion tensor imaging (DTI) has gained much interest recently due to its possible utility in detecting structural integrity of white matter pathways in mild TBI (mTBI) cases. However, the results from recent DTI studies in mTBI patients remain equivocal. Also, there are important shortcomings for DTI such as limited resolution in areas of multiple crossings and false tract formation. The detection of white matter damage in concussion remains challenging, and development of imaging biomarkers for mTBI is still in great need. In this chapter, we discuss our experience with high-definition fiber tracking (HDFT), a diffusion spectrum imaging-based technique. We also discuss ongoing developments and specific advantages HDFT may offer concussion patients. © 2014 S. Karger AG, Basel

Traumatic brain injury (TBI) places a tremendous burden on our society, but the use of imaging modalities has been limited to the more severe forms of TBI. Conventional imaging methods such as computed tomography or T2-weighted magnetic resonance imaging (MRI) with FLAIR may aid in detecting gross abnormalities such as hemorrhagic contusions and chronic atrophy of the brain after injury, but these methods are often insensitive to white matter injury resulting from mild TBI (mTBI) or concussion. For example, 43–68% of mTBI patients will have normal structural findings on MRI [1], and concussion leading to small areas of injury consisting of injured axons surrounded by uninjured axons may be largely undetectable. Functional and cognitive deficits after concussions may be attributed to microscopic disruptions of these important white matter tracts (e.g., corpus callosum, fornix) that are not detected by current imaging techniques.

About 80% of the 2,000,000 annual TBI cases occurring in the USA are mTBI [2]. These cases are commonly found in sports concussion injury, motor vehicle accidents, and assaults. In addition, military blast injury has been a widespread mode of injury among soldiers. This widespread pathology does not have a definitive method of detection, and development of imaging biomarkers to reliably diagnose mTBI is in great need. Such tools will aid in multiple aspects of medical management of TBI patients by predicting long-term outcome of TBI, aiding in directing rehabilitation strategies specific to damage, and differentiating true injury from non-TBI-related disorders such as malingering.

TBI often results in diffuse axonal injury resulting from damage to the axolemma and neurofilament organization, as well as degradation of the myelin sheath [3, 4]. These microstructural damages may not be apparent on conventional imaging. Detection of microstructural damage has been the focus of much recent research given that these injuries are often undetectable with conventional MRI. Diffusion imaging can detect white matter integrity by analyzing the direction of water diffusion. White matter tracts have axonal membranes and myelin that orient the diffusion of water longitudinally along the direction of axonal fiber as long as they are structurally intact. If there is a structural compromise that leads to diffusion in orthogonal direction to the direction of the axon, this change is detectable by diffusion tensor imaging (DTI). In the last few years, DTI has been shown to be sensitive to microstructural axonal injury in several studies [5–7].

However, most of these studies showed either no or only a minority of mTBI patients with structural damage using DTI. Even in a notable study by MacDonald et al. [8], which looked at a large number of blast concussions in military subjects, only 18 of 63 were found with structural damage detected by DTI. Although this was a statistically greater number of detections than by chance alone, the majority of patients were found to have no damage. Thus, a more sensitive method of detection of white matter injury in concussion patients is needed. Imaging methods sensitive to concussion will have an important future role given that persistent neurobehavioral sequelae following mTBI are posited to be due to subtle white matter injury not detectable by current imaging methods [9].

As reviewed by Niogi et al. [10], one of the methods of diffusion imaging analysis is quantitative tractography: demyelination or axonal damage causes discontinuous tracts, intuitively indicating the specific location of damage. Fiber tracking is sensitive to disruptions in connectivity between different regions of the brain, which aids in the understanding of specific cognitive deficits. The use of quantitative tractography in detection of TBI was previously reported using DTI fiber tracking [11–14], but most of these studies were case reports using qualitative assessment such as locations of fiber discontinuations and gross changes in tract volume. However, quantitative characterizations of connectivity and tract volume may give insight into the degree and

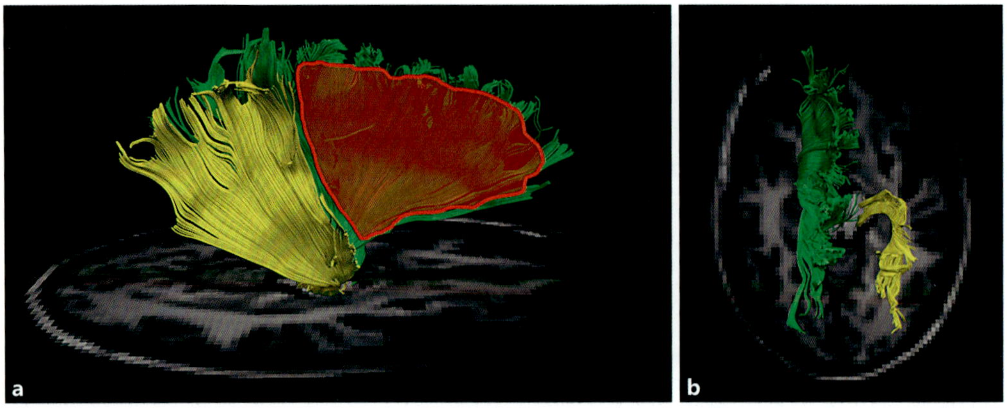

Fig. 1. Lateral (**a**) and top (**b**) view of a TBI subject. A damaged and missing part of the corona radiata on the right side is visible in the red highlighted area.

nature of damage in TBI. For example, alterations in tractography-based parameters such as fiber volume, count, length, etc., in TBI patients were compared to controls [15], and there were significant functional correlations detected by the Extended Glasgow Outcome Score (GOS-E).

Recently, a diffusion spectrum imaging-based technique that combines image processing, reconstruction, and tractography called high-definition fiber tracking (HDFT) has been developed [16]. In this initial report, the utility of HDFT was shown in surgical planning, where images from HDFT accurately predicted the optimal surgical route for dermoid cyst cannulation. In addition, comparison of HDFT and anatomical fiber dissections showed accurate replication of many neuroanatomical features [17]. The resolution of HDFT accurately replicates the somatotopic mapping previously possible only by postmortem histological dissection [18]. This reliable reconstruction of axonal pathways by HDFT potentially allows it to accurately localize the area of damage, as well as to quantify the degree of damage when applied in the setting of TBI [19].

Aside from reliable reconstruction of known white matter pathways, specific methods of quantification have been shown to be useful in understanding the degree of injury in TBI [19]. The first is by comparing the total volume of contralateral fiber tracts in the two hemispheres. The volume of major tracts such as the corona radiata, cingulum, and superior longitudinal fasciculus were compared, and the right corona radiata showed a drastic decrease in the number of fibers and volume as a result of injury. These changes were grossly visible on HDFT images (fig. 1a, b).

Another method of quantification was by comparing the number of fiber termination points. The number of fiber tracts terminating on the cortical surface was compared between the corona radiata of the left and right hemispheres since injury to the white matter tract of the corona radiata would result in degeneration of axons terminating on the cortical surface. A significant decrease (54%) was found among

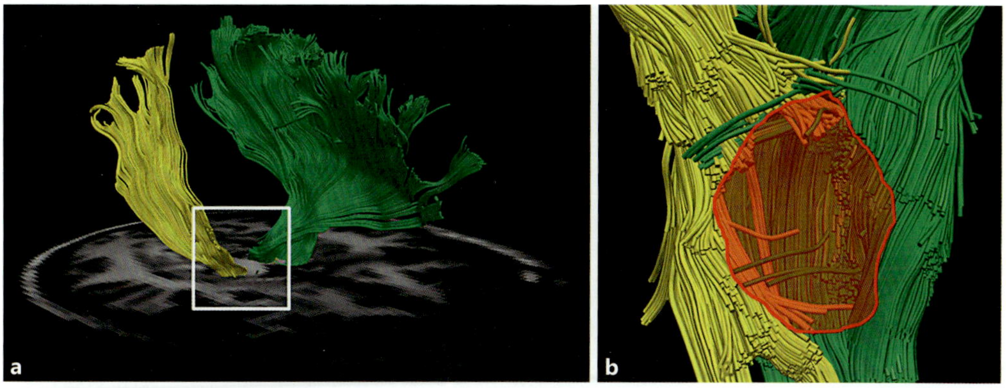

Fig. 2. Closer inspection of the damaged site marked by the white rectangle (**a**) shows specific localization of the site of damage (red outline) in TBI (**b**).

the termination points of the right corona radiata, correlating with the decrease in tract volume.

Visualization of the exact location of fiber breakage can also be helpful in qualitatively assessing the location and nature of axonal injury (fig. 2). By close inspection of the fiber reconstructions, specific areas of fiber breaks can be visualized, showing specific loss of corticospinal fibers originating from the ventrolateral primary motor cortex, but preservation of fibers from the dorsomedial primary motor cortex. Moreover, the specific location of fiber breaks can be found by quantifying the number of fibers along the direction of the fiber tracts from the rostral to caudal direction: fiber counts at the precentral gyrus, internal capsule, and midbrain. Although this is not an example of mTBI, the quantitative methods used here will provide a framework for HDFT studies of mTBI cases in the future.

The limited number of applied diffusion gradients and degrees of freedom makes DTI unable to accurately reconstruct areas where multiple axonal pathways cross [20]. Unlike DTI, which reconstructs average direction of diffusion within a voxel, diffusion spectrum imaging measures multiple pathways within a voxel and accurately reconstructs fiber crossings [21]. This results in superior imaging in areas of multiple fiber crossings: (1) crossing of the middle cerebellar peduncle and corticospinal tract in the pons, and (2) the centrum semiovale where the corticospinal tract, corpus callosum, and arcuate fasciculus cross [20]. DTI also suffers from the problem of artifactual tracts [22, 23]. In comparison, the advantage of HDFT is a reduced number of artifacts such as false continuation and false termination. This is apparent in areas such as the crossings between the corona radiata and corpus callosum: whereas HDFT is able to accurately reconstruct the corona radiata consistent with known anatomy, DTI reconstructs false continuation and turns between the two separate fiber tracts [19]. In addition, these specific advantages of HDFT along with its submillimeter precision will theoretically allow a superior detection of microstructural damage in concussion cases.

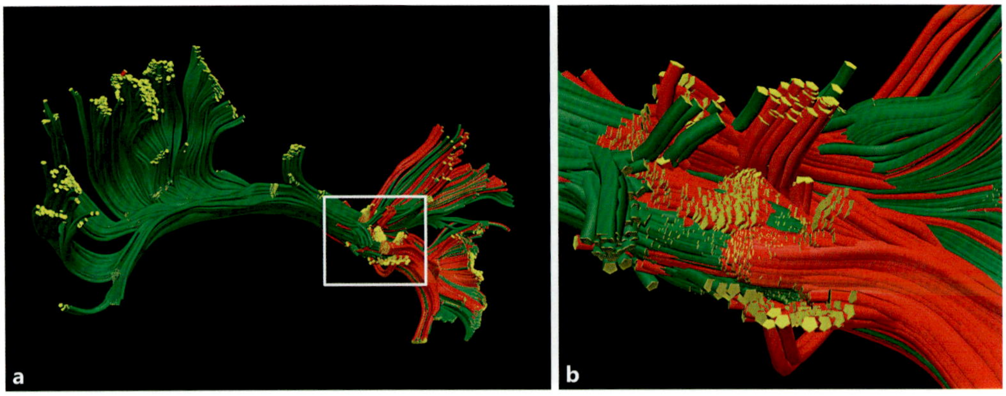

Fig. 3. Cingulum of an mTBI subject (**a**), and the enlarged view of an area marked by the white rectangle (**b**) shows specific fiber tracts that are discontinuous (red tracts).

Since HDFT can accurately reconstruct the known anatomy of major fiber tracts in the human brain, multiple major white matter pathways can be analyzed for each case of TBI. Commonly damaged tracts in mTBI are the frontal white matter pathways such as the corpus callosum, corona radiata, superior longitudinal fasciculus, and uncinate fasciculus [24, 25]. In our current analysis of TBI subjects, we are analyzing 17 major tracts which include commonly damaged tracts such as the corona radiata, corpus callosum, inferior frontooccipital fasciculus, optic radiations, cingulum, and superior longitudinal fasciculus. One method of analyzing TBI-induced damage is by comparing the estimated tract volume between the two hemispheres. This volumetric analysis can be reconstructed with high reliability, as reseeding the tracts multiple times confirmed that the same volume can be generated repeatedly with low variance at 0.3% [19]. In addition, the number of fiber tracts at each point along the anterioposterior axis (y-axis) as well as superior-inferior axis (z-axis) can be compared between the pathways from both hemispheres to localize the area of axonal damage.

One may postulate that detection of significant injury in fiber tracts may be more difficult in mTBI cases, as previously shown in several DTI studies. However, we have identified several subjects with mTBI and evidence of white matter changes based on HDFT analysis. For example, a subject in our database who suffered from repeated concussions showed a noticeable decrease and partial disruption of the cingulum, a major pathway that interconnects frontal, parietal, and temporal mesial regions, with functional implications in the processing of emotions (fig. 3). Future studies will focus on specific quantification of white matter damage in concussion subjects and how they correlate with symptoms.

Similarly, two other patients with mTBI who had HDFT analysis were found to have significant discrepancy between the major tracts of the left and right sides (fig. 4). Although conventional MRI detected no significant alteration, there was a significant

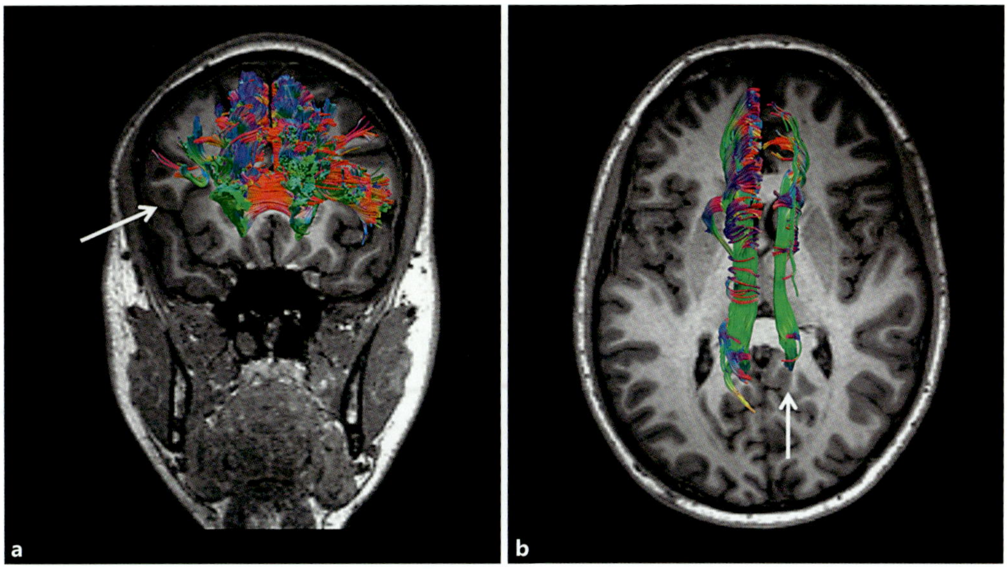

Fig. 4. a Right side of the fiber tracts originating from the corpus callosum shows a significant decrease in volume and extension (arrow). **b** In another subject, the left cingulum shows significant decrease in volume compared to the right (arrow).

decrease in extension and volume of the white matter pathways passing through the genu of the corpus callosum (fig. 4a) and again the cingulum (fig. 4b). Thus far, HDFT analysis for mTBI cases remains largely unexplored. However, we are in the process of developing a more robust accumulation of data, including correlation of fiber tracking findings with behavioral data for mTBI. Previous DTI studies have shown a correlation of injury in the anterior corona radiata with executive function deficits and injury of the uncinate fasciculus to verbal memory deficit [26]. As HDFT can reveal greater detail about the location of damage as well as degree of white matter tract loss, the comparison of imaging analysis to the results of a rigorous battery of cognitive tests in TBI patients will be an exciting opportunity to correlate functional with structural changes after years of using less revealing conventional imaging methods.

Quantitative tractography techniques including HDFT are relatively new, however, and warrant further testing. There are still several limitations to the current analysis methods and room for further development. In our current methods, we normalize the fiber tract counts by using ratios of the left and right sides. Although this reduces the intersubject variability and artifactual differences due to the quality of the scans, this may not be a reliable quantification in cases of severe injury where both coup and contrecoup injuries are present. In addition, the effect of hemorrhage or edema on the quality of HDFT has not been thoroughly analyzed. Since hemosiderin deposition or tissue edema can impede fiber reconstruction by reduction of fractional anisotropy, the presence of these changes in a TBI subject can alter the outcome of HDFT analysis. However, our initial report used a comparison of HDFT at 3 and

8 months to exclude the effects of acute hemorrhage on the quality of diffusion imaging, and reliable reconstruction was repeated at 8 months.

Although HDFT is a new technique in the field of imaging, its unique set of advantages are promising features for its utility in detection of structural damage in mild traumatic brain injury.

References

1 Belanger HG, Vanderploeg RD, Curtiss G, Warden DL: Recent neuroimaging techniques in mild traumatic brain injury. J Neuropsychiatry Clin Neurosci 2007;19:5–20.

2 Kraus J, Nourjah P: The Epidemiology of Mild Head Injury. Oxford, Oxford University Press, 1989.

3 Gennarelli TA, Graham DI: Neuropathology of the head injuries. Semin Clin Neuropsychiatry 1998;3: 160–175.

4 Povlishock JT, Katz DI: Update of neuropathology and neurological recovery after traumatic brain injury. J Head Trauma Rehabil 2005;20:76–94.

5 Niogi SN, Mukherjee P, Ghajar J, Johnson C, Kolster RA, Sarkar R, Lee H, Meeker M, Zimmerman RD, Manley GT, McCandliss BD: Extent of microstructural white matter injury in postconcussive syndrome correlates with impaired cognitive reaction time: a 3T diffusion tensor imaging study of mild traumatic brain injury. AJNR Am J Neuroradiol 2008;29:967–973.

6 Levin HS, Wilde E, Troyanskaya M, Petersen NJ, Scheibel R, Newsome M, Radaideh M, Wu T, Yallampalli R, Chu Z, Li X: Diffusion tensor imaging of mild to moderate blast-related traumatic brain injury and its sequelae. J Neurotrauma 2010;27:683–694.

7 Lipton ML, Gulko E, Zimmerman ME, Friedman BW, Kim M, Gellella E, Gold T, Shifteh K, Ardekani BA, Branch CA: Diffusion-tensor imaging implicates prefrontal axonal injury in executive function impairment following very mild traumatic brain injury. Radiology 2009;252:816–824.

8 MacDonald CL, Johnson AM, Cooper D, Nelson EC, Werner NJ, Shimony JS, Snyder AZ, Raichle ME, Witherow JR, Fang R, Flaherty SF, Brody DL: Detection of blast-related traumatic brain injury in U.S. military personnel. N Engl J Med 2011;364:2091–2100.

9 Shenton ME, Hamoda HM, Schneiderman JS, Bouix S, Pasternak O, Rathi Y, Vu MA, Purohit MP, Helmer K, Koerte I, Lin AP, Westin CF, Kikinis R, Kubicki M, Stern RA, Zafonte R: A review of magnetic resonance imaging and diffusion tensor imaging findings in mild traumatic brain injury. Brain Imaging Behav 2012;6:137–192.

10 Niogi S, Mukherjee P, Ghajar J, McCandliss BD: Individual differences in distinct components of attention are linked to anatomical variations in distinct white matter tracts. Front Neuroanat 2010;4:2.

11 Rutgers DR, Toulgoat F, Cazejust J, Fillard P, Lasjaunias P, Ducreux D: White matter abnormalities in mild traumatic brain injury: a diffusion tensor imaging study. AJNR Am J Neuroradiol 2008;29:514–519.

12 Hashimoto K, Okumura A, Shinoda J, Abo M, Nakamura T: Tensor magnetic resonance imaging in a case of mild traumatic brain injury with lowered verbal intelligence quotient. J Rehabil Med 2007;39: 418–420.

13 Mao H, Polensek SH, Goldstein FC, Holder CA, Ni C: Diffusion tensor and functional magnetic resonance imaging of diffuse axonal injury and resulting language impairment. J Neuroimaging 2007;17:292–294.

14 Le TH, Mukherjee P, Henry RG, Berman JI, Ware M, Manley GT: Diffusion tensor imaging with three-dimensional fiber tractography of traumatic axonal shearing injury: an imaging correlate for the posterior callosal 'disconnection' syndrome: case report. Neurosurgery 2005;56:189.

15 Wang JY, Bakhadirov K, Devous MD Sr, Abdi H, McColl R, Moore C, Marquez de la Plata CD, Ding K, Whittemore A, Babcock E, Rickbeil T, Dobervich J, Kroll D, Dao B, Mohindra N, Madden CJ, Diaz-Arrastia R: Diffusion tensor tractography of traumatic diffuse axonal injury. Arch Neurol 2008;65: 619–626.

16 Fernandez-Miranda JC, Engh JA, Pathak SK, Madhok R, Boada FE, Schneider W, Kassam AB: High-definition fiber tracking guidance for intraparenchymal endoscopic port surgery. J Neurosurg 2010;113: 990–999.

17 Fernandez-Miranda JC, Pathak S, Engh J, Jarbo K, Verstynen T, Yeh FC, Wang Y, Mintz A, Boada F, Schneider W, Friedlander R: High-definition fiber tractography of the human brain: neuroanatomical validation and neurosurgical applications. Neurosurgery 2012;71:430–453.

18 Verstynen T, Jarbo K, Pathak S, Schneider W: In vivo mapping of microstructural somatotopies in the human corticospinal pathways. J Neurophysiol 2011; 105:336–346.
19 Shin SS, Verstynen T, Pathak S, Jarbo K, Hricik AJ, Maserati M, Beers SR, Puccio AM, Boada FE, Okonkwo DO, Schneider W: High-definition fiber tracking for assessment of neurological deficit in a case of traumatic brain injury: finding, visualizing, and interpreting small sites of damage. J Neurosurg 2012;116:1062–1069.
20 Hagmann P, Jonasson L, Maeder P, Thiran JP, Wedeen VJ, Meuli R: Understanding diffusion MR imaging techniques: from scalar diffusion-weighted imaging to diffusion tensor imaging and beyond. Radiographics 2006;26(Suppl 1):S205–S223.
21 Wedeen VJ, Hagmann P, Tseng WY, Reese TG, Weisskoff RM: Mapping complex tissue architecture with diffusion spectrum magnetic resonance imaging. Magn Reson Med 2005;54:1377–1386.
22 Alexander DC, Barker GJ: Optimal imaging parameters for fiber-orientation estimation in diffusion MRI. Neuroimage 2005;27:357–367.
23 Le Bihan D, Poupon C, Amadon A, Lethimonnier F: Artifacts and pitfalls in diffusion MRI. J Magn Reson Imaging 2006;24:478–488.
24 Mayer AR, Ling J, Mannell MV, Gasparovic C, Phillips JP, Doezema D, Reichard R, Yeo RA: A prospective diffusion tensor imaging study in mild traumatic brain injury. Neurology 2010;74:643–650.
25 Kraus MF, Susmaras T, Caughlin BP, Walker CJ, Sweeney JA, Little DM: White matter integrity and cognition in chronic traumatic brain injury: a diffusion tensor imaging study. Brain 2007;130:2508–2519.
26 Niogi SN, Mukherjee P, Ghajar J, Johnson CE, Kolster R, Lee H, Suh M, Zimmerman RD, Manley GT, McCandliss BD: Structural dissociation of attentional control and memory in adults with and without mild traumatic brain injury. Brain 2008;131:3209–3221.

Juan C. Fernandez-Miranda, Assistant Professor
Department of Neurological Surgery
UPMC Presbyterian, Suite B-400
200 Lothrop Street, Pittsburgh, PA 15213 (USA)
E-Mail fernandezmirandajc@upmc.edu

Niranjan A, Lunsford LD (eds): Concussion. Prog Neurol Surg. Basel, Karger, 2014, vol 28, pp 94–111
DOI: 10.1159/000358768

Magnetoencephalography in the Diagnosis of Concussion

Roland R. Lee • Mingxiong Huang

Department of Radiology, VA San Diego Healthcare System, and University of California, San Diego, San Diego, Calif., USA

Abstract

Magnetoencephalography (MEG) is a biomedical technique which measures the magnetic fields emitted by the brain, generated by neuronal activity. Commercial whole-head MEG units have been available for about 15 years, but currently there are only about 20 such units operating in the USA. Here, we review the basic concepts of MEG and list some of the usual clinical indications: noninvasive localization of epileptic spikes and presurgical mapping of eloquent cortex. We then discuss using MEG to diagnose mild traumatic brain injury (mTBI; concussions). Injured brain tissues in TBI patients generate abnormal low-frequency magnetic activity (delta-waves: 1–4 Hz) that can be measured and localized by MEG. These abnormal delta-waves originate from neurons that experience deafferentation from axonal injury to the associated white matter fiber tracts, also manifested on diffusion tensor imaging as reduced fractional anisotropy. Magnetoencephalographic evaluation of abnormal delta-waves (1–4 Hz) is probably the most sensitive objective test to diagnose concussions. An automated MEG low-frequency (slow wave) source imaging method, frequency-domain vector-based spatiotemporal analysis using a L1-minimum norm (VESTAL), achieved a positive finding rate of 87% for diagnosing concussions (blast-induced plus nonblast), 100% for moderate TBI, and no false-positive diagnoses in normal controls. There were also significant correlations between the number of cortical regions generating abnormal slow waves and the total postconcussive symptom scores in TBI patients.
© 2014 S. Karger AG, Basel

Magnetoencephalography (MEG) is a biomedical technique which measures the magnetic fields emitted by the brain. The first magnetoencephalogram measured with a superconducting quantum interference device (SQUID) was obtained by Cohen [1] in 1972. Commercial whole-head MEG units were developed in the mid-1990s (fig. 1). The typical cost of an MEG unit, including its shielded room, is roughly the same as a high-field magnetic resonance imaging (MRI) scanner. There are currently about 20 whole-head MEG units operating in the USA, with several of these having only been installed in the last few years. Outside of the USA, there are about 60 units, many in Japan and Germany.

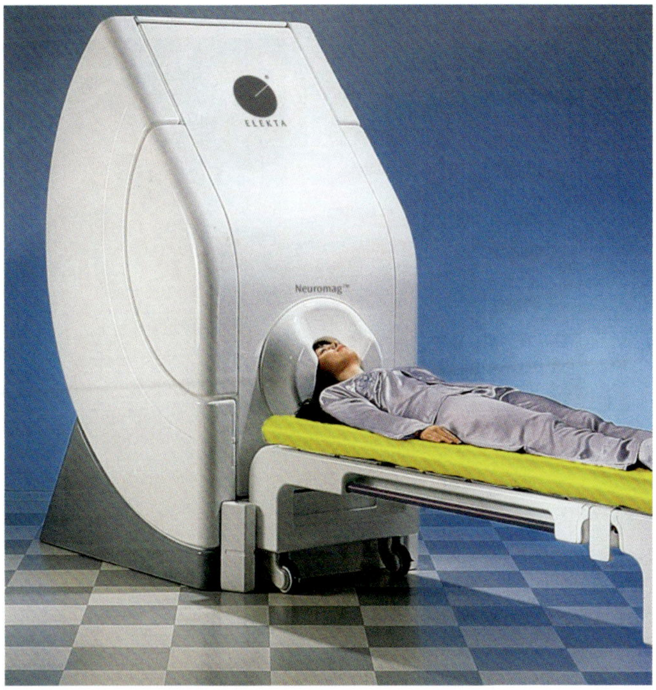

Fig. 1. A modern whole-head MEG system with 306 SQUID measurement channels.

MEG is conceptually similar to the better known and more widely disseminated technique of electroencephalography (EEG), which measures the brain's electrical fields. Both MEG and EEG share excellent submillisecond temporal resolution. This is markedly superior to the temporal resolution of many other functional neuroimaging techniques, such as functional magnetic resonance imaging (100s of ms), or positron emission tomography (PET; min). Moreover, MEG (and EEG) directly samples the electromagnetic fields instantaneously generated by neuronal activity. This is in contrast to functional MRI that measures regional blood flow in the brain or F-18 fluorodeoxyglucose PET that measures regional brain glucose metabolism, both of which are indirect (albeit useful) concomitants of neuronal activity.

The advantage of MEG over EEG is that magnetic fields pass essentially undisturbed through human tissue, unlike electric fields, which are distorted by the differing conductivities of dura, blood, skull, skin, etc., as they pass from the brain to sensors on the scalp [2]. Hence, one may obtain better spatial localization of neuronal sources using MEG (mm) compared to EEG (cm). In a study by Leahy et al. [3], simultaneous whole-head MEG and high-density EEG signals were collected from 32 electric current dipoles in a human skull phantom. Although the signal-to-noise ratio of EEG was better than that of MEG in this phantom study, and the EEG sensor density was slightly higher than that of MEG, the localization error of MEG (approx. 3 mm) was substantially smaller than that of EEG (approx. 8 mm). It was concluded that the reason for EEG's poorer localization accuracy was due to the difficulty of

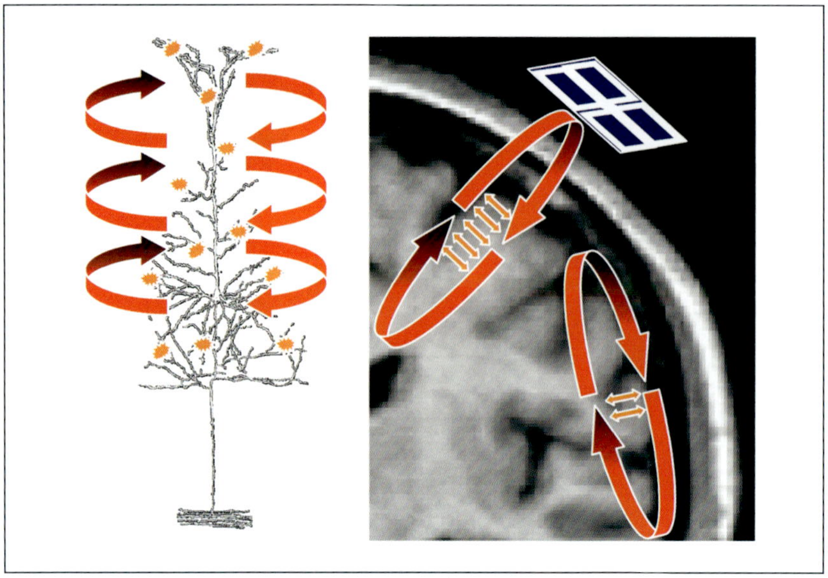

Fig. 2. MEG detection of the neuronal magnetic field depends on orientation of the current dipole. Left: current flow in postsynaptic apical dendrites of pyramidal cells generates a neuronal magnetic field. Right: MEG measurement is sensitive to the magnetic fields generated by the tangentially oriented neuronal current in the wall of the sulcus. The radially oriented neuronal current flow generates a negligible external magnetic field.

estimating and modeling the conductivity profile of the head, especially the substructure of the skull [3]. In that phantom experiment, the conductivity of the human skull phantom was carefully measured, and that value was used in the EEG head modeling. In real-life EEG measurements, the conductivity values of the different compartments of the head are unlikely to be as accurately obtained as in the phantom study, and the typical localization error would be on the order of 10–20 mm [3].

The disadvantages of MEG compared to EEG are: (1) that the brain's magnetic fields are extremely weak compared to other magnetic signals such as the earth's magnetic field and magnetic fields generated by the heart, and (2) it is often difficult or impossible to uniquely determine the neuronal current sources which generate the magnetoencephalographic signals measured at the surface of the head. However, in certain circumstances, such as when the neuronal activity is accurately approximated as a few current dipoles, these sources can be determined uniquely [4].

Basic Principles of Magnetoencephalography

During brain function, such as initiating volitional movement, ensembles of about 10^5–10^6 cortical neurons are activated together, with electrical current (moving electric charges) flowing in the postsynaptic apical dendrites of pyramidal cells [5] (fig. 2). This intracellular electric current generates an associated magnetic field, described by Maxwell's equations of electrodynamics. Although weak (on the order of 10^{-13} T for a typical evoked response such as median nerve stimulation [5]), this magnetic field can be detected by magnetometers composed of extremely sensitive superconducting quantum interference devices (SQUIDs) coupled to 'pick-up coils' (fig. 2) that are embedded in a helmet and mounted in an array around the head. These whole-head helmets typically contain 120–300 small SQUID sensors arranged to cover the surface of the cranium, which is bathed in liquid helium at 4° K because the SQUIDs require such a low temperature to transition to their superconducting state. For comparison, the earth's magnetic field is about 3×10^{-5} T, the magnetic field generated by the heart is 10^{-11} T [5], the baseline electromagnetic noise from the urban environment is in the range of 10^{-6} T (near DC) to 10^{-12} T above 10 Hz [2], and a standard MRI magnet is 1.5 T.

Two techniques are usually employed to successfully measure the brain's weak magnetic fields, despite the presence of such overwhelming magnetic noise. First, the patient and MEG instrument are housed in a shielded room composed of alternating layers of aluminum and mu-metal, which attenuates the external 'noise' of magnetic fields by a factor of about a thousand below 0.1 Hz, and by about 10^6 at 100 Hz [5]. Secondly, most instruments employ spatially closely paired magnetometers (i.e. gradiometers), which are aligned so that their measured signals subtract from one another, thus effectively canceling distant fields of any magnitude [2]. This enables detection only of the magnetic fields originating within a few centimeters of the gradiometers, which are positioned at fixed locations just above the patient's scalp. Hence, although weak, only the fields generated by the adjacent brain neurons are detected.

As a consequence of the geometry of magnetic fields generated by the neuronal currents, and their relationship to the magnetometer/gradiometer pickup coils, only neuronal currents tangential to the brain surface are detectable by MEG; radial fields are essentially invisible to the detectors [5] (fig. 2).

Magnetoencephalography Forward and Inverse Modeling

To localize neuronal sources using MEG, one needs to solve the MEG *forward* and *inverse* problems. In MEG forward models, the magnetic field distribution at MEG sensor sites is calculated from a given neuronal current-source configuration, and the conductivity distribution of different compartments of the head. Typical head models assume that the head contains several homogeneous layers (e.g. scalp, skull, and brain). Most investigators use spherical models that approximate the head (or a part of it) with spheres [6]. The advantage of spherical head models is that the magnetic fields can be solved analytically [6, 7]. A more sophisticated and accurate alternative is to use the boundary element method [8–11]. In this method, the surfaces of the head compartments (e.g. scalp, skull, and brain) are tessellated with small triangles (boundary elements), and the forward magnetic fields are calculated using this realistic head model. The main limitation of the boundary element method is its high computational cost.

With the head model selected, one can examine the recorded magnetic fields and attempt to determine the brain areas responsible for the observed field distribution. This is done by solving the MEG *inverse* problem. If no constraint is imposed, the solution of the MEG inverse problem is nonunique; i.e. there is an infinite set of source configurations that can generate the same magnetic field distribution. To deal with this nonuniqueness, one must impose constraints on the sources by stipulating a source model (which is a concept distinct from the 'head model' described above). The most widely adopted source model for MEG clinical applications is a set of equivalent current dipoles, which assumes that there are multiple focal neuronal current sources that can be modeled by multiple dipoles. In this approach, the equivalent current dipole model is applied to MEG data to describe underlying focal brain sources, and a unique solution (up to the uncertainty of the noise) can be obtained [4]. However, there are other more sophisticated inverse modeling techniques such as vector-based spatiotemporal analysis using a L1-minimum norm (VESTAL) [12], which can obtain distributed rather than discrete dipole sources (discussed later in this report).

Clinical Applications of Magnetoencephalography

In 2002, MEG achieved recognition as a reimbursable clinical procedure by the American Medical Association, with three Current Procedural Technology (CPT) codes including recording and analysis of spontaneous brain magnetic activity (e.g. epileptic cerebral cortex localization, or measurement of brain rhythms) and of evoked magnetic fields (e.g. sensory, motor, language, visual cortex, etc.) [13].

Magnetoencephalography in Epilepsy

MEG has proven to be very useful in localizing interictal spikes in epileptic patients [14–16]. The large focal electromagnetic spikes can be modeled as current dipoles, and their large magnitude makes their detection and localization relatively straightforward. By analyzing brain spontaneous activity epoch by epoch with millisecond temporal resolution, the propagation of the interictal spikes can be modeled temporally as well as spatially. Using MEG, the neuronal dipoles can be localized to within several millimeters, more accurately than with scalp EEG [14–16], since the generated magnetic fields are not spatially blurred by intervening human tissue such as skull or scalp, and the dipole orientation can also be calculated. Figure 3 displays a montage of the raw data from a 122-channel magnetometer demonstrating an epoch containing MEG spikes, the resultant magnetic fields superimposed on the MEG sensors, and the calculated locations of the left temporal spikes in this patient.

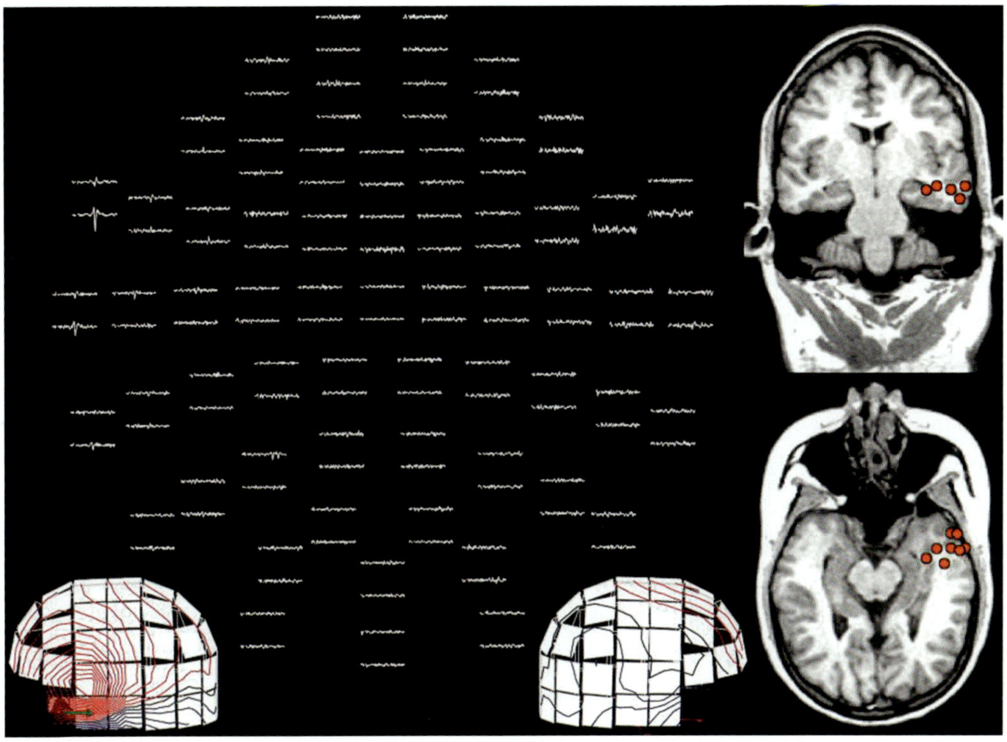

Fig. 3. Interictal spike localization using MEG. The sensor waveform layout demonstrates a spike in the left temporal MEG channels. The contour plots at the bottom of the figure show strong magnetic fields in the sensors above the left temporal region. The red dots on the MRI on the right side of figure show the calculated localization of the spikes in the left medial temporal lobe.

Mapping of Eloquent Cortex Using Magnetoencephalography

MEG is also very useful in presurgical mapping of eloquent cortex such as somatosensory/motor cortex, and correlates well with intraoperative mapping such as electrocorticography [17–19]. The main purpose is to document the location of eloquent cortex with respect to a surgical lesion such as tumor or arteriovenous malformation, in order to determine resectability, or aid in planning the surgical approach to minimize morbidity [17]. In this application (which also has reimbursable CPT codes [13]), evoked neuronal responses are measured to an applied stimulus, such as median-nerve stimulation by electric shock, auditory stimulation by tones, visual stimulation by patterns projected on a computer screen, or finger-tapping time-locked to a visual stimulus. Because the magnetic evoked response is very weak, multiple (about 200) time-locked repetitions are performed, and the responses are averaged together before analysis is performed.

Unlike functional MRI, which measures the blood flow to activated regions of brain, MEG directly measures neuronal magnetic activity. Hence, high-flow arteriovenous malformations can cause artifactual misrepresentation of functional localization in the vicinity of eloquent cortex with fMRI [20], whereas MEG is independent of blood flow and directly demonstrates the site of neuronal activation.

Determination of Hemispheric Language Dominance Using Magnetoencephalography

Determining hemispheric language dominance is crucial in presurgical planning to avoid aphasia after brain surgery. For decades, the gold-standard for determining the language-dominant hemisphere has been the Wada test [21], an invasive technique involving catheterizing the right and left internal carotid arteries and injecting sodium amytal to anesthetize each hemisphere separately, and observing the effects on language and memory. Recently, a number of MEG studies have documented its ability to determine language dominance [22, 23].

MEG activations from language-generating areas (Broca's area) have also been used to determine hemispheric language dominance. Recently, Hirata et al. [24] reported increased beta- and gamma-band MEG signals from the inferior frontal gyrus and middle frontal gyrus during a word-reading test without phonation. The laterality of these signals was used to determine hemispheric dominance, and the MEG measurements correlated well with the Wada test (95% concordance). Language-evoked magnetic field mapping is included in the reimbursable MEG CPT codes [13].

Biomedical Research Applications of Magnetoencephalography

Because of its superb temporal resolution and good spatial resolution in localizing neuronal magnetic activity, and its ability to measure the frequencies/spectra of brain electromagnetic activity, MEG is a valuable tool in biomedical/neuroscience research, including studying patients with schizophrenia, stroke, autism, and many other neurological and psychiatric diseases. Of equal importance, it can elucidate the temporal/spatial activation of the normal brain, as well as its normal rhythms.

Concussions and Conventional Brain Imaging

Traumatic brain injury (TBI) is a leading cause of sustained physical, cognitive, emotional, and behavioral deficits in the civilian population (due to motor vehicle accidents, sports, falls, and assaults) and military personnel (with blast injury as an additional cause). The demographics and natural history of mild TBI (mTBI, i.e. concussion) have been discussed in previous reports.

Conventional neuroimaging techniques have limited sensitivity to detect physiological alterations caused by TBI and are usually not used to assess the efficacy of mTBI treatments. mTBI (and some moderate TBI) can be difficult to detect because the injuries are usually not visible on conventional acute MRI or computed tomography (CT) [25]. Approximately 80% of civilian patients with TBI do not show visible lesions using conventional MRI or CT [26]. For mTBI, intracranial lesions were detected with conventional neuroimaging techniques in only 4, 16, and 28% of patients with Glasgow Coma Scale scores of 15, 14, and 13, respectively [27]. A more recent combat-related TBI study in Operation Iraqi Freedom with 2,074 participants showed that 89% of all TBIs were mild [28]. These examples illustrate the limited diagnostic utility of standard neuroimaging techniques in this population. Furthermore, the absence of abnormalities on conventional neuroimaging techniques in the majority of mTBI patients even with postconcussive symptoms and cognitive and/or behavioral deficits illustrates the limited prognostic value of conventional neuroimaging techniques.

Usually, PCS and cognitive deficits in TBI patients cannot be explained solely by focal pathology; traumatic axonal injury is another major contributor to these deficits. Traumatic axonal injury is commonly induced by sudden acceleration-deceleration or rotational forces. In a rodent TBI model, a silver-staining technique revealed that axonal injury was the most prominent feature following blast exposure [29]. In humans, the subsequent tissue injury is characterized by axonal stretching, inflammation, disruption, and separation of nerve fibers, although axotomy has been found to be relatively rare in even severe TBI [30]. Since conventional CT and MRI are primarily sensitive to blood from nearby torn capillaries and less sensitive to axonal damage itself, they underestimate the presence of traumatic axonal injury, especially in mTBI cases. The limited diagnostic value and poor predictive utility for long-term outcome of the conventional neuroimaging techniques underscores the urgent need for new neuroimaging methods for better diagnosis and longitudinal assessment of mTBI. The availability of neuroimaging techniques with greater sensitivity to the physiological alterations caused by TBI could promote development of treatment interventions for mTBI through an improved understanding of brain mechanisms of injury.

Diffusion tensor imaging (DTI) measures white matter integrity in the brain by measuring the Brownian motion of water through tissues. Information obtained from DTI is representative of the local physical properties of tissue and may be used to estimate the location and orientation of white matter within the brain. Recently, DTI has also been used to examine potential axonal injury in mTBI patients with promising results (discussed in the chapters by Henry, pp. 67–69, and Chamard et al., pp. 80–82, this volume).

Huang et al. [31] reported reduced fractional anisotropy (FA) in a multimodal MEG-DTI study of mTBI (discussed in more detail below). However, increased FA [32] or no change in FA [33] have also been reported in mTBI, indicating that more research is needed to delineate the relationships between DTI parameters and underlying neuropathological processes in mTBI.

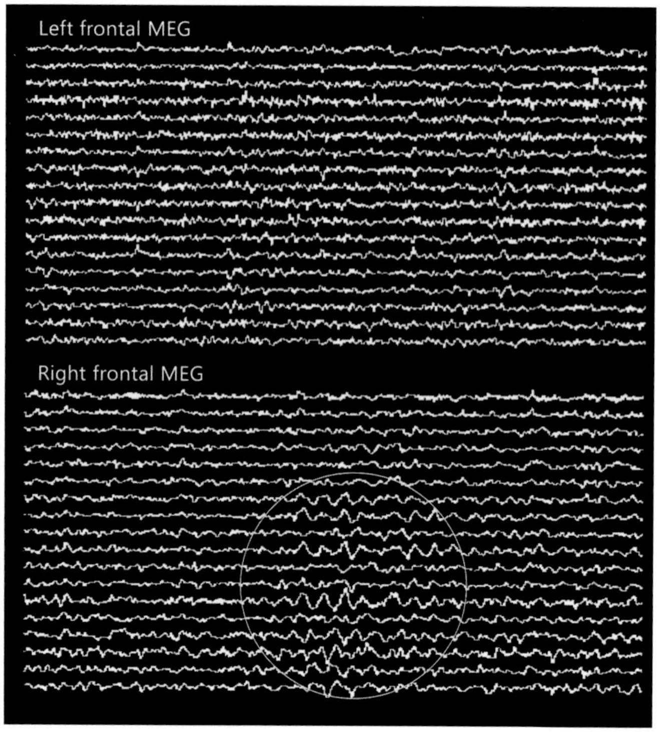

Fig. 4. Abnormal MEG slow-waves (1–4 Hz, delta-waves) in right frontal gray matter are characteristic of neurological injuries in the brain, resulting from axonal injury. Etiologies include infarct, tumor, epilepsy, and TBI, among others.

Concussions and Magnetoencephalography

MEG sensitively demonstrates abnormal neuronal signals resulting from axonal injuries. Unlike *normal* spontaneous MEG data, which is dominated by neuronal activity with frequencies above 8 Hz, injured neuronal tissues (due to head trauma, brain tumors, stroke, etc.) generate abnormal focal or multifocal low-frequency neuronal magnetic signal (delta-band 1–4 Hz, or theta-band 5–7 Hz) that can be directly measured and localized using MEG (fig. 4) [34, 35].

Pioneering studies by Lewine et al. [35, 36] showed that the brains of mTBI patients generate abnormal low-frequency magnetic fields that can be measured and localized by MEG. They also showed that MEG was more sensitive than conventional MRI or EEG for detecting abnormalities in mTBI patients. Studying 20 normal subjects and 20 concussion patients with persistent postconcussive symptoms, Lewine et al. [35] showed that MEG slow waves were 65% sensitive in detecting symptomatic concussions, whereas EEG was only 20–25% sensitive, and MRI was only 20% sensitive in detecting lesions in patients with mild or moderate TBI. None of the 20 normal controls exhibited abnormal MEG slow waves.

In a subsequent paper, Lewine et al. [36] performed a retrospective blinded review of 30 patients with persistent postconcussive symptoms more than 1 year after mild blunt head trauma, comparing the diagnostic utility of MEG, single-photon emission tomography (SPECT), and MRI. They found that MEG demonstrated abnormal dipolar slow-wave activity (DSWA) in 19 patients, compared with abnormal decreased SPECT uptake in 12, and abnormal MRI findings in 4 patients. No definite imaging associations were found with postconcussive *psychiatric* symptoms. However, in the subgroup of patients with postconcussive *cognitive* symptoms, MEG was abnormal in 86% of patients, compared with 40% of patients with abnormal SPECT, and 18% with abnormal MRIs ($p < 0.01$). In addition, MEG showed statistically significant ($p < 0.01$) associations between temporal lobe slow waves (DSWA) and memory problems, parietal DSWA and attention problems, and frontal DSWA and executive function problems.

A recent paper by Huang et al. [31] examined the relationship between DTI abnormalities in white matter fiber tracts and the generation of abnormal MEG slow waves in mTBI in 10 human patients with persistent postconcussive symptoms after mTBI. They found that MEG slow waves in mTBI patients originate from cortical gray matter areas that experience deafferentation due to axonal injuries in the white matter fibers with reduced FA.

All 10 subjects showed abnormal slow waves on MEG, but only one had any lesions on MRI or CT, and only 7 showed abnormalities on DTI. The DTI tractography patterns that link MEG and DTI findings fell into three categories [31]. In category 1 (n = 6 patients), slow-wave-generating gray matter areas were directly linked with nearby nonmajor fiber tracts showing abnormal diffusion (fig. 5). In category 2 (n = 2 patients), multiple slow-wave-generating areas were linked with the same major fiber tracts showing abnormal diffusion (fig. 6). In category 3 (n = 3 patients), abnormal slow waves were observed, but DTI findings were within normal range. One patient showed abnormalities in both categories 1 and 2.

The findings of slow waves in this MEG study are corroborated by prior animal studies of delta-wave generation in gray matter and axonal injuries in white matter, which have established a solid connection between pathological delta-wave generation in gray matter and axonal injuries in white matter. Gloor et al. [37] showed that polymorphic delta-band slow waves produced by white matter axonal lesions in cats are localized to the area of cortex overlying the lesion. They performed a series of experiments using a combination of cortical surface electrodes, microelectrodes, and depth electrodes to identify the generators of the delta-waves and establish their relationship to single-cell discharge of cortical neurons [37, 38]. They found that delta-waves due to white matter lesion formation by thermocoagulation were predominantly generated in pyramidal neurons of layer V or its vicinity, overlying the axonal lesion in the white matter. They also found that delta-waves can be induced by the administration of atropine to block the afferent cholinergic axonal input [39]. These experiments concluded that partial cortical deafferentation (due to axonal injury or disruption of afferent cholinergic axonal input) was an important factor in delta-wave production. The human MEG-DTI results were compatible with this conclusion, showing that MEG delta-waves in TBI patients are generated from gray matter

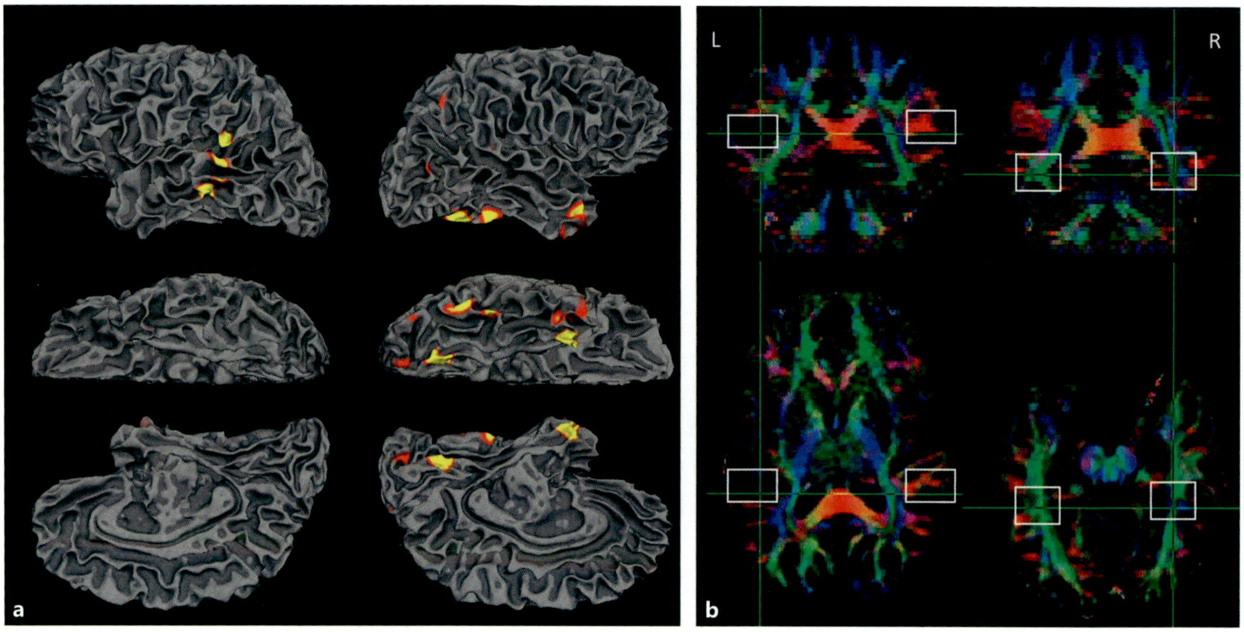

Fig. 5. MEG delta-wave generation and DTI abnormalities in a sport-related concussion patient. **a** Abnormal MEG delta-waves generated from two regions: left column = left lateral superior-posterior temporal region; right column = right inferior temporal-occipital areas. The top, middle, and bottom rows are lateral-view, ventral-view, and middle-view (upside-down), respectively. **b** Abnormally reduced FA-modulated first eigenvector of diffusion tensor from two regions: left column = coronal and axial views show DTI abnormality in left superior-posterior temporal lobe; right column = DTI abnormality in right inferior longitudinal fasciculus.

neurons that experience deafferentation due to axonal injury in the underlying white matter fiber tracts, or blockage of cholinergic transmission [31].

Currently, MEG slow wave detection and localization is usually manually performed by MEG analysts. However, to make MEG low-frequency source imaging an effective clinical tool for assisting in the diagnosis of mTBI, it would be helpful to have an objective, automated, and operator-independent MEG low-frequency source imaging method for detecting and localizing the MEG slow waves.

To this end, VESTAL is a high-resolution time-domain MEG source imaging solution [12]. It (1) can model many dipolar and nondipolar sources, (2) requires no predetermination of the number of sources (model order), and (3) can resolve 100% temporally correlated sources. To more effectively image oscillatory MEG signals such as complicated MEG slow waves, Huang et al. [40] expanded VESTAL from a time domain to a frequency domain.

Using an automated MEG low-frequency source imaging approach (fig. 7), Huang et al. [40] found abnormal delta-waves in 87% of 45 patients with mTBI (23 with blast and 22 with nonblast causes), and 100% of 10 patients with moderate TBI (fig. 8). These positive-finding rates are markedly higher than the approximately 9 and 20%

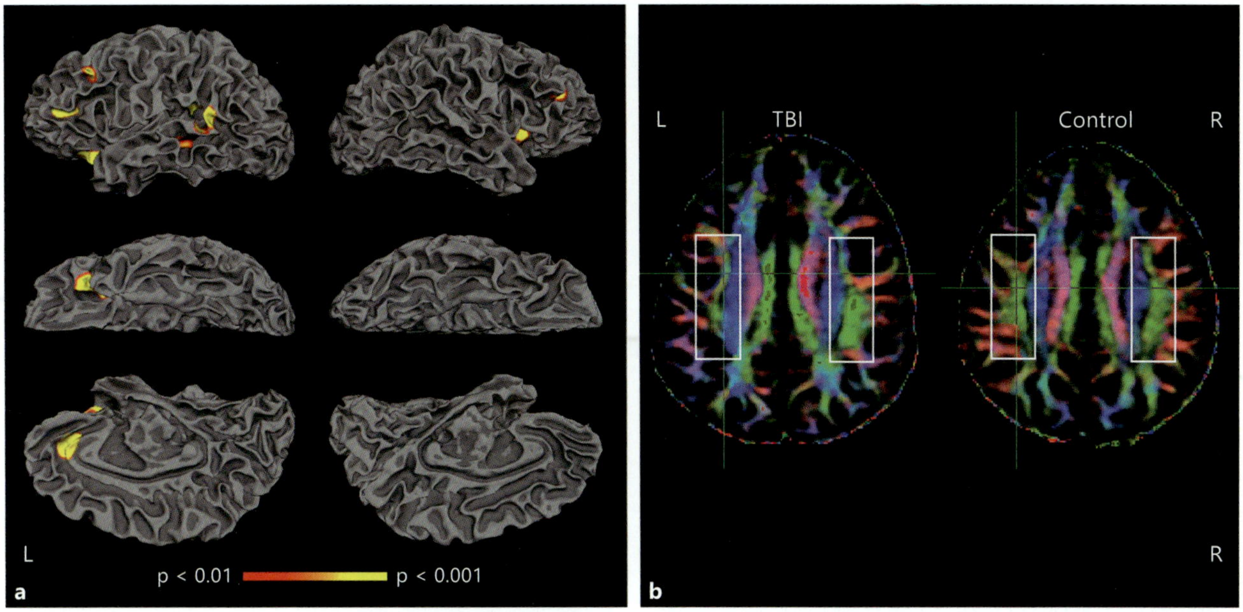

Fig. 6. MEG and DTI findings in a blast-related mTBI patient. **a** Abnormal MEG delta-waves generated from the left lateral prefrontal cortex, orbitofrontal cortex, anterior cingulate cortex, and parietal-temporal junction regions in the left hemisphere (left column) and the lateral prefrontal cortex in the right hemisphere (right column). **b** DTI abnormality was found in the left superior longitudinal fasciculus white matter fiber tract (left column) in this TBI patient, compared with a symmetrical superior longitudinal fasciculus in a typical healthy control subject (right column).

rates using the conventional neuroimaging approaches (i.e. MRI) in the same mild and moderate TBI patients, respectively. We are not aware of any other neuroimaging techniques that are as sensitive as this MEG approach. At the threshold of 4.28 for the Z_{max} which is associated with $p = 0.01$ after Bonferroni correction, none of the 44 normal controls showed abnormal slow waves. This result is consistent with the general conclusion from the MEG concussion studies by Lewine et al. [35, 36], except that the true positive-finding rates in the study by Huang et al. [40] are higher.

Two reasons explain the high positive-finding rates from the new automated MEG low-frequency source imaging approach based on frequency-domain VESTAL. First, the diagnosis in the new approach is based on making an objective comparison with a control normative database containing MEG slow-wave source power from 96 cortical regions. The source imaging analysis is performed by analyzing all the artifact-free epochs from the entire resting state recording. The procedure is objective since no human interaction is involved in manually selecting the epochs. Furthermore, this approach is based on imaging results of slow waves in source space rather than sensor space. This is substantially different from the conventional approaches in which an operator with experience selects the sensor-waveform epochs that he/she considers to demonstrate abnormal low-frequency MEG signals.

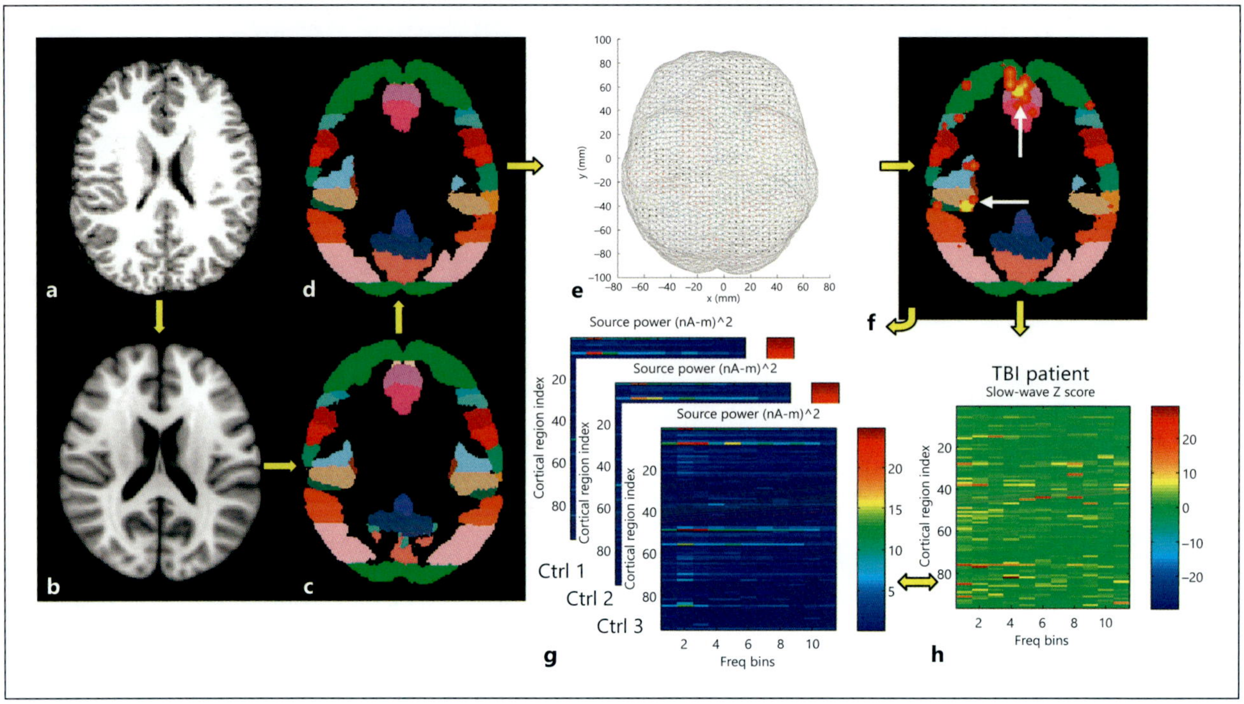

Fig. 7. Processing stream of frequency-domain VESTAL MEG source imaging for slow-wave signals: individual subject's T1-weighted MRI (**a**), MNI-152 brain atlas (**b**), Harvard-Oxford cortical region mask in the MNI-152 coordinate (**c**), cortical region mask is transferred to the individual subject's MRI coordinate (**d**), and cortical regions are resampled to the MEG source grid with a 5-mm grid size for frequency-domain VESTAL (**e**). The gray triangles are the boundary element method mesh. **f** MEG slow-wave activities (hot spots) obtained with frequency-domain VESTAL. A cortical mask is then applied to these slow-wave activities. **g** MEG slow-wave power diagrams (cortical regions vs. frequency bins) for healthy control subjects are used to construct normative database. **h** Comparing the slow-wave power from a TBI patient with the normative database, a Z-score diagram is obtained. Increased slow-wave activities are shown in yellow and red color.

Second, the MEG low-frequency source imaging has the advanced features of frequency-domain VESTAL, which can localize neuronal sources with a variety of spatial profiles such as focal, multifocal, dipolar, and distributed sources, as well as a variety of temporal profiles with uncorrelated, partially correlated, or even 100% correlated source time-courses [12]. It has also been shown that the generators of abnormal slow waves in mTBI patients can possess one or more of the above spatial and temporal profiles [31], which is ideal for the VESTAL approach. In contrast, the conventional MEG slow-wave source analysis used a single dipole fit [35, 36], limiting its ability to analyze MEG signals with complicated neuronal source configurations, which may include some cases of abnormal slow waves in TBI patients.

An additional advantage of the neuroimaging approach described above, which is shared with other MEG protocols that detect delta slow waves, is that the resting-state

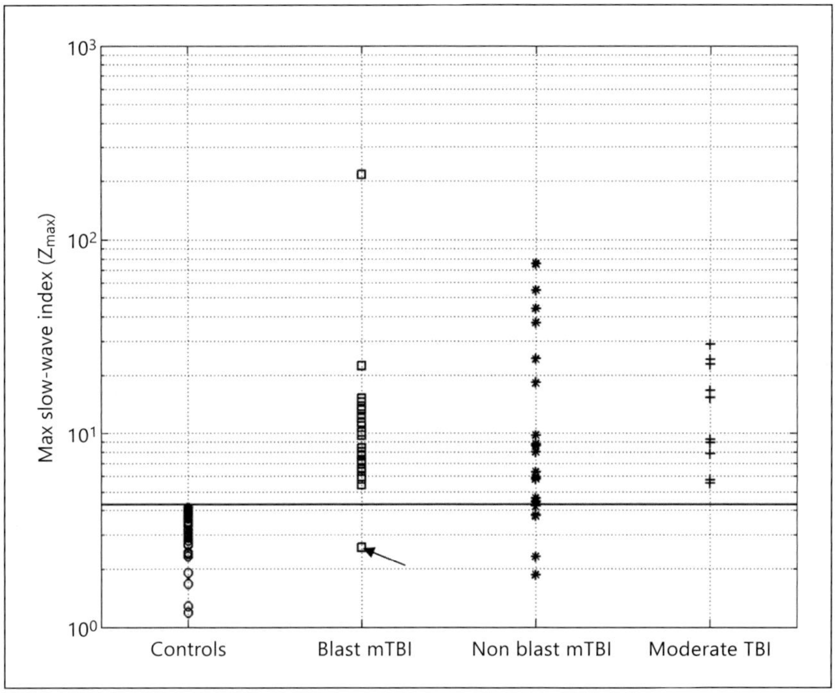

Fig. 8. Z_{max} values obtained from frequency-domain VESTAL low-frequency source imaging are plotted separately for (1) healthy control, (2) blast-induced mTBI, (3) nonblast-induced mTBI, and (4) moderate TBI groups. The y-axis is a logarithmic scale. Z_{max} values from all healthy control subjects are below the solid horizon line indicating the threshold of 4.28 for $p = 0.01$ with Bonferroni correction. The arrow points to a blast-induced TBI patient with probable malingering.

MEG recording procedure is spontaneous, requiring almost no effort from TBI patients, and is thus independent of patients' performance and effort. With the wide availability of information about TBI symptomatology and commonly used psychometric tests on the Internet, and the variety of motivations (i.e. legal, financial, healthcare factors, etc.) for patients to exaggerate/understate symptoms and deficits, more objective diagnostic tests such as this resting-state MEG exam, which cannot be easily manipulated or 'gamed', are invaluable.

Note that abnormal slow/delta-waves are not specific to, nor pathognomonic of, TBI [35], and are also found in neurological/psychiatric disorders such as infarcts, epilepsy, brain tumors, Alzheimer's disease [41], schizophrenia [42–44], and other organic brain disease. Hence, in patients with these serious but readily diagnosable conditions, MEG cannot readily diagnose concussions, as distinguished from their other underlying serious brain disease. Also, the factors that may increase slow-wave power must be controlled in this MEG exam. These factors include neuroleptic, sedative, and hypnotic medications, as well as sleep deprivation.

The 2012 study by Huang et al. [40] also revealed the diffuse nature of the neuronal injuries in TBI patients (fig. 9). On average, approximately 4–8 cortical gray matter

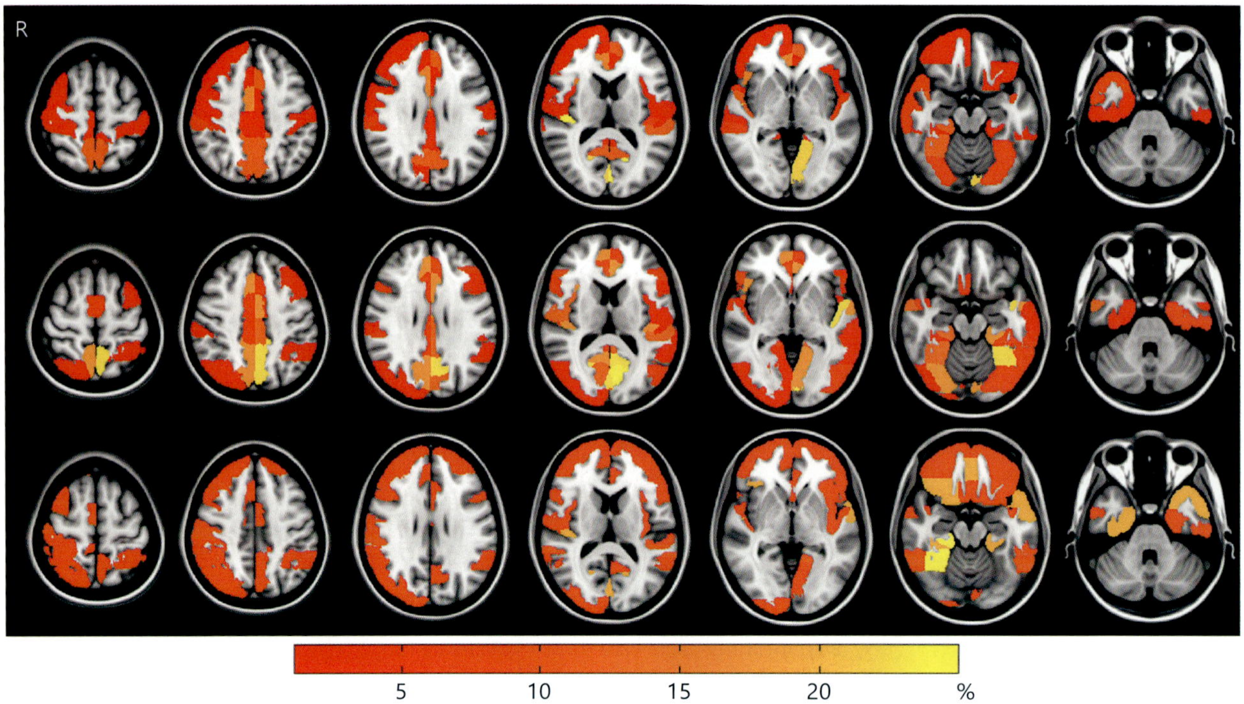

Fig. 9. Percent-likelihood of MEG abnormal slow-wave generation (in MNI-152 atlas space) from blast-induced mTBI (top row), nonblast mTBI (middle row), and moderate TBI (bottom row) groups.

areas showed abnormal slow-wave generation in each TBI patient using the automated MEG low-frequency source imaging. Such findings are consistent with the mechanism of diffuse axonal injury in TBI due to a combination of linear and rotational acceleration and deceleration [30, 45, 46]. The findings are also consistent with Huang's 2009 MEG-DTI study in mTBI [31], in which they found that abnormal MEG slow waves are generated from cortical gray matter areas that connect to white matter fibers with reduced DTI FA due to axonal injury in patients with mTBI. Specifically, the reduced DTI FA in local white matter fiber tracts led to focal abnormal MEG slow waves from neighboring gray matter in mTBI. On the other hand, reduced anisotropy in major white matter fiber tracts led to multifocal or distributed patterns of abnormal slow waves generated from cortical gray matter areas that can be remote in location, but functionally and structurally linked by the injured major/long white matter fiber tracts [31]. The diffuse nature of MEG slow-wave generation is also consistent with a recent DTI study in blast mTBI subjects which showed reduced FA in a diffuse, widespread, and spatially variable pattern [47].

The diffuse nature of abnormal MEG slow-wave generation in TBI also raises questions about the conventional neuroimaging analysis of group averaging of source locations in space. Unlike abnormal slow-wave generation in patient populations with specific psychiatric and neurological disorders such as schizophrenia [42–44] and

Alzheimer's disease [41] where group averaging of source locations in space yielded meaningful information about dysfunctional neuronal networks, the loci that showed abnormal slow-wave generations in TBI patients tend to be highly variable in location. Hence, group averaging of MEG slow-wave source locations in space is unlikely to be the most effective way to detect brain injuries. Instead, analyses of the MEG slow-wave generation characteristics of individual patients, such as that introduced in the study by Huang et al. [40] likely will provide more insights about the neuronal injuries in TBI.

In summary, MEG evaluation of abnormal brain slow delta-waves (1–4 Hz) is probably the most sensitive objective test to diagnose concussions. An automated MEG low-frequency (slow-wave) source imaging method, frequency-domain VESTAL achieves a positive-finding rate of 87% for diagnosing concussions/mTBI (blast-induced plus nonblast) and 100% for the moderate TBI group, with the threshold chosen at $p < 0.01$ level, and no false-positive diagnoses in the normal controls. That study also showed that the characteristics of slow-wave generation in blast-induced mTBI and nonblast mTBI patients are significantly correlated. There were also significant correlations between the number of cortical regions that generate abnormal slow waves and the total postconcussive symptom scores in TBI patients.

Acknowledgements

Portions of the text and figures 7–9 were previously published in the journal *Neuroimage* (reference 40), and are reprinted with permission of the publisher. Portions of the text and figures 5 and 6 were previously published in the *Journal of Neurotrauma* (reference 31), and are reprinted with permission of the publisher. We thank Michael Weisend, PhD, for figures 2 and 3. Veterans Affairs (VA) Merit Review Grants provided financial support.

References

1 Cohen D: Magnetoencephalography: detection of the brain's electrical activity with a superconducting magnetometer. Science 1972;175:664–666.
2 Hamalainen MS, Hari R, Ilmoniemi RJ, Knuutila J, Lounasmaa OV: Magnetoencephalography – theory, instrumentation, and applications to noninvasive studies of the working human brain. Rev Mod Phys 1993;65:413–497.
3 Leahy RM, Mosher JC, Spencer ME, Huang MX, Lewine JD: A study of dipole localization accuracy for MEG and EEG using a human skull phantom. Electroencephalogr Clin Neurophysiol 1998;107: 159–173.
4 Huang M, Aine CJ, Supek S, Best E, Ranken D, Flynn ER: Multi-start downhill simplex method for spatio-temporal source localization in magnetoencephalography. Electroencephalogr Clin Neurophysiol 1998; 108:32–44.
5 Lewine JD, Orrison WW: Magnetoencephalography and magnetic source imaging; in Orrison WW, Lewine JD, Sanders JA, Hartshorne MF (eds): Functional Brain Imaging. St. Louis, Mosby, 1995, pp 369–417.
6 Sarvas J: Basic mathematical and electromagnetic concepts of the biomagnetic inverse problem. Phys Med Biol 1987;32:11–22.
7 Cuffin BN, Cohen D: Magnetic fields of a dipole in special volume conductor shapes. IEEE Trans Biomed Eng 1977;24:372–381.

8 Hamalainen MS, Sarvas J: Realistic conductivity geometry model of the human head for interpretation of neuromagnetic data. IEEE Trans Biomed Eng 1989;36:165–171.
9 Ferguson AS, Zhang X, Stroink G: A complete linear discretization for calculating the magnetic field using the boundary element method. IEEE Trans Biomed Eng 1994;41:455–460.
10 Schlitt HA, Heller L, Aaron R, Best E, Ranken DM: Evaluation of boundary element methods for the EEG forward problem: effect of linear interpolation. IEEE Trans Biomed Eng 1995;42:52–58.
11 Meijs JW, Bosch FG, Peters MJ, Lopes da Silva FH: On the magnetic field distribution generated by a dipolar current source situated in a realistically shaped compartment model of the head. Electroencephalogr Clin Neurophysiol 1987;66:286–298.
12 Huang MX, Dale AM, Song T, Halgren E, Harrington DL, Podgorny I, Canive JM, Lewis S, Lee RR: Vector-based spatial-temporal minimum L1-norm solution for MEG. Neuroimage 2006;31:1025–1037.
13 American Medical Association. Current Procedural Technology (CPT) 2004. Chicago, AMA Press, 2003.
14 Knowlton RC, Elgavish RA, Bartolucci A, Ojha B, Limdi N, Blount J, Burneo JG, Ver Hoef L, Paige L, Faught E, Kankirawatana P, Riley K, Kuzniecky R: Functional imaging: II. Prediction of epilepsy surgery outcome. Ann Neurol 2008;64:35–41.
15 Knowlton RC, Elgavish RA, Limdi N, Bartolucci A, Ojha B, Blount J, Burneo JG, Ver Hoef L, Paige L, Faught E, Kankirawatana P, Riley K, Kuzniecky R: Functional imaging: I. Relative predictive value of intracranial electroencephalography. Ann Neurol 2008;64:25–34.
16 Sutherling WW, Mamelak AN, Thyerlei D, Maleeva T, Minazad Y, Philpott L, Lopez N: Influence of magnetic source imaging for planning intracranial EEG in epilepsy. Neurology 2008;71:990–996.
17 Alberstone CD, Skirboll SL, Benzel EC, Sanders JA, Hart BL, Baldwin NG, Tessman CL, Davis JT, Lee RR: Magnetic source imaging and brain surgery: presurgical and intraoperative planning in 26 patients. J Neurosurg 2000;92:79–90.
18 Roberts TP, Ferrari P, Perry D, Rowley HA, Berger MS: Presurgical mapping with magnetic source imaging: comparisons with intraoperative findings. Brain Tumor Pathol 2000;17:57–64.
19 Castillo EM, Simos PG, Wheless JW, Baumgartner JE, Breier JI, Billingsley RL, Sarkari S, Fitzgerald ME, Papanicolaou AC: Integrating sensory and motor mapping in a comprehensive MEG protocol: clinical validity and replicability. Neuroimage 2004;21:973–983.
20 Ulmer JL, Hacein-Bey L, Mathews VP, Mueller WM, DeYoe EA, Prost RW, Meyer GA, Krouwer HG, Schmainda KM: Lesion-induced pseudo-dominance at functional magnetic resonance imaging: implications for preoperative assessments. Neurosurgery 2004;55:569–579.
21 Wada J, Rasmussen T: Intracarotid injection of sodium amytal for the lateralization of cerebral speech dominance: experimental and clinical observations. J Neurosurg 1960;17:266–282.
22 Papanicolaou AC, Simos PG, Castillo EM, Breier JI, Sarkari S, Pataraia E, Billingsley RL, Buchanan S, Wheless J, Maggio V, Maggio WW: Magnetocephalography: a noninvasive alternative to the Wada procedure. J Neurosurg 2004;100:867–876.
23 Simos PG, Papanicolaou AC, Breier JI, Fletcher JM, Wheless JW, Maggio WW, Gormley W, Constantinou JE, Kramer L: Insights into brain function and neural plasticity using magnetic source imaging. J Clin Neurophysiol 2000;17:143–162.
24 Hirata M, Kato A, Taniguchi M, Saitoh Y, Ninomiya H, Ihara A, Kishima H, Oshino S, Baba T, Yorifuji S, Yoshimine T: Determination of language dominance synthetic aperture magnetometry: comparison with the Wada test. Neuroimage 2004;23:46–53.
25 Bigler ED, Orrison WW: Neuroimaging in sports-related brain injury; in Lovell MR, Echemendia RJ, Barth JT, Collins MW (eds): Traumatic Brain Injury in Sports: An International Perspective. Lisse, Swets and Zeitlinger, 2004, pp 71–94.
26 Alexander MP: Mild traumatic brain injury: pathophysiology, natural history, and clinical management. Neurology 1995;45:1253–1260.
27 Culotta VP, Sementilli ME, Gerold K, Watts CC: Clinicopathological heterogeneity in the classification of mild head injury. Neurosurgery 1996;38:245–250.
28 MacGregor AJ, Dougherty AL, Galarneau MR: Injury-specific correlates of combat-related traumatic brain injury in Operation Iraqi Freedom. J Head Trauma Rehabil 2010;25:1–8.
29 Garman RH, Jenkins LW, Switzer RC III, Bauman RA, Tong LC, Swauger PV, Parks SA, Ritzel DV, Dixon CE, Clark RS, Bayir H, Kagan V, Jackson EK, Kochanek PM: Blast exposure in rats with body shielding is characterized primarily by diffuse axonal injury. J Neurotrauma 2011;28:947–959.
30 Adams JH, Doyle D, Ford I, Gennarelli TA, Graham DI, McLellan DR: Diffuse axonal injury in head injury: definition, diagnosis and grading. Histopathology 1989;15:49–59.
31 Huang MX, Theilmann RJ, Robb A, Angeles A, Nichols S, Drake A, D'Andrea J, Levy M, Holland M, Song T, Ge S, Hwang E, Yoo K, Cui L, Baker DG, Trauner D, Coimbra R, Lee RR: Integrated imaging approach with MEG and DTI to detect mild traumatic brain injury in military and civilian patients. J Neurotrauma 2009;26:1213–1226.

32 Henry LC, Tremblay J, Tremblay S, Lee A, Brun C, Lepore N, Theoret H, Ellemberg D, Lassonde M: Acute and chronic changes in diffusivity measures after sports concussion. J Neurotrauma 2011;28: 2049–2059.
33 Messe A, Caplain S, Paradot G, Garrigue D, Mineo JF, Soto AG, Ducreux D, Vignaud F, Rozec G, Desal H, Pelegrini-Issac M, Montreuil M, Benali H, Lehericy S: Diffusion tensor imaging and white matter lesions at the subacute stage in mild traumatic brain injury with persistent neurobehavioral impairment. Hum Brain Mapp 2011;32:999–1011.
34 Vieth JB, Kober H, Grummich P: Sources of spontaneous slow waves associated with brain lesions, localized by using the MEG. Brain Topogr 1996;8:215–221.
35 Lewine JD, Davis JT, Sloan JH, Kodituwakku PW, Orrison WW Jr: Neuromagnetic assessment of pathophysiologic brain activity induced by minor head trauma. AJNR Am J Neuroradiol 1999;20:857–866.
36 Lewine JD, Davis JT, Bigler ED, Thoma R, Hill D, Funke M, Sloan JH, Hall S, Orrison WW: Objective documentation of traumatic brain injury subsequent to mild head trauma: multimodal brain imaging with MEG, SPECT, and MRI. J Head Trauma Rehabil 2007;22:141–155.
37 Gloor P, Ball G, Schaul N: Brain lesions that produce delta waves in the EEG. Neurology 1977;27:326–333.
38 Ball GJ, Gloor P, Schaul N: The cortical electromicrophysiology of pathological delta waves in the electroencephalogram of cats. Electroencephalogr Clin Neurophysiol 1977;43:346–361.
39 Schaul N, Gloor P, Ball G, Gotman J: The electromicrophysiology of delta waves induced by systemic atropine. Brain Res 1978;143:475–486.
40 Huang MX, Nichols S, Robb A, Angeles A, Drake A, Holland M, Asmussen S, D'Andrea J, Chun W, Levy M, Cui L, Song T, Baker DG, Hammer P, McLay R, Theilmann RJ, Coimbra R, Diwakar M, Boyd C, Neff J, Liu TT, Webb-Murphy J, Farinpour R, Cheung C, Harrington DL, Heister D, Lee RR: An automatic MEG low-frequency source imaging approach for detecting injuries in mild and moderate TBI patients with blast and non-blast causes. Neuroimage 2012; 61:1067–1082.
41 Fernandez A, Maestu F, Amo C, Gil P, Fehr T, Wienbruch C, Rockstroh B, Elbert T, Ortiz T: Focal temporoparietal slow activity in Alzheimer's disease revealed by magnetoencephalography. Biol Psychiatry 2002;52:764–770.
42 Canive JM, Lewine JD, Edgar JC, Davis JT, Torres F, Roberts B, Graeber D, Orrison WW Jr, Tuason VB: Magnetoencephalographic assessment of spontaneous brain activity in schizophrenia. Psychopharmacol Bull 1996;32:741–750.
43 Rockstroh BS, Wienbruch C, Ray WJ, Elbert T: Abnormal oscillatory brain dynamics in schizophrenia: a sign of deviant communication in neural network? BMC Psychiatry 2007;7:44.
44 Wienbruch C, Moratti S, Elbert T, Vogel U, Fehr T, Kissler J, Schiller A, Rockstroh B: Source distribution of neuromagnetic slow wave activity in schizophrenic and depressive patients. Clin Neurophysiol 2003; 114:2052–2060.
45 Basser PJ: Inferring microstructural features and the physiological state of tissues from diffusion-weighted images. NMR Biomed 1995;8:333–344.
46 Xu J, Rasmussen IA, Lagopoulos J, Haberg A: Diffuse axonal injury in severe traumatic brain injury visualized using high-resolution diffusion tensor imaging. J Neurotrauma 2007;24:753–765.
47 Davenport ND, Lim KO, Armstrong MT, Sponheim SR: Diffuse and spatially variable white matter disruptions are associated with blast-related mild traumatic brain injury. Neuroimage 2012;59:2017–2024.

Roland R. Lee, MD
Department of Radiology, VA San Diego Healthcare System
University of California, San Diego
3350 La Jolla Village Drive, MC 114, San Diego, CA 92161 (USA)
E-Mail rrlee@ucsd.edu

Niranjan A, Lunsford LD (eds): Concussion. Prog Neurol Surg. Basel, Karger, 2014, vol 28, pp 112–127
DOI: 10.1159/000358769

Evidence-Based Management of Sport-Related Concussion

Michael McCrea[a–c] · Kevin Guskiewicz[d]

Departments of [a]Neurosurgery and [b]Neurology, Medical College of Wisconsin, and [c]Clement Zablocki VA Medical Center, Milwaukee, Wis., and [d]Department of Exercise and Sport Science, University of North Carolina at Chapel Hill, Chapel Hill, N.C., USA

Abstract

Concussion is not only one of the most common injuries encountered by athletes participating in contact and collision sports, but also among the most complex injuries to manage in a sports medicine setting. Over the past two decades, we have made great progress in advancing the basic and clinical science of concussion. These advances have had enormous clinical translational value for developing evidence-based guidelines for management of concussion in sports. Applied clinical research has clarified the defining characteristics of sport-related concussion (SRC) that support new diagnostic criteria. At the same time, major advancements have been realized in the development and validation of clinical tools that allow a more objective and accurate assessment of concussion and performance-based measures of recovery. These tools provide clinicians with a more informed basis for determining an athlete's cognitive and physical fitness to return to competition after concussion. Standardized injury management protocols that systematically prescribe rest, graded activity, and return to play have been adopted in nearly all clinical settings. Herein, we briefly summarize the findings and recommendations from several national and international consensus guidelines and position statements on best practice in the evaluation and management of SRC.

© 2014 S. Karger AG, Basel

It is now widely recognized that concussion is not only one of the most common injuries encountered by athletes participating in contact and collision sports, but also among the most complex injuries to manage in a sports medicine setting [1, 2]. A combination of factors often presents the clinician with a unique set of challenges in the diagnoses, evaluation, and management of sport-related concussion (SRC). First, we know that athletes commonly do not report concussive events, either because they do not recognize the signs of injury, they do not consider the injury serious enough to warrant medical attention, or they purposefully mask their injury in order to avoid any lost time from participation [3]. Second, even when reported by the athlete, the clinical effects of concussion are often subtle and difficult to detect on common assessment tools. Third, athletes commonly underreport their postinjury symptoms, falsely inflating their level of recovery in hopes of being more rapidly cleared for return to competition. Fourth, to complicate matters further, 'signal detection' on clinical measures (e.g. cognitive and balance testing) often diminishes rapidly in the acute setting of early recovery, making it difficult to precisely determine the athlete's level of recovery and fitness to resume participation after concussion [4]. Finally, there is now recognition that our clinical assessment of concussion merely represents a surrogate index of recovery, but not a direct measure of the integrity of brain structure and function after concussion. Historically, this set of challenges has hampered the front-line clinician responsible for evaluating athletes with suspected concussion on the sports sideline and objectively determining when the athlete is fit to resume participation.

Over the past two decades, we have made enormous strides toward advancing the basic and clinical science of concussion. In doing so, a new evidence base now informs us on the magnitude of this problem, including large-scale epidemiologic studies indicating the frequency of concussion in contact and collision sports at all competitive levels, including youth sports. We now have a new understanding of the defining characteristics of concussion, on which current definitions of injury and diagnostic criteria are based [5]. Several large prospective studies have described the true natural history of acute clinical effects and recovery, including detailed evidence on the time course in recovery of symptoms, cognitive functioning, balance, and other functional capacities in athletes affected by SRC [4, 6–8]. From the basic science arena, major scientific breakthroughs have shed light on the underlying pathophysiology of concussion, which in turn has implications on our understanding of the time course of physiological effects and recovery after injury [9].

In the spirit of true clinical translation, these research advances have directly impacted the development of evidence-based best practice guidelines for the diagnosis, assessment, and management of SRC, including protocols that drive the decision-making process on an athlete's fitness to return to participation after concussion. In essence, translational research over the past 20 years has delivered several key findings that to a large extent take the guess work out of concussion management and provide the clinician with parameters for best practice. Several professional organizations have conducted extensive reviews of the existing literature relevant to SRC and developed consensus guidelines based on the available evidence [1, 2, 5, 10]. As would be expected based on their empirical foundation, there is a great deal of consistency and overlap among the current consensus guidelines and position statements.

While the published consensus guidelines and position statements provide a lengthy and detailed set of evidence-based recommendations, our chapter is intended as a brief, high-level summary of the state of the evidence and international consensus on best practice in management of SRC. The publications principally relied on for the purpose of this brief review include those from the American Academy of Neurology (AAN) [5], American Medical Society for Sports Medicine (AMSSM) [2], National

Athletic Trainers Association (NATA) [10], and 4th International Consensus Conference on Concussion in Sport [1]. We recommend that clinicians caring for athletes affected by SRC become directly familiar with these specific guidelines statements. Similarly, several accompanying papers in this special issue provide a more detailed and substantive review of the existing literature within specific topic areas (e.g. diagnosis, pathophysiology, neurocognitive testing, special populations, postconcussion syndrome, rehabilitation, etc.), extending beyond the scope of this more global review on evidence-based injury management of SRC.

Evidence-Based Concussion Evaluation and Management

Defining and Recognizing Concussion

One of the major challenges associated with SRC over the years has been the degree of heterogeneity in the clinical presentation of this injury. There has been a fair amount of variability in various concussion definitions developed over the past 30 years, but thankfully with a movement toward greater consensus based on the latest evidence. The Zurich 2012 statement defines concussion as a brain injury characterized by a complex pathophysiological process affecting the brain, induced by biomechanical forces [1]. In a similar vein, the AMSSM defines concussion as a traumatically induced transient disturbance of brain function involving a complex pathophysiological process [2]. In basic terms, all definitions of concussion reference a central tenet of injury to the brain that results in temporary loss of normal brain function. Current guidelines indicate that concussion may be caused either by a direct blow to the head or by forces elsewhere to the body that transmit force to the head.

Central to the concussion definition is the rapid onset of short-lived impairment of neurologic function, which most often and typically resolves spontaneously over a short time frame. What is most evident from research over the past two decades is that unconsciousness, once considered a defining characteristic of concussion, is a relatively infrequent occurrence in a sports settings, with only approximately 10% of athletes having any period of witnessed unconsciousness associated with their injury [4]. Similarly, posttraumatic amnesia is observed in less than 50% of all SRCs. Retrograde amnesia is relatively less common, occurring in less than 25% of athletes [4].

Current guidelines stipulate that concussion is a clinical diagnosis based on the combination of injury mechanism and acute symptoms and signs [1, 2, 5]. In other words, the clinical diagnosis of concussion is based largely on what happened to the athlete at the time of the injury event. The mechanism of injury is an important consideration in ruling out other causes of nonspecific signs or symptoms. Once the mechanism is better delineated, then the astute clinician surveys for a constellations of common signs and symptoms indicative of concussion. Ideally, the diagnosis is formulated by a healthcare provider with expertise and knowledge in the recognition and evaluation of concussion.

Table 1. Common signs and symptoms of concussion

Physical	Cognitive	Emotional	Sleep
Headache	Feeling mentally 'foggy'	Irritable	Drowsiness
Nausea	Feeling slowed down	Sadness	Sleep more than usual
Vomiting	Difficulty concentrating	More emotional	Sleep less than usual
Balance problems	Difficulty remembering	Nervousness	Difficulty falling asleep
Dizziness	Forgetful of recent information and conversations		
Visual problems	Confused about recent events		
Fatigue	Answers questions slowly		
Sensitivity to light	Repeats questions		
Sensitivity to noise			
Numbness/tingling			
Dazed			
Stunned			

Adapted from AMSSM position statement, 2013 [2].

Concussion often produces a common set of physical, cognitive, behavioral, and other symptoms. Table 1 lists common signs and symptoms observed in the setting of SRC [11]. Along with the established mechanism of injury, these signs and symptoms essentially represent the clinical criteria used to diagnose concussion. It should be noted that several symptoms of concussion are considered nonspecific, meaning that they commonly occur in the context of health conditions other than concussion that are commonly encountered by athletes. Further, certain symptoms may also be common in other comorbid conditions, such as mood disorders, learning disabilities, or other developmental cognitive disorders other than concussion. Therefore, it is essential for the clinician to link the onset of suspected concussion signs and symptoms with an apparent mechanism of injury in order to more precisely isolate concussion as the probable cause of those signs and symptoms. Infrequently, there may be delayed onset of symptoms after concussion, but most often these abnormalities manifest immediately after the head impact in question.

Concussion symptom checklists can provide the clinician with a systematic way to document the presence and severity of concussion symptoms, as well as a method for tracking changes in symptom levels on serial assessment over the course of the athlete's postinjury recovery [11]. These tools should not, however, be used as the sole basis to diagnose concussion.

Acute Concussion Assessment and Management

Both consensus guidelines and legislation in most states indicate that any athlete suspected of having a concussion should be immediately removed from play and assessed by a qualified healthcare provider who is knowledgeable in the evaluation and management of concussion. Any athlete with suspected concussion is prohibited from returning to competition or participation on the same day of injury [1].

During the acute injury phase, the first priority is to rule out the occurrence of a more severe injury (i.e. cervical spine injury, severe brain injury, airway obstruction, etc.) that may represent a medical emergency [12]. Regardless of the setting, an emergency action plan is critical. The emergency action plan should spell out in a detailed progression the protocol for management of acute injuries, including SRC. The emergency action plan should clearly indicate the protocol for emergency transport to a local hospital when there are signs or suspicion of a more severe underlying brain injury [12].

Once other or more severe injuries have been ruled out and all first aid issues have been addressed, a formal concussion assessment should then be initiated. Concussion clearly produces a constellation of symptoms and functional impairments during the acute phase (e.g. initial 24 h). Therefore, the immediate or 'sideline' evaluation of athletes with suspected concussion should, at a minimum, include a survey of common concussion signs, assessment of symptoms, and objective testing of cognition, balance, and other functional capacities [11].

Over the past 10 years or more, several standardized tests have been developed to aid in acute concussion assessment. A basic premise of this standardization movement has been that performance-based assessment measures may be superior to an athlete's self-reporting of symptoms, which might be unreliable due to athletes' tendency to underreport or fail to recognize their symptoms. Standardized tests are intended to provide a more objective, performance-based method of measuring postinjury recovery and determining an athlete's fitness to return to play. In most cases, these tests assess single domains of concussion effects (e.g. postconcussion symptoms, neurocognitive functioning, and postural stability).

We now know that the effects of concussion are not confined to one domain (e.g. cognitive functioning). That is, athletes, to varying degrees, experience a complex combination of symptoms and exhibit deficits across multiple domains of functioning. As a result, reliance on a single test or multiple measures in a single assessment domain will likely be less accurate than a multimodal assessment. A multidimensional approach that integrates assessment of self-reported symptoms and other functional domains known to be affected by concussion is recommended. This approach includes formal symptom assessment and standardized testing of cognitive ability and balance.

Several tests and measures are appropriate for use in the assessment of acute concussion in the competitive sporting environment [11]. These tests provide important data on symptoms and functional impairments that clinicians can incorporate into their diagnostic formulation, but should not solely be used to diagnose concussion. The specific tests selected to form the multidimensional assessment approach not only need to be reliable and valid, but also may vary depending on the situational constraints of the sporting environment, athlete population, and the experience of the assessor. Based on their review of the evidence, the AAN recently identified a number of clinical tools to help identify individuals with concussion and assess their level of injury, including a symptom checklist, the Standardized Assessment of Concussion (SAC), neuropsychological testing, and the Balance Error Scoring System (BESS) [5].

The recently-revised Sports Concussion Assessment Tool – Third Edition (SCAT3) involves a multimodal assessment model that integrates several of the AAN-recommended assessments into a singular assessment package (see Appendix A) [1]. SCAT3 has a graded symptom checklist, SAC, and BESS all embedded in a unified, multidimensional assessment tool appropriate for use in a competitive sporting environment. The individual components of SCAT3 (symptom checklist, SAC, and BESS) have all been well validated in the acute assessment of athletes affected by sports concussion, but further research is required to determine the overall utility of the integrated SCAT3 [11]. Likewise, in 2012 the National Football League's (NFL) Head Neck and Spine Committee introduced mandatory use of the Sideline Assessment Tool for physicians and athletic trainers. This instrument includes many of the same components in the SCAT3, with the inclusion of a series of 'no-go' or disqualification questions to assist clinicians (see Appendix B).

Far and away, the vast majority of athletes with SRC do not require or undergo neuroimaging studies. As in the case of civilian brain injury, computed tomography is the preferred technology to rule out structural or more severe underlying brain injury that may represent or escalate to a neurosurgical emergency (i.e. skull fracture, intracranial bleed, contusion, cerebral swelling, brain stem herniation, etc.). In the subacute setting, brain magnetic resonance imaging may be helpful in identifying any underlying structural abnormalities that correlate with persistent symptoms, prolonged recovery, or poor outcome. Newer, innovative neuroimaging technologies such as diffusion tensor imaging, functional magnetic resonance imaging, positron emission tomography, single-photon emission tomography, and others show promise in identifying changes in brain structure and function associated with concussion, but require further study before being considered a central component of best practice for evaluating athletes with SRC.

Subacute Concussion Evaluation and Management

Research over the last decade has demonstrated that the overwhelming majority of athletes achieve a complete recovery in symptoms, cognitive functioning, postural stability, and other functional impairments over a period of 1–3 weeks following concussion [7, 13–16]. The rate of recovery will vary among athletes and may be modified by several factors, including severity of injury, athlete age and gender, prior concussion and health history, presence of comorbidities, sport and level of participation, and other factors. Over the past decade, we have seen a major paradigm shift away from injury management strategies based on the 'grade' of injury severity to a new approach that emphasizes the monitoring and measurement of clinical recovery in the individual athlete. In fact, concussion grading scales have essentially fallen away from use during this paradigm shift. Current guidelines for tracking recovery and decision-making on return to play are based on this new approach rather than prescriptive or 'cookbook' recommendations based largely on concussion grade.

To that end, athletes with concussion should have medical follow-up with a qualified healthcare professional knowledgeable in the evaluation and management of SRC. Follow-up should include serial monitoring of postconcussive symptoms, in addition to performance-based measures of recovery at the appropriate point in the athlete's recovery. Ideally, a standardized symptom checklist, such as that included in SCAT3 or the NFL Sideline Assessment Tool, should be used to quantify the presence and severity of common postconcussive symptoms, which also allows the clinician to then quantitatively track the athlete's level of symptom recovery over time. Although a rare occurrence, any indication of rapidly worsening symptoms or deterioration in the athlete's neurologic status should obviously prompt emergent medical evaluation and workup.

Current consensus guidelines recommend the introduction of performance-based measures of recovery once an athlete has reached or is closely approximating the point of being completely symptom free [1]. The basis for this approach is that there is no clinical decision to be made regarding the athlete's readiness to return to participation until they are symptom free. At the point in which an athlete is reportedly symptom free, performance-based measures of recovery can then be used to substantiate the athlete's self-reported recovery. In essence, the clinician can then utilize the results of performance-based testing to objectively determine the athlete's level of recovery and fitness to resume participation. Several modalities of performance-based testing have emerged as central components to most concussion evaluation programs, primarily involving neurocognitive testing, balance testing, and other functional assessment measures.

Neurocognitive testing has been demonstrated to be a valuable component of the multidimensional approach to concussion evaluation [17]. In addition to cognitive screening tools such as SCAT3 that are intended for use during the acute postinjury phase, neuropsychological testing can provide a more objective and sensitive measure of subtle changes in memory, cognitive processing speed, working memory, executive functioning, and other cognitive functions during the subacute phase after SRC.

International consensus guidelines indicate that formal neuropsychological testing is not required for all athletes with concussion and that most concussions can be managed appropriately without the use of a neuropsychological testing [1]. Objective cognitive testing may, however, prove valuable in instances of complicated recovery or in cases where there are questions about the reliability of a player's reported level of symptom recovery. In any case, neuropsychological testing should not be the sole basis of management decisions, but instead be used only as part of a comprehensive multidimensional concussion management strategy, and should not be used in isolation [1, 2, 17, 18].

A combination of both conventional (paper-and-pencil) and computerized neuropsychological testing modules have been utilized in the setting of sport concussion assessment. In recent years, there has been a major increase in the utilization of computerized neurocognitive testing at all competitive levels in the USA and worldwide. Among expert neuropsychologists involved in the assessment of SRC, there is often a strong preference toward a 'hybrid approach' that combines the benefits of both conventional and computerized neuropsychological testing. The AMSSM indicates that 'paper and pencil neuropsychological tests can be more comprehensive, test different domains and assess for other conditions which may masquerade as or complicate assessment of concussion' [2]. At present, international guidelines state that there is 'insufficient evidence to recommend a widespread routine use of baseline neuropsychological testing' [1].

A 'one size fits all' solution when it comes to neurocognitive testing of athletes affected by SRC is unlikely. In the acute setting (sideline), brief cognitive screening tools are likely to be the most effective and practical for gathering immediate assessment of an athlete's level of cognitive functioning, which can be incorporated into the overall diagnostic formulation. Tools such as SCAT3 are valuable in this regard. During the subacute phase, brief neuropsychological test batteries are most appropriate to conduct a more detailed assessment of subtle cognitive impairments that may linger over the course of clinical recovery. Many customized batteries are in use at various competitive levels, which are able to assess multiple domains of cognitive functioning in 30 min or less. In cases of complex recovery or where comorbidities are evident, a more comprehensive neuropsychological evaluation may be more appropriate.

International guidelines recommend that neuropsychological testing be used to assist in return-to-play decisions once an athlete is clinically asymptomatic [1]. In some instances, neuropsychological assessment may provide helpful information during earlier stages of recovery, particularly with respect to an athlete's fitness to return to normal academic activities. While it may be practically necessary for other qualified healthcare providers to administer neuropsychological tests, particularly in the setting of computerized neurocognitive assessment tools, test results ideally should be interpreted by a trained neuropsychologist [17, 18].

There is now a growing body of literature indicating that balance is typically affected in concussed athletes in the early postinjury period [4, 19–24]. As such, clinical balance testing is also now considered a central component to most concussion evaluation programs. Recent consensus guidelines and evidence-based reviews support the use of BESS to evaluate athletes during the acute and subacute recovery periods following SRC. A clinical assessment for postural stability, BESS has been found to be sensitive in detecting acute postural stability alterations up to postconcussion day 3 and can be used to assist clinicians in evaluating concussion when laboratory force platforms are unavailable or impractical [4, 19, 25].

BESS is comprised of a series of clinical balance tests that progressively challenge the sensory systems through variations in stance (double-leg, single-leg, and tandem) and surface (firm and foam) (fig. 1). The double-leg stance is performed with the feet touching at the arches, creating a small base of support. During the single-leg stance, the patient is asked to maintain the on-stance leg in 20–30° of hip flexion and 40–50° of knee flexion. The tandem stance is performed with the patient standing with one

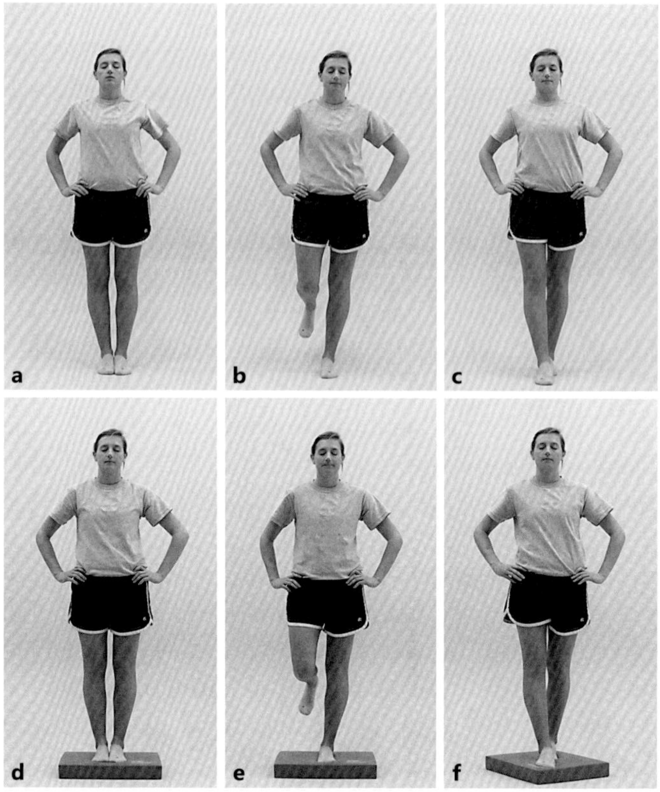

Fig. 1. BESS performed on a firm surface (**a–c**) and a foam surface (**d–f**).

Table 2. Types of errors for BESS

Lifting hand off iliac crest(s)
Opening eyes
Step, stumble, or fall
Moving hip into more than 30° of flexion or abduction
Lifting the forefoot or heel
Remaining out of the test position for greater than 5 s
The BESS score is calculated by adding one error point for each error committed during each of the six 20-second trials.

foot in front of the other so that the heel of the front foot and the toes of the rear foot are in contact. Patients are asked to stand quietly in the required test position with their hands on their hips. Once the eyes are closed the 20-second trial begins. During each condition, patients are told that upon losing their balance they should return to the starting position as quickly as possible and continue balancing until asked to stop.

Table 2 presents the scored BESS errors, which are summed at the conclusion of the 6 trials resulting in a total BESS score. If a patient is unable to remain in the proper

Table 3. Graduated return-to-play protocol

Rehabilitation stage	Functional exercise at each stage of rehabilitation	Objective of each stage
1. no activity	symptom limited physical and cognitive rest	recovery
2. light aerobic exercise	walking, swimming, or stationary cycling keeping intensity <70% maximum permitted heart rate; no resistance training	increase heart rate
3. sport-specific exercise	skating drills in ice hockey, running drills in soccer; no head impact activities	add movement
4. noncontact training drills	progression to more complex training drills, e.g. passing drills in football and ice hockey; may start progressive resistance training	exercise, coordination, and cognitive load
5. full-contact practice	following medical clearance participate in normal training activities	restore confidence and assess functional skills by coaching staff
6. return to play	normal game play	

From 4th International Consensus Conference on Concussion in Sport [1].

stance for at least 5 s during a trial, the trial is considered to be incomplete and a maximum error score of 10 is assigned. BESS requires minimal equipment, is portable, and has been demonstrated as a useful and cost-effective sideline evaluation technique to evaluate postural stability following concussion. BESS has been shown to have low to high inter- and intratester reliability, depending on the source of the study [26–29].

A small number of recent studies have provided preliminary data regarding the use of electrophysiological and other measures in the acute evaluation of concussion [30, 31]. Although these methods show promise, further research is required to support their use in the clinical setting.

Graduated Exertion and Return to Play

Across all consensus guidelines, two standards are consistently evident. First, current guidelines universally recommend that no athlete should return to play if still experiencing symptoms or exhibiting signs of concussion. Second, an initial period of physical and cognitive rest is a cornerstone of concussion management. Although there is a dearth of empirical research in this area, it is thought that an initial period of rest in the order of 24–48 h may be of benefit to the athlete [32, 33]. At the same time, lengthy or indefinite periods of complete rest are not supported by the literature and believed by some to even be detrimental to the athlete's overall recovery.

Following the initial rest period, the prevailing approach to injury management calls for a graded return to activity and sports participation. The Zurich consensus statement outlines a graded exertion protocol specifically designed for athletes that has become the standard in the field (table 3) [1]. This approach provides the combined advantages of allowing adequate time for recovery, enabling the athlete to reacclimate to demanding physical activity, and reducing the known risk of reinjury. With this stepwise progression, the athlete should continue to proceed to the next level as long as they are able to remain asymptomatic during activities at the prescribed level. In most cases, each step requires a minimum of 24 h for the athlete to acclimate to the level of exertion, without any recurrent or worsening symptoms. With older elite athletes, two steps may be conducted on the same day. Typically, athletes are able to progress through all stages of the rehabilitation process within 5–7 days; however, they should begin the process only after they have become asymptomatic. Should the athlete experience any recurrent or worsening symptoms or other setbacks once the process has begun, they are then recommended to throttle back to the prior rehabilitation stage for another 24-hour trial before graduating to the next stage of exertion.

In instances of atypical or prolonged recovery, or in cases of athletes with a history of multiple prior concussions, a lengthier rehabilitative process may be recommended. In these situations, an adaptation to the Zurich graded exertion protocol may be appropriate. The authors have commonly utilized such an approach, typically extending the trial period of each rehabilitative stage from a minimum of 24 h to 3–5 days, on average. An example of this modified graded exertion protocol is contained in table 4.

Conclusion

Major advances in the basic and clinical science of concussion over the past 20 years have taken much of the guesswork out of this injury and now provide clinicians with a fairly mature evidence base to guide the diagnosis, evaluation, and management of SRC. While some questions remain about certain nuances of concussion evaluation (e.g. which tests are most sensitive and specific in detecting clinicallymeaningful change resulting from concussion) and management (e.g. how long an athlete should observe total rest after concussion) of SRC, there is a great deal of agreement on the general principles of injury management recommendations across current consensus guidelines that are based on the latest evidence. Clinicians charged with the care of athletes are encouraged to become familiar with the latest evidence-based guidelines for the evaluation and management of SRC, which provide detailed recommendations well beyond this high-level review.

The most critical element to effective concussion management is having a well-designed plan that is in alignment with the current consensus guidelines. All institutions and clinicians should have a systematic protocol that spells out the plan for preparticipation screening or baseline testing of athletes, acute injury evaluation and management, tracking and determining an athlete's level of postinjury recovery, and criteria for clearing an athlete for return to participation. In addition, general guidelines for managing complex cases (e.g. athletes with a history of multiple concussion, cases of prolonged recovery, etc.) should also be well defined. While the specific details

Table 4. Modified return-to-play protocol for prolonged or atypical recovery athletes

Rehabilitation stage	Objective	Activity examples and exertional range	Activity duration	Restrictions	Predicted time line, days	Indicator to proceed to next stage
Light, low-intensity aerobic exercise	Gradually increase heart rate as tolerated without symptoms	Walking, elliptical machine, or stationary bike up to 60% of MPHR[a]	15 min maximum	No contact or head impact activities (e.g. treadmill, etc.) No loud or hectic environments (sporting events, dances, etc.)	3–5	Tolerating this level of activity without symptoms for 3 days
Moderate-intensity aerobic exercise	Gradually increase heart rate as tolerated without symptoms	Walking, elliptical machine, or stationary bike up to 70% of MPHR[a]	30 min maximum	No contact or head impact activities No loud or hectic environments (sporting events, dances, etc.)	3–5	Tolerating this level of activity without symptoms for 3 days
High-intensity aerobic exercise	Gradually increase heart rate as tolerated without symptoms	Jogging, elliptical machine, or stationary bike up to 80% of MPHR[a]	30 min maximum	No head impact activities Limited social activity, as tolerated	3–5	Tolerating this level of activity without symptoms for 3 days
Non-contact training drills	Progression to normal sporting activity without symptoms	Volleyball-specific drills without risk of head impact	60 min	No head impact activities	3–5	Tolerating this level of activity without symptoms for 3 days
Full participation	Full participation without symptoms	Normal sport-related activities	N/A	None	N/A	N/A

Adapted from 4th International Consensus Conference on Concussion in Sport [1]. MPHR = Maximum predicted heart rate. [a] The predicted timeline for this graduated program is extended from a minimum of 24 h per stage to 3–5 days per stage to allow adequate accommodation without symptoms at each rehabilitation stage. N/A = Not applicable.

of a concussion management protocol will vary to some degree among clinicians and institutions, the key is for all care providers to be well-prepared and familiar with their respective concussion protocol. This advanced preparation will go a long way in maximizing the consistency, efficiency, and effectiveness of care delivery to protect the health and safety of athletes affected by SRC.

Beyond the scope of conventional concussion assessment and management, future research should explore new frontiers in treatment interventions to facilitate recovery and prevent poor outcome after SRC. Although a number of treatment and rehabilitation modalities (e.g. vestibular therapy, multimodal rehabilitation, cognitive behavioral therapy, and pharmacologic agents) are often employed in various clinical settings, the efficacy of these methods remains unclear. Similarly, the future should also bring greater emphasis on the development of strategies to reduce or prevent the incidence of SRC in contact and collision sports. A multidimensional approach to injury prevention that dually focuses on changes in policy, protective equipment, and the culture of sports is likely to be more effective than any singular solution. Collectively, scientific advances that drive evidence-based approaches to injury assessment, diagnosis, treatment, and prevention are in the best interest of protecting the health of young athletes and preserving the richness of competitive sports.

Appendix A

Sports Concussion Assessment Tool – 3rd Edition (SCAT3) [1]

This tool does not constitute, and is not intended to constitute, a standard of medical care. It is a guide derived from the Standardized Concussion Assessment Tool 2 (SCAT2) (McCrory, et al, BJSM '09) and represents a standardized method of evaluating NFL players for concussion consistent with the reasonable, objective practice of the healthcare profession. This guide is not intended to be a substitute for the clinical judgment of the treating healthcare professional and should be interpreted based on the individual needs of the patient and the specific facts and circumstances presented.

NFL Sideline Concussion Assessment Tool: Completed by healthcare professional. Athlete completes symptoms at bottom.

Athlete __________________ **Position** ______________ **Team** ______________ **Evaluator** _____________ ATC / MD / DO

Evaluation date____ **time** ____am / pm **Injury date** ____ **time** ____ am / pm **during** ☐ Game ☐ Practice ☐ Other ________

How was the injury identified (check all that apply) ☐ if game, call by ATC spotter ☐ medical staff ☐ self report ☐ teammate ☐ coach ☐ referee ☐ other ___________ Penalty called ☐ Yes ☐ No Other circumstances ____________________

Mechanism of injury ☐ head to head ☐ elbow to head ☐ knee to head ☐ ground to head ☐ blow to body ☐ unknown ☐ other mechanism or comments ______________________________

This concussion assessment tool contains an assessment of orientation, memory, concentration, balance & symptoms. This tool is intended to be used in conjunction with your clinical judgment. If ANY significant abnormality is found, a conservative, safety first approach should be adopted. An athlete suspected of sustaining a concussion is a "No Go" and does not return to play in the same game or practice.

ANY OF THE FOLLOWING ARE OBVIOUS SIGNS OF DISQUALIFICATION (i.e. "No Go"):

1)	**LOC or unresponsiveness?** (for any period of time) If so, how long? _____________	☐	Y	N
2)	**Confusion?** (any disorientation or inability to respond appropriately to questions)	☐	Y	N
3)	**Amnesia (retrograde / anterograde)?** If so, how long? ______________	☐	Y	N
4)	**New and/or persistent symptoms: see checklist?** (e.g. headache, nausea, dizziness)	☐	Y	N
5)	**Abnormal neurological finding?** (any motor, sensory, cranial nerve, balance issues, seizures) **or**	☐	Y	N
6)	**Progressive, persistent or worsening symptoms? If so, consider cervical spine and/or a more serious brain injury (See box below)**	☐	Y	N

Other ______________________ **Total Physical Signs Score: (total above ☐ Yes scores) of 6 =** _____

Neurological Screen for Cervical Spine and/or More Serious Brain Trauma

Deteriorating mental status?	**Y**	**N**
Any reported neck pain, cervical spine tenderness or decreased range of motion?	**Y**	**N**
Pupil reaction abnormal or pupils unequal?	**Y**	**N**
Extra-ocular movements abnormal and/or cause double vision? (difficulty tracking and/or reading)	**Y**	**N**
Asymmetry or abnormalities on screening motor or sensory exam?	**Y**	**N**

SAC / ORIENTATION	**of 5 =** ____	
What month is it?	0	1
What is the date today?	0	1
What is the day of the week?	0	1
What year is it?	0	1
What time is it right now? (within an hour)	0	1

ORIENTATION / Maddock's Questions	**of 5 =** ____	
Where are we?	0	1
What quarter is it right now?	0	1
Who scored last in the practice / game?	0	1
Who did we play last game?	0	1
Did we win the last game?	0	1

SAC / Word Recall: Read list of 5 words 1 per second, ask athlete to repeat list, in any order. (Use of specific lists below optional). For Trial 2 & 3, read the same list of words again and have athlete repeat them back, in any order. One point for each word remembered. You must conduct all 3 trials regardless of their success on trial 1. **Do not tell athlete that delayed recall will be tested**

List 1	**Immediate Recall Trials #1**	**#2**	**#3**	**Alternative Lists**		**Delayed recall (perform at end of all sideline testing, at least > 5 minutes)**
elbow	_______	_______	_______	candle	baby	_________
apple	_______	_______	_______	paper	monkey	_________
carpet	_______	_______	_______	sugar	perfume	_________
saddle	_______	_______	_______	sandwich	sunset	_________
bubble	_______	_______	_______	wagon	iron	_________

Total of all three immediate word recalls: out of 15 = _____ **Total delayed recall: out of 5 =** _____

Appendix B

NFL Sideline Assessment Tool

Downloaded from bjsm.bmj.com on March 12, 2013 - Published by group.bmj.com

SCAT3™

FIFA® IIHF FEI

Sport Concussion Assessment Tool – 3rd Edition

For use by medical professionals only

Name

Date/Time of Injury:
Date of Assessment:

Examiner:

What is the SCAT3?[1]

The SCAT3 is a standardized tool for evaluating injured athletes for concussion and can be used in athletes aged from 13 years and older. It supersedes the original SCAT and the SCAT2 published in 2005 and 2009, respectively[2]. For younger persons, ages 12 and under, please use the Child SCAT3. The SCAT3 is designed for use by medical professionals. If you are not qualified, please use the Sport Concussion Recognition Tool[1]. Preseason baseline testing with the SCAT3 can be helpful for interpreting post-injury test scores.

Specific instructions for use of the SCAT3 are provided on page 3. If you are not familiar with the SCAT3, please read through these instructions carefully. This tool may be freely copied in its current form for distribution to individuals, teams, groups and organizations. Any revision or any reproduction in a digital form requires approval by the Concussion in Sport Group.

NOTE: The diagnosis of a concussion is a clinical judgment, ideally made by a medical professional. The SCAT3 should not be used solely to make, or exclude, the diagnosis of concussion in the absence of clinical judgement. An athlete may have a concussion even if their SCAT3 is "normal".

What is a concussion?

A concussion is a disturbance in brain function caused by a direct or indirect force to the head. It results in a variety of non-specific signs and/or symptoms (some examples listed below) and most often does not involve loss of consciousness. Concussion should be suspected in the presence of **any one or more** of the following:

- Symptoms (e.g., headache), or
- Physical signs (e.g., unsteadiness), or
- Impaired brain function (e.g. confusion) or
- Abnormal behaviour (e.g., change in personality).

SIDELINE ASSESSMENT

Indications for Emergency Management

NOTE: A hit to the head can sometimes be associated with a more serious brain injury. Any of the following warrants consideration of activating emergency procedures and urgent transportation to the nearest hospital:

- Glasgow Coma score less than 15
- Deteriorating mental status
- Potential spinal injury
- Progressive, worsening symptoms or new neurologic signs

Potential signs of concussion?

If any of the following signs are observed after a direct or indirect blow to the head, the athlete should stop participation, be evaluated by a medical professional and **should not be permitted to return to sport the same day** if a concussion is suspected.

Any loss of consciousness?	Y	N
"If so, how long?"		
Balance or motor incoordination (stumbles, slow/laboured movements, etc.)?	Y	N
Disorientation or confusion (inability to respond appropriately to questions)?	Y	N
Loss of memory:	Y	N
"If so, how long?"		
"Before or after the injury?"		
Blank or vacant look:	Y	N
Visible facial injury in combination with any of the above:	Y	N

1 Glasgow coma scale (GCS)

Best eye response (E)	
No eye opening	1
Eye opening in response to pain	2
Eye opening to speech	3
Eyes opening spontaneously	4
Best verbal response (V)	
No verbal response	1
Incomprehensible sounds	2
Inappropriate words	3
Confused	4
Oriented	5
Best motor response (M)	
No motor response	1
Extension to pain	2
Abnormal flexion to pain	3
Flexion/Withdrawal to pain	4
Localizes to pain	5
Obeys commands	6
Glasgow Coma score (E + V + M)	of 15

GCS should be recorded for all athletes in case of subsequent deterioration.

2 Maddocks Score[3]

"I am going to ask you a few questions, please listen carefully and give your best effort."

Modified Maddocks questions (1 point for each correct answer)

What venue are we at today?	0	1
Which half is it now?	0	1
Who scored last in this match?	0	1
What team did you play last week/game?	0	1
Did your team win the last game?	0	1
Maddocks score		of 5

Maddocks score is validated for sideline diagnosis of concussion only and is not used for serial testing.

Notes: Mechanism of Injury ("tell me what happened"?):

Any athlete with a suspected concussion should be REMOVED FROM PLAY, medically assessed, monitored for deterioration (i.e., should not be left alone) and should not drive a motor vehicle until cleared to do so by a medical professional. No athlete diagnosed with concussion should be returned to sports participation on the day of Injury.

© 2013 Concussion in Sport Group

References

1 McCrory P, et al: Consensus statement on concussion in sport: the 4th International Conference on Concussion in Sport held in Zurich, November 2012. Br J Sports Med 2013;47:250–258.

2 Harmon KG, et al: American Medical Society for Sports Medicine position statement: concussion in sport. Br J Sports Med 2013;47:15–26.

3 McCrea M, et al: Unreported concussion in high school football players: implications for prevention. Clin J Sport Med 2004;14:13–17.

4 McCrea M, et al: Acute effects and recovery time following concussion in collegiate football players: the NCAA Concussion Study. JAMA 2003;290:2556–2563.

5 Giza CC, et al: Summary of evidence-based guideline update: evaluation and management of concussion in sports: report of the Guideline Development Subcommittee of the American Academy of Neurology. Neurology 2013;80:2250–2257.

6 McCrea M, et al: An integrated review of recovery after mild traumatic brain injury (mTBI): implications for clinical management. Clin Neuropsychol 2009;23:1368–1390.

7 Belanger HG, Vanderploeg RD: The neuropsychological impact of sports-related concussion: a meta-analysis. J Int Neuropsychol Soc 2005;11:345–357.

8 McCrea M, et al: Acute effects and recovery after sport-related concussion: a neurocognitive and quantitative brain electical activity study. J Head Trauma Rehabil 2010;25:283–292.

9 Giza CC, Hovda DA: The neurometabolic cascade of concussion. J Athl Train 2001;36:228–235.

10 Guskiewicz KM, et al: National Athletic Trainers' Association position statement: management of sport-related concussion. J Athl Train 2004;39:280–297.

11 McCrea M, et al: Day of injury assessment of sport-related concussion. Br J Sports Med 2013;47:272–284.

12 Putukian M, et al: Onfield assessment of concussion in the adult athlete. Br J Sports Med 2013;47:285–288.

13 Collins MW, et al: Relationship between concussion and neuropsychological performance in college football players. JAMA 1999;282:964–970.

14 Guskiewicz KM, et al: Cumulative effects associated with recurrent concussion in collegiate football players: the NCAA Concussion Study. JAMA 2003;290:2549–2555.

15 Macciocchi SN, et al: Neuropsychological functioning and recovery after mild head injury in collegiate athletes. Neurosurgery 1996;39:510–514.

16 Broglio SP, Puetz TW: The effect of sport concussion on neurocognitive function, self-report symptoms and postural control: a meta-analysis. Sports Med 2008;38:53–67.

17 Echemendia RJ, et al: Advances in neuropsychological assessment of sport-related concussion. Br J Sports Med 2013;47:294–298.

18 Echemendia RJ, et al: Role of neuropsychologists in the evaluation and management of sport-related concussion: an inter-organizational position statement. Clin Neuropsychol 2011;25:1289–1294.

19 Guskiewicz KM: Postural stability assessment following concussion: one piece of the puzzle. Clin J Sport Med 2001;11:182–189.

20 Peterson CL, et al: Evaluation of neuropsychological domain scores and postural stability following cerebral concussion in sports. Clin J Sport Med 2003;13:230–237.

21 Broglio SP, Macciocchi SN, Ferrara MS: Sensitivity of the concussion assessment battery. Neurosurgery 2007;60:1050–1057, discussion 1057–1058.

22 Guskiewicz KM, Perrin DH, Gansneder BM: Effect of mild head injury on postural stability in athletes. J Athl Train 1996;31:300–306.

23 Guskiewicz KM, et al: Alternative approaches to the assessment of mild head injury in athletes. Med Sci Sports Exerc 1997;29(7 Suppl):S213–S221.

24 Riemann BL, Guskiewicz KM: Effects of mild head injury on postural stability as measured through clinical balance testing. J Athl Train 2000;35:19–25.

25 McCrea M, et al: Incidence, clinical course, and predictors of prolonged recovery time following sport-related concussion in high school and college athletes. J Int Neuropsychol Soc 2013;19:22–33.

26 Bell DR, et al: Systematic review of the balance error scoring system. Sports Health 2011;3:287–295.

27 Broglio SP, et al: Generalizability theory analysis of balance error scoring system reliability in healthy young adults. J Athl Train 2009;44:497–502.

28 Finnoff JT, et al: Intrarater and interrater reliability of the Balance Error Scoring System (BESS). PM R 2009;1:50–54.

29 Hunt TN, et al: The reliability of the modified Balance Error Scoring System. Clin J Sport Med 2009;19:471–475.

30 Prichep LS, et al: Time course of clinical and electrophysiological recovery after sport-related concussion. J Head Trauma Rehabil 2013;28:266–273.
31 Barr WB, et al: Measuring brain electrical activity to track recovery from sport-related concussion. Brain Inj 2012;26:58–66.
32 Schneider KJ, et al: The effects of rest and treatment following sport-related concussion: a systematic review of the literature. Br J Sports Med 2013;47:304–307.
33 Silverberg ND, Iverson GL: Is rest after concussion 'the best medicine?': recommendations for activity resumption following concussion in athletes, civilians, and military service members. J Head Trauma Rehabil 2013;28:250–259.

Michael McCrea, PhD, Professor and Director of Brain Injury Research
Medical College of Wisconsin
9200 W. Wisconsin Avenue
Milwaukee, WI 53226 (USA)
E-Mail mmccrea@mcw.edu

Niranjan A, Lunsford LD (eds): Concussion. Prog Neurol Surg. Basel, Karger, 2014, vol 28, pp 128–138
DOI: 10.1159/000358770

In-Office Management of Sport-Related Concussion

Erin Reynolds[a, b] · Michael W. Collins[a, b]

[a]University of Pittsburgh Medical Center, Sports Medicine Concussion Program, and [b]University of Pittsburgh School of Medicine, Department of Orthopaedic Surgery, Pittsburgh, Pa., USA

Abstract

The field of sport-related concussion has grown exponentially over the past decade, with more concussion-specific clinics being identified in major hospital systems as well as independent practitioner's offices. To date, there is no standardized in-office protocol for managing ongoing symptoms. The University of Pittsburgh Medical Center (UPMC) Sports Concussion Program, established in 2000, is one of the largest programs in the USA, pioneering the way in clinical management, research, and education of sport-related concussion. This report will outline the essential components of a successful concussion clinic, using the UPMC Sports Concussion Program as a case example of best practice. We will share several case studies illustrating the individualized and complex nature of this injury, as well as review important rehabilitation components. © 2014 S. Karger AG, Basel

The field of sport-related concussion has grown rapidly over the past decade. With growing concerns among athletes, coaches, and parents, developments in the field have tended to focus on sideline assessments. The on-field assessment of concussion continues to evolve and has been met with a host of challenges, including the lack of a consistently utilized standardized assessment tool and reliance on clinical diagnostic impression [1]. While acute management of injury is critical in ruling out more serious intracranial pathology and preventing the cumulative effects of concussion, ongoing in-office management is essential to returning athletes back to play once an on-field diagnosis is made. Traditionally, concussion management has occurred primarily in pediatric and primary care offices. Given new state laws mandating that medical clearance must be given by a provider trained in concussion management, concussion-specific clinics are becoming more commonplace. While pediatricians and primary care physicians continue to treat a large number of these patients, the number of clinics specializing in concussion is increasing. Given the ongoing development of this relatively new, subspecialized field, there is a lack of information available regarding best practices for care. This report will outline the essential components of a comprehensive multidisciplinary treatment model for the diagnosis and rehabilitation of sport-related concussion. Using the University of Pittsburgh Medical Center (UPMC) Sports Concussion Program as an example, we will examine the essential components of a clinical team, as well as walk through an established in-office protocol for concussion management. We will conclude with several case examples from our clinic illustrating the complex and individualized nature of this injury.

Establishing a Clinical Team

In order to establish a comprehensive clinical team for the management of sport-related concussion, one must understand the individual roles clinicians may play and how these roles work together. Establishing a centralized 'point guard' for clinical management will help to streamline care and facilitate communication. Clinical team point guards may be neuropsychologists, physiatrists, primary care physicians, pediatricians, neurosurgeons, neurologists, or other medical professionals trained in the diagnosis and management of sport-related concussion. The designated clinician should conduct an initial evaluation, incorporate information gathered from the treatment team, and make decisions regarding referrals and treatment planning. It is then this clinician's role to disseminate clinical information and facilitate communication among providers.

The UPMC Sports Concussion program places neuropsychologists in the point guard position. The neuropsychologist oversees each athlete's care from the initial evaluation through the final clearance appointment. Primary referral sources include emergency departments, primary care physicians, pediatricians, and athletic trainers. After undergoing an initial evaluation with the neuropsychologist, a number of other assessments or treatment referrals may be made, including vestibular therapy, vision therapy, exertion therapy, cervicogenic physical therapy, neuroradiology, or neurosurgery. The UPMC Sports Concussion Program has developed an extensive network of providers who specialize in postconcussion rehabilitation protocols. Currently, the program includes over 40 physical therapists specializing in either vestibular or exertion therapy, with over 100 athletic trainers in over 45 contracted high schools and colleges/universities. All providers are expected to communicate on a regular basis and provide feedback to the treatment team regarding an athlete's progress; it is the neuropsychologist's role to disseminate this information accordingly.

There are a host of challenges in organizing a treatment team of this magnitude. Vestibular therapists should have some training in neurorehabilitation and not simply a generalized orthopedic background. Vision therapy providers should be able to

Table 1. Signs and symptoms of concussion

Signs observed by staff	Symptoms reported by athlete
Appears dazed or stunned	Headache
Is confused about assignment	Nausea
Forgets plays	Balance problems
Is unsure of game, score, or opponent	Dizziness
Moves clumsily	Double or blurred vision
Answers questions slowly	Sensitivity to light and/or noise
Loses consciousness (even temporarily)	Feeling sluggish
Shows behavior or personality change	Feeling foggy
Forgets events prior to hit (retrograde)	Change in sleep patterns
Forgets events after hit (anterograde)	Concentration or memory problems

Table 2. Brief on-field cognitive screening

Orientation	What stadium are you in? What city are you in? What team are you playing? What day is it?
Anterograde amnesia	Ask the athlete to repeat the following words: girl, dog, green
Retrograde amnesia	What happened in the prior quarter/period? What do you remember just prior to the hit? What was the score of the game prior to the hit? Do you remember the hit?
Concentration	Repeat the days of the week backward Repeat these numbers backward: 36 *(63 is correct)*, 419 *(914 is correct)*
Retention	Repeat the three words from earlier

demonstrate measurable outcomes with concussion patients. Athletic trainers should be educated in proper concussion management and should be able to demonstrate a working knowledge of exertion protocols and return-to-play guidelines. It is the point guard's job to ensure that all members of the treatment team are qualified and properly educated prior to engaging in patient care.

In addition to educating the treatment team, it is important to expand this network to include coaches, team physicians, student assistants, and even players themselves, in regard to proper education. Ensuring that these individuals are able to accurately identify a concussive event will reduce the potential for cumulative events and may reduce the occurrence of postconcussion syndrome. Providing a checklist of signs and symptoms (table 1), as well as a brief cognitive screening tool (table 2), to on-field personnel is recommended.

Table 3. Essential components of a clinical interview

Mechanism of injury
Acute symptoms
Chronic symptoms
Medications
Biopsychosocial history
Premorbid risk factors
Education history
Family medical history
History of prior concussions
Sports played (including position)

In-Office Protocol

Once the essential members of the treatment team have been identified, it is necessary to develop an in-office assessment protocol. The UPMC Sports Concussion Program utilizes a three-pronged approach to assessment, which includes a detailed clinical interview, vestibular/ocular motor screening, and computerized neurocognitive testing. All three components are critical in providing comprehensive care and none may be used in isolation for diagnosis or treatment planning.

Clinical Interview

The clinical interview serves as the gateway in which information is gathered. It is through this process that the clinician begins to understand the athlete as an individual and the nature of the athlete's injury. Concussion is an individualized injury and an understanding of the mechanism of injury, coupled with the course of acute and chronic symptoms, is critical. The clinical interview also allows the clinician to build a relationship with the athlete and to establish a therapeutic alliance, which becomes valuable in ensuring treatment compliance and in communicating openly about ongoing concerns. Table 3 outlines the essential components of a comprehensive clinical interview.

In conducting a clinical interview, it is clinically useful to begin conceptualizing symptoms within clusters. Traditionally, concussion symptoms have been categorized within four generalized symptom clusters: cognitive, neuropsychiatric, physical (migraine), and sleep [2]. A 2012 factor analysis of the 22-item Post-Concussion Symptom Scale (PCSS) revealed four new postconcussion factors: cognitive-fatigue migraine, affective, somatic, and sleep, with the cognitive-fatigue migraine factor demonstrating strong cross-loadings on all other factors [3]. The authors of this study felt that this might suggest a 'global concussion' factor that exists within the first 7 days

Table 4. Examples of clinical interview queries

Instead of:	Ask:
Do you have a headache?	Where is the headache located? Can you characterize the pain? What time of day is the headache at its worst? What activities will definitely trigger a headache?
Are you dizzy?	Do you feel dizzy when standing/rising from bed/rolling over in bed/looking up or down? Do you feel dizzy in complex visual environments? Does moving quickly make you feel dizzy? Do you experience motion sickness?
Do you have cognitive difficulties?	Do you feel more distractible than usual? Do you feel more fatigued than normal at the end of the day? Give me an example of a 'memory problem' that you might have

of injury. This global factor includes a compilation of symptoms from all four factors that may begin to break down into more finite symptom clusters after the acute (>7 days) stage of injury [3]. Identifying the acute symptom presentation and reevaluating an athlete after this initial 7-day period will help the clinician to understand the trajectory of symptoms and the course of the athlete's injury, thus leading to an individualized rehabilitation plan.

One important goal of the clinical interview is to determine whether the athlete has become asymptomatic. Current return-to-play guidelines specify that an athlete must be asymptomatic at rest, asymptomatic with exertion, and demonstrate neurocognitive test data that is commensurate with baseline expectations [4]. Determining whether an athlete is asymptomatic requires a sophisticated style of questioning in which one does not simply ask blanket questions (i.e. do you have a headache?), but rather a series of more detailed, explicit questions (table 4). It is important that the interviewer is aware of the subtleties of the injury and the many ways in which symptoms may present.

Vestibular/Ocular-Motor Screening

Research suggests that up to 50% of athletes report dizziness and 43% report balance difficulties as initial postconcussive symptoms [5]. In addition, a 2007 retrospective analysis to determine the frequency of occurrence of ocular-motor dysfunction in concussed individuals found that 90% demonstrated ocular-motor dysfunction, with accommodative and convergence insufficiencies being the most common [6]. Given these statistics, it is important to screen for potential vestibular/ocular-motor

Table 5. UPMC Sports Concussion Program vestibular/ocular-motor screening evaluation

Ocular-motor	Vestibular-ocular	Balance examination
Smooth pursuits ('H-Test') Saccades (vertical/horizontal) Any dizziness, blurriness, over/under shoots?	Gaze stability (vertical/horizontal) Any observable nystagmus, provocative dizziness/blurriness, slowed movements? Vestibulo-ocular reflex cancellation (vertical/horizontal) Near point convergence Accommodation	Romberg, compliant foam – eyes open/eyes closed, feet together

dysfunction and to refer patients to appropriate providers for treatment. The UPMC Sports Concussion Program has developed a vestibular/ocular-motor screening assessment that can be administered in less than 5 minutes by any trained medical professional (table 5). This screening tool allows the neuropsychologist, or other managing provider, to screen for provocation of symptoms, as well as assess for overt abnormal findings. This information is then utilized to determine the appropriate rehabilitation referral and to inform treatment planning. As noted, having a network of vestibular therapists trained in neurorehabilitation is an essential component of a comprehensive multidisciplinary treatment team.

Neurocognitive Assessment

Neuropsychological testing has been identified as the gold standard in managing sport-related concussion, with computer-based neurocognitive testing quickly becoming the preferred method of evaluation [7–10]. While there are a number of programs available, Immediate Post-Concussion Assessment and Cognitive Testing (ImPACT) is widely used among high school, collegiate, and professional athletic organizations. Extensive data has been published regarding ImPACT's reliability and validity. A recent study revealed ImPACT to have a sensitivity of 94.6% and a specificity of 97.3% in detecting concussion in an otherwise asymptomatic population [11]. Preseason baseline testing of all athletes is recommended; however, it is possible to interpret postinjury data without a baseline for comparison. Without a formal baseline available for comparison, an athlete's academic history, including grade point average and performance on standardized tests, may be used to estimate premorbid neurocognitive abilities. All postinjury data should be interpreted by a trained neuropsychologist, particularly when baseline data is unavailable.

Utilizing computer-based neurocognitive test data in a comprehensive assessment protocol allows the clinician to make better informed decisions regarding an athlete's treatment plan and ultimate return to play. Research shows that athletes typically report symptom resolution several days prior to resolution of neurocognitive deficits [10, 12, 13]. A 2013 study revealed that when asked to estimate the percentage in which athletes aged 12–18 years felt 'back to normal', low correlations were demonstrated between the subjective report and objective neurocognitive test data [13]. Meehan et al. [10] found that when computer-based neurocognitive test data were utilized, high school athletes were less likely to return to play within 10 days of injury, even after controlling for duration of symptoms. This suggests that the use of computer-based neurocognitive testing provides information regarding cognitive deficits that are not otherwise detected. In addition, neurocognitive test data may lend support when making more complicated return-to-play decisions, particularly when the symptom profile is ambiguous.

Case Studies

The successful management of sport-related concussion is contingent upon the understanding that concussion is an individualized injury. Each athlete will present with his or her own individual presentation and treatment course. Being attuned to individual differences will allow the managing provider to make informed treatment decisions and should improve the efficiency of rehabilitation. The following case studies illustrate the individual nature of this injury and the potential rehabilitation pathways one may seek.

Case 1

Kate is a 15-year-old female who sustained a cerebral concussion while at cheerleading practice. Kate was a base cheerleader and was kicked in the head by a teammate, which caused her to fall and strike her face on the floor. While there was no loss of consciousness or retrograde amnesia, Kate did report approximately 30 s of confusion and anterograde amnesia. Acute symptoms included bilateral blurred vision, dizziness, nausea, headache, and fatigue. Kate's mother was called and she was taken to the emergency room, where a CT scan was unremarkable. During the car ride home, Kate experienced an increase in headaches and fatigue, as well as fogginess and anxiety. She was subsequently managed by her pediatrician for 4 weeks, during which time she was provided with light academic accommodations and was not allowed to participate in cheerleading or other sports. Kate did not experience any improvement in symptoms and was therefore referred to our clinic for evaluation.

Kate's initial evaluation occurred 5 weeks after the injury. At that time, she reported a daily headache at an 8/10 in intensity, as well as photo- and phonosensitivity, dizziness, nausea, dysregulated sleep, and fatigue. Her vestibular/ocular-motor screening exam revealed provocation of symptoms with horizontal saccades, as well as horizontal gaze stability and visual suppression. Near point convergence was measured at 11 cm. Neurocognitive test data revealed verbal memory within the average range, with visual memory, processing speed, and reaction time all within the impaired range. Kate was referred to vestibular therapy and was instructed to avoid busy environments, long car rides, and heavy ocular activity. She was placed on half days of school with full academic accommodations based on her vestibular and ocular-motor dysfunction. Kate was instructed to return for follow-up in 3 weeks.

She returned 1 month later (2 months after the injury) and reported that she had attended one session of vestibular therapy and discontinued, as she did not feel that it was helpful. She remained on half days of school and felt that the accommodations were helpful in that regard. She reported minimal symptoms including headaches approximately twice per week and mild fatigue. Her vestibular exam was improved with only mild provocation of symptoms; near point convergence was within normal limits (WNL). Neurocognitive test scores were improved, with all scores within the average to high average ranges. Our recommendations included full days of school and the introduction of physical exertion. She was instructed to begin working through a 5-stage exertion progression with her athletic trainer and to return for a clearance appointment in 1 month.

Kate returned 6 weeks later and reported that she was 'back to normal'. She was experiencing approximately one headache every 2 weeks and denied other symptoms. She had fully exerted with no return of symptoms. Neurocognitive test data was stable with the exception of a decrease in reaction time to the low average range, which was consistent with a mild relative deficit. Given this, Kate was given clearance for low-risk activities (no stunting or tumbling in cheer) and was asked to return in 1 month for a final clearance appointment.

Kate did not follow up as asked and never returned for her clearance appointment. She returned to the clinic 3 months later due to a 'new' injury. Kate had been participating fully in cheerleading and was reportedly struck in the larynx by a teammate while cheering. She denied any acute mental status changes, but did report immediate headache, dizziness, and nausea. She had been attending school full time and reported a marked increase in headaches, as well as dizziness, nausea, fogginess, and anxiety while in school. Her sleep was extremely dysregulated, as she reported staying up until 2 a.m. and sleeping approximately 4 h per night. Her vestibular exam was highly provocative for dizziness with both horizontal and vertical gaze stability, as well as vestibulo-ocular reflex cancellation. Near point convergence was measured at 20 cm. Vestibular exam also provoked an increase in anxiety. Neurocognitive test scores revealed verbal memory within the low average range, with all other scores within the impaired range. Kate was immediately taken out of school for 10 days. She was referred back to vestibular therapy, as well as vision therapy, and was explicitly instructed to abstain from cheerleading. Kate was counseled on the importance of behavioral regulation and was instructed to have a regulated sleep schedule, as well as maintain a healthy diet, stay hydrated, and manage stress. She was instructed to return in 1 month for reevaluation.

Kate returned 6 weeks later. She reported that she completed both vestibular therapy and vision therapy. She was reportedly 100% symptom free for over 2 weeks. She reported excellent compliance with her behavioral modifications. Vestibular exam was WNL and neurocognitive test data ranged from the average to superior ranges. Kate was instructed to begin physically exerting through the 5-stage exertion protocol and was cleared back to play once she completed this task approximately 1 week later.

Discussion

This case highlights the importance of treatment compliance. Despite an improvement in her overall presentation, it is clear that Kate had not fully rehabilitated her vestibular system after her initial injury. Athletes may begin to feel better soon after initiating therapy and may then become noncompliant in completing treatment recommendations. Computerized neurocognitive test data, though improved, was consistent with mild relative deficits and indicated that full recovery had yet to occur. Moreover, there was likely some underlying vestibular dysfunction that was unaddressed. Given this, it required less biomechanical force for reinjury to occur and more severe postconcussive symptoms to ensue. Once appropriate compliance to treatment occurred (in this instance vestibular therapy), neurocognitive and vestibular recovery was complete and a full return to cheerleading and academic activity was possible with normal risk.

Case 2

Taylor is a 17-year-old female who sustained a cerebral concussion while playing in a soccer game. She reportedly headed the ball awkwardly, at which time she reportedly 'saw stars' and experienced a headache. These symptoms abated quickly. The next day, during practice, she was struck in the head with a ball and her symptoms returned. At this time, she reported experiencing retrograde amnesia (<5 min), headache (7/10 in intensity), nausea, dizziness, balance problems, fatigue, photo- and phonosensitivity, emotional lability, fogginess, and difficulties concentrating. She also reported feeling slowed down and hypersomnic. She was taken to the emergency room, where a CT scan was unremarkable. Taylor rested over the weekend, with symptoms waxing and waning. The symptoms improved over the next few days. Taylor attended school and immediately experienced an increase in symptoms. Specifically, she experienced an increase in photosensitivity and difficulty reading. She was sent home after two periods and slept for an extended period of time.

Taylor was evaluated in our clinic 4 days after the injury. Her initial evaluation revealed a number of symptoms (PCSS Total Symptom Score = 57), with her top three symptoms being fogginess, mental slowing, and fatigue. Neurocognitive testing revealed three out of four clinical composites below baseline, with verbal memory and reaction time within the impaired range. Vestibular exam was WNL. Recommendations included several days out of school, which Taylor refused. She did, however, agree to modified days with heavy academic accommodations and a focus on her core/advanced placement classes. We provided a significant amount of education regarding the importance of both physical and cognitive rest, behavioral management (i.e. regulation of schedule), and sleep hygiene. Follow-up was scheduled for 2 weeks.

Taylor returned to the clinic 2 weeks later and reported some improvement, with essentially all symptoms remaining. Headaches were occurring at least 5 days per week, mostly when in school. Taylor reported that she was not taking breaks in school and that she needed significantly more time to complete her homework and class assignments. She admitted to pushing herself with a rigorous academic course load. She was resting more on the weekends and noticed a significant difference with her symptom presentation on those days. Her parents were concerned that she always appeared fatigued. Taylor's ImPACT scores revealed verbal memory and reaction time within the impaired range (both well below baseline), with processing speed improved to the average range (commensurate with baseline). Her vestibular exam remained WNL. Recommendations included a referral to physical medicine and rehabilitation for a medication consultation and instruction to begin taking a daily walk. We also reinforced behavioral management in school in the form of frequent breaks and compliance with academic accommodations.

Taylor returned 2 weeks later. She had started taking amantadine 100 mg 10 days earlier and noticed a slight improvement, with a significant improvement 5 days later when she increased to 200 mg. While all symptoms remained at a low level, she continued to experience an increase in symptoms with cognitive exertion. She reported that she no longer felt foggy, but still experienced cognitive slowing and fatigue. She reported minimal use of accommodations and breaks while in school. Regarding physical exertion, Taylor had started using a stationary bike, light strength training, and light soccer drills without an increase in symptoms. Taylor's neurocognitive test scores were all back to baseline with a PCSS score of 12. Recommendations included ongoing, but basic, academic accommodations, continued light exertion until symptom free and then progressing to the 5-stage exertion protocol, and follow-up with physical medicine and rehabilitation.

One month later, Taylor returned and was reportedly symptom free for over 2 weeks. She was not utilizing any academic accommodations and all grades were WNL. She had weaned off of amantadine with no return of symptoms. She completed the 5-stage exertion protocol with no difficulties other than being deconditioned physically. ImPACT scores were stable at baseline. At this time, Taylor did meet return-to-play criteria and was cleared to resume soccer.

Discussion

This case illustrates the occurrence of cognitive fatigue after cerebral concussion. This case also highlights the importance of compliance regarding both cognitive and physical rest. Students who are identified as high achievers, or who tend to push themselves academically, often have significant difficulty following treatment recommendations when asked to reduce their workload. Providing education to both the student and the parents regarding behavioral management is critical in this case, as it allows the student to understand the rationale behind the recommendations.

Conclusion

The ongoing, in-office management of sport-related concussion is a relatively new specialty area and parameters regarding the appropriate structure of the clinic and in-office protocols have not yet been fully delineated. Due to the individualized nature of the injury, there is no 'cook book' regarding treatment protocols and each athlete must be conceptualized according to his or her specific symptom presentation, neurocognitive test data, and clinical trajectory. Given the complexity of treatment, it is essential that the clinic designate a 'point guard' to oversee treatment planning and manage communication amongst team members. This organization will not only improve the quality of care, but will also streamline rehabilitation plans and allow for a deeper understanding of the treatment goals by both the patient and the clinical providers.

References

1. Putukian M, Raftery M, Guskiewicz K, Herring S, Aubry M, Cantu R, Molloy M: Onfield assessment of concussion in the adult athlete. Br J Sports Med 2013; 47:285–288.
2. Pardini J, Stump J, Lovell MR, Collins MW, Moritz K, Fu F: The Post-Concussion Symptom Scale (PCSS): a factor analysis (abstract). Br J Sports Med 2004;38:661–662.
3. Kontos AP, Elbin RJ, Schatz P, Covassin T, Henry L, Pardini J, Collins MW: A revised factor structure for the post-concussion symptom scale: baseline and postconcussion factors. Am J Sports Med 2012;40: 2375–2384.
4. McCrory P, Meeuwisse WH, Aubry M, et al: Consensus statement on concussion in sport: the 4th International Conference on Concussion in Sport held in Zurich, November 2012. Br J Sports Med 2013;47: 250–258.
5. Hoffer ME, Gottshall KR, Moore R, Balough BJ, Wester D: Characterizing and treating dizziness after mild head trauma. Otol Neurotol 2004;25:135–138.
6. Ciuffreda KJ, Kapoor N, Rutner D, Suchoff IB, Han ME, Craig S: Occurrence of oculomotor dysfunctions in acquired brain injury: a retrospective analysis. Optometry 2007;78:155–161.
7. Lovell MR, Collins MW, Fu F: New technology and sports-related concussion. Orthop Technol Rev 2003;5:35–37.

8 McClincy MP, Lovell MR, Pardini J, Collins MW, Spore MK: Recovery from sports concussion in high school and collegiate athletes. Brain Inj 2006;20:33–39.

9 Van Kampen DA, Lovell MR, Pardini J, Collins MW, Fu F: The 'value added' of neurocognitive testing after sports-related concussion. Am J Sports Med 2006;34:1630–1635.

10 Meehan WP 3rd, d'Hemecourt P, Collins CL, Taylor AM, Comstock RD: Computerized neurocognitive testing for the management of sport-related concussion. Pediatrics 2012;129:38–44.

11 Schatz P, Sandel N: Sensitivity and specificity of the online version of ImPACT in high school and collegiate athletes. Am J Sports Med 2012;41:321–326.

12 Lovell MR, Collins MW, Iverson GL, Field M, Maroon JC, Cantu R, Podell K, Powell JW, Belza M, Fu F: Recovery from mild concussion in high school athletes. J Neurosurg 2003;98:296–301.

13 Sandel NK, Lovell MR, Kegel NK, Collins MW, Kontos AP: The relationship of symptoms and neurocognitive performance to perceived recovery from sports-related concussion among adolescent athletes. Appl Neuropsychol Child 2013;2:64–69.

Erin Reynolds, PsyD
University of Pittsburgh Medical Center, Sports Medicine Concussion Program
3200 S. Water St.
Pittsburgh, PA 15203 (USA)
E-Mail Reynoldse2@upmc.edu

Niranjan A, Lunsford LD (eds): Concussion. Prog Neurol Surg. Basel, Karger, 2014, vol 28, pp 139–148
DOI: 10.1159/000358771

Treating Prolonged Symptoms of Mild Traumatic Brain Injury: Neuropharmacology

Kirk Lercher[a] · Cara Camiolo Reddy[b]

[a]Mount Sinai Hospital New York, New York, N.Y., and [b]University of Pittsburgh Medical Center, Pittsburgh, Pa., USA

Abstract

The clinical presentation of concussion can vary widely as patients experience any number of symptoms including headache, dizziness, cognitive symptoms of difficulty with concentration and memory, sleep dysregulation, and mood disturbances. The variability in clinical presentation underscores the importance of thorough history-taking to clearly understand the clinical picture and to allow individualization of the treatment plan. Most postconcussive symptoms are transient in nature and respond to conservative measures, including education of the patient and their caregivers. For those individuals whose symptoms persist or significantly impair quality of life, pharmacologic intervention may be warranted. Though few studies have investigated the use of pharmacology for treatment of postconcussion syndrome specifically, targeted treatment of medications known to improve selected symptoms can be considered. © 2014 S. Karger AG, Basel

Concussion and mild traumatic brain injury (mTBI) can result in a myriad of postinjury consequences that vary in duration and severity. The complexity and variability of the clinical presentation highlights the importance of obtaining a thorough history and physical examination in order to develop an individualized treatment plan. Furthermore, education is paramount to the rehabilitation process so as to prevent further injury and provide patients an understanding of the injury and ways in which they may facilitate recovery. Concussion management, as discussed in other reports of this work, remains centered upon physical and cognitive rest with a graduated return to activity. When conservative measures fail to adequately control postconcussive symptoms, pharmacologic intervention can be considered.

There is a relative paucity of studies that validate the pharmacologic management of postconcussive symptoms, with the majority of recommendations derived from accepted interventions for similar neurologic impairments. When considering pharmacologic intervention, it is imperative that clear outcome measures be identified prior to treatment and that regular follow-up is established to determine the efficacy of any medication in treating the targeted symptoms. This report will review the common symptoms that result from concussion and will discuss the pharmacologic treatment options and strategies.

Headaches

Headaches are one of the most commonly reported symptoms following mTBI, reported to occur in more than 85% of people who have sustained a concussion [1]. Complicating the diagnosis of posttraumatic headaches (PTH) is the lack of defining characteristic features. Most patients will describe either tension-type or migraine headaches; however, the nature of the trauma itself may also influence the headache characteristics related to cervical or other concomitant injury. As a result, PTH may fit into multiple subtypes of headache classification. Other complicating factors related to the trauma, including medication overuse, emotional distress, myofascial pain, occipital neuralgia, cervical referred pain, and vascular etiologies can also influence the presentation of PTH [2].

As with traditional headache management, care must be given to provide education regarding proper sleep hygiene, exercise, and dietary considerations. In addition, when PTH result from or worsen with cognitive and/or physical activity, this overexertion must be adequately addressed before pharmacologic intervention can be effective. As the presentation of PTH is complicated, the pharmacologic management strategy is similarly difficult, in part due to the lack of randomized controlled trials. The focus of pharmacologic treatment has relied on the use of well-accepted migraine-preventative medications such as antidepressants, anticonvulsants, β-blockers, and calcium channel blockers. When choosing an appropriate agent one must be cognizant of the side-effect profile of the given medication, especially as it pertains to cognitive impairment that may impede recovery from the concussion itself.

Intervention with preventative medications is indicated when PTH are reported as disabling, occurring more than 4–5 times per month, and persist despite use of acute abortive medications [3]. Preventative treatments may decrease headache frequency, severity, and duration, in addition to improving the response to acute therapies [4]. Of particular consideration when deciding to initiate preventative treatments is the frequency with which the patient has been taking acute medications, including over-the-counter pain relievers and migraine abortive medications. Frequent use of acute medications, usually greater than 3 days per week, can hasten the onset of rebound headaches, further complicating the management of PTH.

As noted above, preventative medications used in the treatment of PTH include β-blockers, antidepressants, and antiepileptic medications [5]. Efficacy has been shown in the treatment of PTH with use of propranolol, amitriptyline, and valproate, alone and in combination with each other [5]. One study showed improvement in 21 of 30 patients, including those involved with litigation, with posttraumatic migraine treated with propranolol or amitriptyline (either alone or in combination) [6]. A retrospective review of 100 patients with PTH found improvement in 60% of those treated for at least 1 month with divalproex sodium [7]. In a retrospective study of US Army soldiers with PTH, topiramate was found to be an effective prophylactic agent as well [8].

The exact mechanism of action of these preventative treatments is unknown, though it has been hypothesized to involve modulation of neurotransmitter pathways and receptors [3]. β-Blockers, such as propranolol, have been suggested to exert benefit through their effect on vascular dilation, prevention of platelet adhesion and aggregation, and through reduction of catecholamine central activity [9]. Tricyclic antidepressants, including amitriptyline and nortriptyline, are commonly used in the treatment of PTH with benefit likely due in part to alteration of central monoamines, specifically serotonin, and an effect on the opioid systems [9]. Anticonvulsants, such as divalproex and topiramate, exert benefit through facilitating neuronal inhibition, via γ-aminobutyric acid (GABA) potentiation and thereby managing neuronal hyperexcitability [10], though cognitive slowing may limit their use.

Overall, the treatment of PTH is complex due to the diversity of symptom presentation and presence of associated complicating factors. It is because of this that a comprehensive approach should be taken in order to structure an individualized treatment plan when pursuing pharmacologic management. At this time, the mainstays in treatment is to taper down the use of acute medications in favor of initiating preventative treatments to minimize the occurrence of rebound headaches.

Cognitive Symptoms

Cognitive symptoms, including impaired memory, concentration, processing speed, and mental 'fogginess', are common sequelae of concussion. Though the extent of these impairments may vary with severity of injury, neuropsychological testing facilitates qualitative assessment of these deficits. Prevalence of cognitive impairment has been reported to be 40–60% in TBI patients at 1–3 months following their injury [11]. The majority of patients who sustain a concussion show complete resolution of cognitive symptoms within a few weeks of injury; however, a subgroup of patients will have symptoms that persist beyond this period [12]. It is this group, with persistent symptomatology, who may benefit from pharmacologic intervention to address these cognitive deficits.

Through an understanding of neurotransmitters and their neurobiological activity regulating cognitive activity, emerging evidence supports the use of neurostimulants in the treatment of cognitive deficits following TBI. Few randomized controlled studies have been executed to date; however, pharmacologic research has been identified as a key area of needed study.

Dopamine is a neurotransmitter involved in the transmission of signals linked to executive function, arousal, and memory. Dopaminergic agonists have been targeted for their potential in neurorecovery and are frequently used to address cognitive deficits following TBI. Amantadine, originally developed as an antiviral agent, has been utilized for its dopaminergic properties to manage Parkinson's disease and the cognitive impairments following TBI. Acting both pre- and postsynaptically, amantadine increases the concentration of dopamine in the synaptic cleft and modulates the postsynaptic dopamine receptors [13]. Additionally, amantadine acts as an antagonist at N-methyl-D-aspartate (NMDA) glutamate receptors, a property which is believed to be neuroprotective [13, 14]. Studies have shown amantadine to be a generally well-tolerated and effective treatment of cognitive impairments following moderate-to-severe TBI with improvements in attention, processing speed, and overall cognitive function. In a study of concussed adolescent athletes, treatment with amantadine was associated with improvements in verbal memory and reaction time on computerized neurocognitive testing, as well as improvements in reported symptoms [15].

Medications traditionally used in the treatment of attention-deficit and hyperactivity disorder, namely methylphenidate and dextroamphetamine, have also been under consideration in the treatment of concussion-related cognitive deficits. These medications target both dopamine and norepinephrine neurotransmitter activity in pre- and postsynaptic mechanisms. Randomized studies have endorsed the use of methylphenidate to address cognitive impairments, particularly deficits in attention and processing speed in patients with moderate-to-severe TBI [16, 17]; however, there have been no randomized placebo-controlled studies that have investigated its use in the setting of concussion.

Medications with cholinergic properties, facilitating activity of acetylcholine activity in cognitive pathways, may also warrant consideration in the treatment of cognitive deficits secondary to TBI. Donepezil, a long-acting acetylcholinesterase inhibitor, has been shown to help improve short- and long-term memory in patients with mTBI [12]. Cytidine diphosphate-choline, a precursor in the synthesis of phosphatidylcholine, acts to increase acetylcholine levels. There has been one double-blinded placebo-controlled study which showed that cytidine diphosphate-choline showed a greater reduction in postconcussion symptoms, including improved memory [18]. Again, limited research exists to make any formal assessments of the efficacy of these medications to treat concussion-related impairments.

The majority of patients with concussion-related cognitive impairment will show relatively complete resolution of symptoms in a short time; however, it is in those patients with protracted recovery who may endorse and display cognitive impairments that negatively affect their quality of life. It is for these patients that a consideration of pharmacologic intervention should be considered. Neurostimulant medications have shown potential, particularly in studies of amantadine and methylphenidate. That said, further studies are needed to confirm the efficacy of neurostimulant medications in the treatment of cognitive symptoms following concussion.

Emotional Symptoms

The prolonged cognitive and somatic impairments that follow a concussion can include depression, anxiety, and disorders of adjustment. Treatment recommendations following a concussion, specifically physical and cognitive rest, may lead to social isolation and exacerbation of the patient's perception of their cognitive or somatic complaints. In the case of traumatic events, recovery may be further complicated by the development of posttraumatic stress disorder. Generally, depressive symptoms that follow concussion are short-lived and are best managed conservatively with coping strategies, support from family and friends, and counseling by trained psychologists [19].

In patients with persistent postconcussive emotional symptoms, pharmacological treatment should be considered. Selective serotonin reuptake inhibitors (SSRIs) are often used as a first-line treatment due to their perceived efficacy and tolerance in this population [12]. Preferred agents with short half-lives and lacking antimuscarinic effects should be most strongly considered, specifically sertraline, citalopram, or escitaolpram [20].

Sertraline has been shown to improve depressive symptoms in patients with mTBI [21]. Notably, in a single-blinded trial involving mTBI patients with depression 3–24 months following their injury, sertraline showed improvement in depressive symptoms and self-reported postconcussive symptoms, as well as improvement in cognitive function at follow-up [22]. An open-label study examined the effectiveness of citalopram over 6 or 10 weeks in the treatment of depression after mild-to-moderate TBI [23]. Those patients who completed the 10-week course had a response rate that was comparable to the report of the largest effectiveness trial of citalopram for patients with major depression in the absence of TBI.

Other SSRIs have been considered as well. One study found paroxetine to be as effective as citalopram in the treatment of emotional symptoms in patients with TBI [24]. Paroxetine, however, may impair cognitive function, believed to be due to its antimuscarinic effects, and therefore caution should be taken if considering this in the treatment of postconcussive depression [25]. Fluoxetine has also been considered as well as it is generally well tolerated and effective; however, it has significant cytochrome P450 inhibition and therefore has a higher propensity for drug-drug interactions or metabolism-related adverse effects than other SSRIs [25].

Tricyclic antidepressants, such as amitriptyline, have also been considered in the treatment of TBI-related depression. While considered effective in the treatment of primary depression and helpful in the management of other postconcussion sequelac such as PTH, evidence showing its efficacy in TBI-related depression is lacking [11].

The majority of patients who experience emotional symptoms following concussion will show resolution with coping strategies, support of friends and family, and counseling. Those with prolonged symptoms may benefit from initiation of pharmacologic management. SSRIs are most commonly used in the treatment of TBI-related depression due to perceived efficacy and tolerance. Special considerations, especially in the adolescent population, should be taken when initiating antidepressants as they may increase the risk of suicidality.

Sleep Disorders

Sleep disorders, including difficulties initiating or maintaining sleep, are common following TBI, reported in as many as 70% of patients [26]. Sleep disruption can in turn adversely affect the patient's recovery due to further exacerbations of their cognitive function, fatigue, and increased irritability. As a result, impaired sleep can lead to significant morbidity and impair return to normal daily activities.

The initial treatment should be nonpharmacologic with a focus on improvement of sleep hygiene. Patient education should emphasize the importance of creating an environment conducive to sleep promotion, such as maintaining consistent times for sleep and waking up, engaging in relaxing activities within 1 h of their set bed time, avoiding day time naps, keeping a quiet and dark sleep environment that is free of distractions, and avoiding alcohol, nicotine, or caffeine within a few hours of going to bed [27]. Maintenance of sleep hygiene is a particularly challenging task in today's society, which thrives on immediate connections to technology, especially with the adolescent population. It is suggested that items such as televisions, computers, cell phones, and video games should be removed from the bedroom environment of patients recovering from concussion. A return to daytime physical and mental activities may also help promote a regular sleep-wake cycle [12]. Cognitive behavioral therapy and education in relaxation techniques is sometimes beneficial and important adjuncts for patients with particularly problematic sleep impairments [2, 27].

If conservative measures fail to adequately address sleep impairments following TBI, careful considerations must be made when deciding to utilize pharmacologic interventions. There is limited data available regarding pharmacologic measures to address sleep impairments after TBI specifically. Therefore most recommendations for sleep medications are devised from information regarding treatment of insomnia in the general population [28]. When initiating pharmacologic agents in a patient with TBI, it is important to ensure that any underlying psychiatric or medical conditions are adequately treated. It is also important to consider that these patients may require lower doses of medications and that cognitive side effects are common with these medications. As such, these patients should be started on low doses and titrated up slowly.

Antidepressants are commonly utilized in the treatment of sleep impairment following TBI. Trazodone, a serotonin reuptake inhibitor, is one of the most common medications used in this population, despite limited research supporting its efficacy in patients with sleep impairments secondary to conditions other than depression. It has anxiolytic and hypnotic effects, with fewer anticholinergic side effects as compared to other classes of antidepressants [12]. Adverse effects to be aware of include dry mouth, dizziness, nausea, priapism, and headache [29].

Melatonin is an endogenous hormone produced by the pineal gland from serotonin. Its production is highest at night and lowest during the daytime hours [30]. Endogenous levels of melatonin are highest in adolescence and begin to decrease in the third decade of life; during this period in life a concurrent rise in insomnia has also been observed, supporting its theoretical benefit in treating sleep disorders. There are three hypotheses regarding its mechanism of action in promoting sleep, which include regulation of the body's circadian rhythm, reduction in core temperature, and/or direct action on structures of the brain responsible for sleep [12, 30]. Melatonin has been shown to be relatively safe and nontoxic. In addition, it is a potent antioxidant and free-radical scavenger which could help protect the central nervous system from inflammatory damage sustained in a traumatic injury [31, 32].

Interestingly, an observational study examined veterans returning from Iraq and Afghanistan who sustained blast-related mTBI and compared a 9-week treatment with prazosin, an α_1-blocker, in conjunction with sleep hygiene counseling to treatment with counseling alone [33]. The study showed improvements in sleep, headaches, and cognition. The authors believe that prazosin helped promote sleep by decreasing sleep latency and prevented nocturnal arousals.

Traditional hypnotic agents such as benzodiazepines should be used very cautiously in patients with TBI. The potential for cognitive impairment, anterograde amnesia, daytime sleepiness, and impaired neuronal recovery make this class of medication potentially detrimental to patients recovering from a concussion [2, 28]. Nonbenzodiazepine hypnotics, such as zolpidem, are preferred by some practitioners as their mechanism of action may decrease the risk of daytime sleepiness or impairing cognitive recovery; however, there are no studies examining the side effects of this medication in patients with concussions and therefore should be used with caution, starting at the lowest effective dose [28]. Despite a favorable side-effect profile when compared to traditional benzodiazepines, nonbenzodiazepine hypnotics can cause somnambulation as well as cognitive impairments; therefore, caution is strongly advised with the recommendation to start at the lowest effective doses to minimize adverse effects.

Studies that investigate the use of sleep medications in patients with TBI are relatively limited. As a result, medication should only be given to those with severe sleep-cycle impairment that has been refractory to more conservative measures including environmental changes, attention to sleep hygiene, and cognitive behavioral therapy. Once the decision is made to initiate medication management, the lowest effective doses should be utilized and close monitoring for adverse effects and dependency is essential.

Vestibular Impairments

Subjective dizziness is another common somatic symptom following a concussion, reported to occur in more than 30% of patients [12]. Further, it is the on-field symptom most closely associated with a prolonged recovery time [34]. The underlying etiology of dizziness is difficult to assess by subjective reports alone and thorough investigation is required in order to determine an appropriate plan of care [12].

Following a concussion, patients can present with symptoms consistent with either central or peripheral causes of dizziness. The pathology of peripheral dizziness involves the vestibular end organs, including the semicircular canals, otolith organs, and the vestibular component of the eighth cranial nerve. In addition to the subjective report of dizziness, patients with peripheral dizziness may report the sensation of spinning, severe nausea/vomiting, and hearing impairments. Benign paroxysmal positional vertigo is a common cause of peripheral vertigo and responds well to repositioning maneuvers such as the Epley maneuver.

In contrast, central dizziness results from pathology involving the central vestibular system including the vestibular nuclear complex, which is essential in sensory integration and spatial orientation [35]. Patients with central dizziness will often have severe imbalance and visual disturbances often in association with migranious symptoms. For these patients, vestibular therapy is the mainstay of treatment. One study demonstrated a benefit in the treatment of persistent dizziness following a concussion, with improvement noted on self-reported dizziness severity, dizziness handicap, balance confidence, and functional balance performance [36].

Patients with vestibular symptoms may also frequently describe an associated sensation of anxiety. This relationship between situational anxiety and vestibular disorders is known as space and motion discomfort [37], and refers to a disorder in sensory integration from vestibular, somatosensory, and visual inputs responsible for maintaining balance, leading to worsening of anxiety symptoms. This may be provoked by situational stimuli including moving crowds, supermarkets, and moving floors, among other environmental triggers. Treatment for this includes vestibular rehabilitation and the use of low-dose anxiolytics, such as clonazepam.

If symptoms of vestibular impairment are significant enough to limit progress in therapies or adversely affect the patient's quality of life, a brief trial of vestibular suppressant medications may be considered. Meclizine, one of the most commonly used vestibular suppressants, can limit the brain's ability to compensate for centrally mediated vestibular disorders through its vestibular suppression; therefore, its role in post-concussion-related dizziness may be quite limited. Though pharmacologic agents that act as vestibular suppressants have been shown to be effective in the acute treatment of vestibular disorders [38], these medications have not been studied following concussion and their efficacy is questionable.

Conclusion

The clinical presentation following concussion can vary significantly among patients. A thorough history and physical examination is essential for development of an individualized treatment plan. These symptoms are transient in nature and generally respond well to conservative measures, including physical and cognitive rest. For those patients whose symptoms persist, pharmacologic interventions should be considered. Special consideration is essential to minimize the risk of adverse effects that may ultimately inhibit recovery or worsen cognitive symptoms. Randomized controlled studies are needed to further investigate these potential treatment options following concussion.

References

1 Guskiewicz KM, Weaver NL, Padua DA, Garrett WE: Epidemiology of concussion in collegiate and high school football players. Am J Sports Med 2000; 28:643–650.
2 Reddy CC: Postconcussion syndrome: a physiatrist's approach. PM R 2011;3(10 suppl 2):S396–S405.
3 Lucas S: Headache management in concussion and mild traumatic brain injury. PM R 2011;3(10 suppl 2): S406–S412.
4 Silberstein SD: Practice parameter: evidence-based guidelines for migraine headache (an evidence-based review): report of the Quality Standards Subcommittee of the American Academy of Neurology. Neurology 2000;55:754–762.
5 Seifert TD: Sports concussion and associated post-traumatic headache. Headache 2013;53:726–736.
6 Weiss HD, Stern BJ, Goldberg J: Post-traumatic migraine: chronic migraine precipitated by minor head or neck trauma. Headache 1991;31:451–456.
7 Packard RC: Treatment of chronic daily posttraumatic headache with divalproex sodium. Headache 2000;40:736–739.
8 Erickson JC: Treatment outcomes of chronic post-traumatic headaches after mild head trauma in US soldiers: an observational study. Headache 2011;51: 932–944.
9 Bell KR, Kraus EE, Zasler ND: Medical management of posttraumatic headaches: pharmacological and physical treatment. J Head Trauma Rehabil 1999;14: 34–48.
10 Lane JC, Arciniegas DB: Post-traumatic headache. Curr Treat Options Neurol 2002;4:89–104.
11 Warden DL, Warden B, McAllister TW, Silver JM, Barth JT, Bruns J, Drake A, Gentry T, Jagoda A, Katz DI, Kraus J, Labbate LA, Ryan LM, Sparling MB, Walters B, Whyte J, Zapata A, Zitnay G: Guidelines for the pharmacologic treatment of neurobehavioral sequelae of traumatic brain injury. J Neurotrauma 2006;23:1468–1501.
12 Petraglia AL, Maroon JC, Bailes JE: From the field of play to the field of combat: a review of the pharmacological management of concussion. Neurosurgery 2012;70:1520–1533, discussion 1533.
13 Zafonte RD, Lexell J, Cullen N: Possible applications for dopaminergic agents following traumatic brain injury: part 2. J Head Trauma Rehabil 2001;16:112–116.
14 Meythaler JM, Brunner RC, Johnson A, Novak TA: Amantadine to improve neurorecovery in traumatic brain injury-associated diffuse axonal injury: a pilot double-blind randomized trial. J Head Trauma Rehabil 2002;17:300–313.
15 Reddy CC, Collins MW, Lovell M, Kontos AP: Efficacy of amantadine treatment on symptoms and neurocognitive performance among adolescents following sports-related concussion. J Head Trauma Rehabil 2013;28:260–265.
16 Whyte J, Hart T, Vaccaro M, Grieb-Neff P, Risser A, Polansky M, Coslett HB: Effects of methylphenidate on attention deficits after traumatic brain injury: a multidimensional, randomized, controlled trial. Am J Phys Med Rehabil 2004;83:401–420.
17 Plenger PM, Dixon CE, Castillo RM, Frankowski RF, Yablon SA, Levin HS: Subacute methylphenidate treatment for moderate to moderately severe traumatic brain injury: a preliminary double-blind placebo-controlled study. Arch Phys Med Rehabil 1996; 77:536–540.

18 Levin HS: Treatment of postconcussional symptoms with CDP-choline. J Neurol Sci 1991;103(suppl): S39–S42.
19 Meehan WP 3rd: Medical therapies for concussion. Clin Sports Med 2011;30:115–124, ix.
20 Arciniegas DB, Anderson CA, Topkoff J, McAllister TW: Mild traumatic brain injury: a neuropsychiatric approach to diagnosis, evaluation, and treatment. Neuropsychiatr Dis Treat 2005;1:311–327.
21 Fann JR, Uomoto JM, Katon WJ: Sertraline in the treatment of major depression following mild traumatic brain injury. J Neuropsychiatry Clin Neurosci 2000;12:226–232.
22 Fann JR, Uomoto JM, Katon WJ: Cognitive improvement with treatment of depression following mild traumatic brain injury. Psychosomatics 2001; 42:48–54.
23 Rapoport MJ, Chan F, Lanctot K, Herrmann N, McCullagh S, Feinstein A: An open-label study of citalopram for major depression following traumatic brain injury. J Psychopharmacol 2008;22:860–864.
24 Müller U, Murai T, Bauer-Wittmund T, von Cramon DY: Paroxetine versus citalopram treatment of pathological crying after brain injury. Brain Inj 1999; 13:805–811.
25 Silver JM, McAllister TW, Arciniegas DB: Depression and cognitive complaints following mild traumatic brain injury. Am J Psychiatry 2009;166:653–661.
26 Ouellet MC, Savard J, Morin CM: Insomnia following traumatic brain injury: a review. Neurorehabil Neural Repair 2004;18:187–198.
27 Morin AK, Jarvis CI, Lynch AM: Therapeutic options for sleep-maintenance and sleep-onset insomnia. Pharmacotherapy 2007;27:89–110.
28 Rao V, Rollings P: Sleep disturbances following traumatic brain injury. Curr Treat Options Neurol 2002; 4:77–87.
29 Flanagan SR, Greenwald B, Wieber S: Pharmacological treatment of insomnia for individuals with brain injury. J Head Trauma Rehabil 2007;22:67–70.
30 Rogers NL, Dinges DF, Kennaway DJ, Dawson D: Potential action of melatonin in insomnia. Sleep 2003;26:1058–1059.
31 Samantaray S, Das A, Thakore NP, Matzelle DD, Reiter RJ, Ray SK, Banik NL: Therapeutic potential of melatonin in traumatic central nervous system injury. J Pineal Res 2009;47:134–142.
32 Reiter RJ, Korkmaz A: Clinical aspects of melatonin. Saudi Med J 2008;29:1537–1547.
33 Ruff RL, Ruff SS, Wang XF: Improving sleep: initial headache treatment in OIF/OEF veterans with blast-induced mild traumatic brain injury. J Rehabil Res Dev 2009;46:1071–1084.
34 Lau BC, Kontos AP, Collins MW, Mucha A, Lovell MR: Which on-field signs/symptoms predict protracted recovery from sport-related concussion among high school football players? Am J Sports Med 2011;39:2311–2318.
35 Furman JM, Whitney SL: Central causes of dizziness. Phys Ther 2000;80:179–187.
36 Alsalaheen BA, Mucha A, Morris LO, Whitney SL, Furman JM, Camiolo-Reddy CE, Collins MW, Lovell MR, Sparto PJ: Vestibular rehabilitation for dizziness and balance disorders after concussion. J Neurol Phys Ther 2010;34:87–93.
37 Jacob RG, Redfern MS, Furman JM: Space and motion discomfort and abnormal balance control in patients with anxiety disorders. J Neurol Neurosurg Psychiatry 2009;80:74–78.
38 Zee DS: Perspectives on the pharmacotherapy of vertigo. Arch Otolaryngol 1985;111:609–612.

Cara Camiolo Reddy, MD
University of Pittsburgh Medical Center
1400 Locust Street, D-G103
Pittsburgh, PA 15219 (USA)
E-Mail camice@upmc.edu

Niranjan A, Lunsford LD (eds): Concussion. Prog Neurol Surg. Basel, Karger, 2014, vol 28, pp 149–160
DOI: 10.1159/000358775

Rehabilitation from Postconcussion Syndrome: Nonpharmacological Treatment

Amelia L. Nelson Sheese[a] · Thomas A. Hammeke[b, c]

[a]Nebraska Medical Center, Omaha, Nebr., and [b]Clement J. Zablocki Veterans Administration Medical Center and [c]Medical College of Wisconsin, Milwaukee, Wis., USA

Abstract

Following mild traumatic brain injury (mTBI), one or more symptoms commonly occur that are known as the postconcussion syndrome (PCS). While PCS typically resolves within a few weeks of injury for most concussed patients, some patients have a more prolonged or otherwise adverse recovery course. There is relatively little systematic research on the treatment of PCS. This report offers strategies for nonpharmacological treatment of PCS during the acute, subacute, and chronic stages of recovery following mTBI. The treatment strategies are supported by clinical consensus and the limited evidence-based research wherever possible. Core treatment strategies emphasize (1) education about mTBI, PCS, and the natural recovery course, (2) reassurance of a good outcome, (3) reduction in activity level and refrain from hazardous behaviors during the acute phase, (4) gradual return to lifestyle activities as symptoms permit, (5) careful monitoring and early intervention for adverse emotional responses, (6) symptom-specific treatment when needed, and (7) ready access to providers during acute and subacute recovery periods.

© 2014 S. Karger AG, Basel

Each year in the USA, an estimated 1.7 million traumatic brain injuries (TBIs) occur [1], most of which are classified as mild TBI (mTBI) or concussion. A significant portion of individuals with mTBI develop one or more symptoms that have been referred to as the postconcussion syndrome (PCS). Common symptoms of PCS are headache, cognitive complaints (i.e., memory or concentration problems, slowed thinking), sleep disturbance, fatigue, irritability, dizziness, and/or blurred vision [2]. Reduced tolerance to alcohol or noises, anxiety, depression, apathy, and/or personality changes are also identified as possible symptoms [3, 4]. Fortunately, no permanent disability is expected after uncomplicated mTBI, and the vast majority of concussed individuals spontaneously achieve full recovery within days or weeks after the injury. However, a small portion of individuals, aptly described by some as the 'miserable minority' [5, 6], continue to report postconcussive symptoms months or even years after sustaining an mTBI despite having no identifiable neurologic cause for their complaints. In such cases, postconcussion disorder (PCD) or persistent PCS [7] may be diagnosed when symptoms become chronic, i.e., continue for longer than 3 months after the injury [3].

The prevalence of PCD or persistent PCS has been historically cited as 15% of individuals who sustain mTBI; however, recently this figure has been disputed and attributed to misinterpretation of results from early studies [4, 8]. Leading TBI researchers argue that the prevalence rate is likely less than 5% of the mTBI population [4, 8]. The lower estimated prevalence rate in part relates to the fact that a substantial portion of mTBI cases never seek medical attention and, thus, are often not counted in the prevalence estimations.

A majority of studies indicate that chronic symptoms after mTBI are most likely attributed to factors other than the TBI itself (e.g., preexisting or concurrent psychiatric problems, musculoskeletal or peripheral nervous system injuries acquired concurrently with the TBI, chronic pain) [5, 9, 10]. Thus, accurate diagnosis and specific treatment of reported symptoms are important to expedite recovery.

The purpose of this report is to assist clinicians in minimizing the risk of PCD/persistent PCS through early identification and nonpharmacological intervention of postconcussive symptoms. Recent literature suggests that early interventions optimize the odds of a normal and complete recovery [4, 11].

Diagnosis and Nonspecificity of Symptoms

Although the term 'postconcussion syndrome' is often used to summarize any combination of the common aforementioned symptoms following mTBI, formal attempts to operationalize a diagnosis for *persistent* (i.e., extending beyond the expected time frame for recovery) postinjury symptoms have not been made. Proposed research criteria for PCD are included in the DSM-IV [3]. This diagnosis may be assigned when 3 or more designated symptoms persist for more than 3 months after injury and result in impairment in functioning. The ICD-10 [12] also includes diagnostic criteria for 3 or more persistent symptoms under the diagnosis of PCS, with the provision that symptom onset occurred within 1 month of a head trauma accompanied by an associated loss of consciousness.

The diagnoses of PCD and PCS are controversial, in part because symptoms are based on the patient's subjective report, and particularly because of the symptom nonspecificity. That is, each of the PCS symptoms (e.g., headache, dizziness, sleep disturbance, etc.) tend to occur at high rates in other medical or psychological disorders and even with regularity in the normal population [13, 14]. Research suggests that in many cases, longstanding or evolving symptoms following mTBI are most likely etiologically related to, or exacerbated by, factors other than the brain trauma itself, such as preexisting or concurrent psychiatric problems, environmental stressors, medications, associated physical injuries, and/or litigation/compensation issues [4, 8–10, 15]. Recent studies have shown that preinjury physical or psychological problems, but not mTBI, predicted postconcussive symptoms at 3 months after injury [10]. Other possible predictors of prolonged symptoms may include female gender, older age (i.e., over 40 years), and psychosocial stressors [2, 9].

The 'Biopsychosocial Approach' to Treatment

Because of the complex nature of persistent postconcussive symptoms, many researchers and clinicians have proposed a biopsychosocial approach to conceptualization and treatment [4, 16]. The biopsychosocial approach recognizes that early clinical symptoms certainly may manifest along with the pathophysiological result of neurologic injury. As previously mentioned, head injury symptoms can be related to or exacerbated by psychological, social, medical, and/or motivational factors, and many persistent symptoms may be completely unrelated to the head injury. The biopsychosocial approach recognizes that the treatment of PCD needs to be diverse and include an integrated model of care [8] to determine the etiology and best course of treatment for protracted symptoms. Consultation with specialists may be necessary to evaluate and treat specific complaints that may not be a result of the TBI itself.

Nonpharmacological Treatment of Postconcussion Symptoms

The remainder of this report focuses on nonpharmacological treatments for postconcussion symptoms. Because treatment strategies and recommendations for specific symptoms vary depending on how much time has elapsed since the injury, they will be discussed within the context of the acute (<1 week), subacute (1 week to 3 months), and chronic (>3 months) periods of recovery from mTBI. Also, recognizing that there is a considerable range of severity embedded within the spectrum of mTBI, it is important for the clinician to make corresponding adjustments in his or her expectations for the patient's speed of recovery. For example, if an mTBI was extremely mild as indicated by no loss of consciousness and perhaps only a momentary interval of posttraumatic amnesia, then expected recovery might include only what has been identified here as the acute phase and perhaps a week or two into the subacute phase. Alternatively, if the mTBI was at the more severe end of the mTBI spectrum as might be indicated by a loss of consciousness of 20 min and posttraumatic amnesia of 20 h, then a more prolonged recovery course would be expected with full resolution of symptoms requiring 2–3 months.

Currently, there is only limited empirical evidence to guide specific nonpharmacological treatment strategies for prevention and management of PCD. However, education and reassurance of a good outcome have been shown to have positive effects on outcome regardless of the stage of recovery [11, 17]. The discussion of treatment that follows incorporates available literature and consensus clinical practices guidelines. Recommended guidelines are primarily focused on individuals who have sustained an uncomplicated mTBI, as more severe head injuries may require a different course of treatment. Treatment recommendations for various therapies (e.g., psychotherapy and psychoeducation, vestibular therapy, cognitive rehabilitation techniques, etc.) will be discussed within a timeline of possible persistent symptoms after injury.

Clinical History and Diagnosis for Treatment Planning

Regardless of stage of recovery, once the diagnosis of mTBI has been established based on careful review of injury characteristics, a comprehensive review of lingering symptoms should be conducted. Clinicians should inquire about the onset and course of reported symptoms and note whether any of the complaints predated the head injury. Particular emphasis should be given to complaints of headaches and other pain, dizziness/vertigo, sleep disturbance, concentration and memory problems, and emotional adjustment, as these symptoms are quite common and often are most disruptive to overall functioning.

Additionally, a thorough clinical history should be conducted, including information about the patient's physical injuries and medical history. Clinicians should determine if there is a prior history of TBI, as well as a preexisting psychiatric condition or substance abuse/dependence, which often complicate recovery from mTBI and signal the need for additional intervention [2, 8]. Further, psychosocial history is relevant to explore in order to uncover any social issues that may predict an adverse recovery (e.g., poor social support or unstable relationships) [2, 8].

Acute Recovery Period: Education, Reassurance, and Symptomatic Treatment

Intervention for postconcussive symptoms should begin as early as feasible, including during an initial evaluation in the emergency room or primary care clinic. For most individuals with mTBI, PCS will resolve within the acute period or shortly thereafter. Thus, the primary focus of early intervention is *education* about the normal course of recovery from mTBI, and *reassurance* that permanent brain injury has not occurred [17]. Moreover, patients should be instructed about coping strategies for current symptoms, prevention of further injury, and gradual resumption of activities [17].

Concerning education, patients should be informed of possible symptoms that result from concussion, as well as the normal course of improvement in symptoms. Clinicians should emphasize the expectation that symptoms will likely remit in the initial days or weeks following injury. Upon review of current symptoms, specific suggestions for coping strategies should be given. Both the Centers for Disease Control and Prevention (CDC) and the Defense and Veterans Brain Injury Center (DVBIC) websites provide consensus management guidelines. For example, rest and relaxation techniques may help to decrease symptoms such as headaches, fatigue, and irritability. Patients should be advised to reduce the usual functional expectations during the recovery window and to make adjustments in their schedule to accommodate the functional limitations during this time. Often, brief absences from work or school immediately after the injury due to symptoms are appropriate. Because there are few research studies to consult regarding rest after mTBI, a gradual return to normal lifestyle is recommended [11]. As individuals resume their usual activities, providers should address any symptoms or difficulties they may have as soon as they arise. Patients should be advised to take precautions to reduce the risk of reinjury. Additionally, they should be instructed not to consume alcohol, drive motorized vehicles, ride bicycles, or operate machinery. If vertigo or balance problems are prominent, use of support during ambulation will be important.

Education about symptom recovery and coping techniques may be provided either verbally to patients by a healthcare provider or through written educational materials [17, 18]. When written materials are given, providers should attempt to ensure that patients read and review them when necessary [11].

As for reassurance and support, it is important that providers convey their sensitivity and understanding of their patients' acute condition. Specifically, the provider should convey to his/her understanding that the patients' complaints represent the effects of disruption of typical physiological functioning and that their emotional experiences reflect a normal reaction to concussion. The difference between brain *injury* and brain *damage* may be explained, with emphasis that a mild injury will heal with time. Patients should keep their providers informed of their symptom status, and patients should be assured that if their symptoms do not resolve, their providers will be actively involved in reassessing their symptoms and adjusting treatment plans. This will be especially important during the graduated return to normal lifestyle as symptoms are often transiently aggravated during these times. Contact information for the clinician should be provided.

While research on the specific timing of intervention is lacking, the professional consensus is that the earlier the intervention occurs, the better [11, 19]. Studies show that intervention within the initial weeks or months after the injury leads to fewer and less severe postconcussive symptoms [20]. Moreover, the intervention may be brief. According to Paniak et al. [20], a single-session treatment involving education and reassurance reduces later symptoms as effectively as more intensive treatment-as-needed approaches (e.g., additional neuropsychological assessment, physical therapy consultation, and/or other treatments).

Subacute Recovery Period

In the subacute phase of recovery (i.e., approx. 7–90 days after mTBI), treatment shifts to focus on specific treatment for residual symptoms. Symptoms that persist into the subacute window may be a direct result of the mTBI, injuries to other organ systems that occurred concurrently with the mTBI, or may represent preexisting health problems. Thus, more in-depth evaluation may be necessary, and symptoms should be tracked over time. Clinicians should continue to educate patients with complaints within this time frame that they are not yet outside of the window of recovery. Continued improvement is likely. Further, patients should continue to feel reassured that their providers are active in the management of their symptoms. Below are examples of the more common residual symptoms during the subacute period of recovery and possible treatment recommendations.

Persistent Pain: Head and Neck Pain

Headaches are a common complaint following mTBI and may be associated with abnormal brain or cerebrovascular function during the acute phase. Often headaches that persist or occur after the acute period are due to a previously unidentified musculoskeletal injury rather than the brain concussion. Comprehensive evaluation by a physiatrist may help to identify and address such injuries. Head and neck pain are common symptoms of whiplash or other cervical spine injury. Generally, pain from whiplash remits in the initial weeks following injury; however, if pain persists, referral to a physiatrist and a physical therapist may be beneficial for specific recommendations for exercise and manual therapy [4].

Vertigo and Disequilibrium

Vertigo and disequilibrium can be functionally debilitating symptoms, particularly when persistent. Vertigo is often described as dizziness, but entails a false sense of 'spinning', which is qualitatively different from the sensation of 'lightheadedness'. If vertigo persists into the subacute phase of recovery, further evaluation should be conducted to determine whether central or peripheral pathology is the cause and if onset coincides with the injury. If a central vestibular disorder is suspected (e.g., due to a central lesion), a neurologic exam is warranted as the vestibular problem is often associated with other cranial nerve injuries. In many cases, especially in cases associated with blunt trauma to the head that conveys vibratory force through the skull, the mechanism is injury to organs in the middle ear. Examples include labyrinthine concussion, perilymphatic fistula, or benign paroxysmal positional vertigo – all of which may or may not improve in the initial weeks after the injury. Referral to an otolaryngologist for evaluation is recommended for patients with persistent vertigo and or disequilibrium complaints. This may well lead to referral for physical therapy that includes a canalith reposition maneuver (for benign paroxysmal positional vertigo) and/or vestibular rehabilitation.

Vision Problems

While the complaint of blurred vision after mTBI is often transient, the complaint of photosensitivity occasionally evolves and persists longer. A subset of patients report being hypersensitive to specific frequencies of light (e.g., fluorescents, halogen, or LED computer or TV screens) that are said to precipitate a sense of visual distress or dizziness. Prolonged exposure to these stimuli often are said to precipitate a migrainous-type headache. The mechanism of this light sensitivity is poorly understood and needs further study. Often times the offending light frequency can be filtered with appropriately tinted glasses, or blocked by the use of brimmed hats. Ongoing complaints of light sensitivity or other vision difficulties warrant referral to a specialist, such as an ophthalmologist, neuro-ophthalmologist, or headache specialist for further evaluation.

Sleep Difficulties

Sleep difficulties are particularly important to address, as restorative sleep plays a significant role in general mental health and cognition. While disturbances of circadian rhythm due to physiological disruption are common in the acute recovery phase, during the subacute phase, sleep problems often evolve out of maladaptive behavioral and emotional adjustments arising from the symptoms in the acute period. Clinicians should assess the nature of the patient's sleep problems (i.e., initial, middle, or late insomnia, poor sleep maintenance due to nightmares or pain, etc.). Techniques for improving sleep hygiene may be discussed such as establishing a regular schedule for bedtime and rising, avoiding stimulants and heavy exercise late in the day, avoiding spending time in bed awake, and working to improve sleep consolidation [21]. Referral to a behavioral health psychologist may be helpful for assistance in determining if the cause of the sleep difficulties is psychological in nature (e.g., anxiety) and for implementation of sleep hygiene techniques. In the event that sleep difficulties persist, a referral for a polysomnogram may be warranted for a better understanding of factors contributing to the insomnia.

Mood Complaints

Depression and increased irritability are commonly experienced following mTBI. Depression, often associated with a reduction in motivation to participate in rehabilitation, particularly complicates recovery. Education and reassurance that mTBI symptoms are generally time-limited can help. Minimizing responsibilities and demands, allowing frequent rest breaks during activities, and implementing relaxation strategies (e.g., deep breathing, progressive muscle relaxation, etc.) in the initial days and weeks after the trauma may help to reduce frustration levels. A gradual increase in activity levels often improves mood. Generally, mood complaints improve with time, but if they persist for weeks, referral to a mental health professional for further treatment is recommended. Furthermore, clinicians should be vigilant of signs of acute stress disorder (ASD) [3] in the initial days and weeks following a trauma. In such cases, patients may report anxiety symptoms or panic episodes as well as a feeling of 'unreality' or feeling detached or outside of their bodies. They may also experience intrusive thoughts or nightmares about the trauma, and they may avoid reminders of the event. Manifestation of ASD necessitates referral to a mental health provider as ASD often evolves into posttraumatic stress disorder (PTSD). Cognitive behavioral therapy effectively reduce symptoms for

ASD and PTSD by using techniques that involve cognitive processing and prolonged exposure to the traumatic stimuli. These evidence-based therapies are more effective when applied early in the recovery rather than after symptoms have become chronic [15].

Cognitive Complaints
Slowed information processing speed and memory and concentration difficulties are common deficits on neuropsychological testing in the initial days after injury [2]. Headache and musculoskeletal pain, emotional distress, and sleep disturbance also contribute to initial cognitive complaints [2] as coping with each of these symptoms makes significant demands on limited attentional resources. Patients with vertigo and vestibular problems commonly report concentration problems presumably for similar reasons. Most neuropsychological studies show resolution of cognitive deficits within 3 months after injury [2, 4, 8, 11]. In the meantime, cognitive rehabilitation and compensation strategies may be utilized. For example, compensatory techniques such as employing a single memory notebook and to-do list may be used to assist with memory and organization. Also, a digital alarm may be set for reminders for tasks and medications. Use of mobile electronic devices should be encouraged (i.e., the digital calendar or to-do lists on cell phones). Additionally, individuals should be encouraged to pace their activities and to frequently take breaks during cognitively demanding tasks.

Chronic Recovery Period

If postconcussive symptoms persist more than 3 months following injury, mechanisms for symptoms other than posttraumatic brain dysfunction are most likely and should be considered. Patients should again be reassured and reminded that non-TBI etiologies for their persistent symptoms are likely. Developing differential diagnoses for each lingering symptom and orchestration of relevant referrals and diagnostic evaluations are appropriate. The interventions will depend on the specific diagnostic results; however, interventions for many specific complaints are likely to be similar to those detailed for the subacute recovery period. Below are additional recommendations for specific symptoms that may be reported several months after an injury.

Headaches
If no improvement in headaches is seen by 3 months after the injury, consultation by a neurologist for evaluation of migraines versus muscle tension headaches (e.g., due to possible neck or scalp injury or stress and anxiety) may be warranted. Additionally, referral to a behavioral psychologist for psychological treatment may be beneficial. Such treatment may involve behavioral relaxation strategies (e.g., pro-

gressive muscle relaxation and/or biofeedback) that target muscles of the neck and scalp, or stress inoculation techniques (e.g., identifying stressors and learning effective stress-coping strategies). Counseling about lifestyle changes that lower overall stress levels may be appropriate (e.g., changes in job, work schedules, and diet and activity levels).

Vertigo and Disequilibrium
As previously mentioned, if complaints of vertigo and balance unsteadiness have persisted chronically, referral to a physical therapist is warranted to determine the etiology of the complaint and to decide whether vestibular training could be beneficial. Patients may benefit from health exercises that emphasize balance (e.g., yoga, Tai Chi).

Cognitive Complaints
Persistent cognitive complaints beyond 3 months after mTBI are unlikely to be related to brain dysfunction [2]. There are many possible underlying factors for persistent cognitive complaints including psychological distress (e.g., depression, anxiety, PTSD), sleep disturbance and fatigue, chronic pain, and/or effects of medications. Referral to a neuropsychologist for further evaluation and treatment planning is recommended. In many cases, appropriate treatment and improvement of underlying causes may lead to improvements in cognition. Additionally, speech therapy may be beneficial for individuals whose cognitive difficulties are adversely affecting their school or work performance, regardless of the etiology of their complaints.

Mood Complaints
If patients experience persistent mood complaints, such as depression, general anxiety, irritability, and/or posttraumatic symptoms, referral to mental health providers (i.e., psychologist, counselor, or psychiatrist) is recommended. Nonpharmacological treatment of persistent mood symptoms may include psychotherapy or counseling. In a specific type of psychotherapy, cognitive behavioral therapy, the therapist and client work together to address and challenge negative or maladaptive thoughts that may lead to depressed or anxious mood [22]. In some cases, therapists may focus specifically on correcting misattributions about symptom recovery from concussion [17]. Behavioral strategies may also be warranted, such as implementing relaxation techniques or increasing exposure to positive activities (i.e., behavioral activation), which may in turn improve affect. Efficacious therapeutic treatments for PTSD include cognitive processing and/or prolonged exposure where the patient learns how to effectively manage distress associated with the previous trauma. A regular exercise program and restful sleep also are known to improve mood and general psychological adjustment.

Other Factors Underlying Persistent Symptoms after Mild Traumatic Brain Injury

It should be noted that in a few cases, individuals may experience chronic symptoms that they attribute to their uncomplicated mTBI, despite attempts at treatment by specialists. This happens with some regularity in patients who have injuries to other organ systems that occurred concurrently with the mTBI that are associated with unresolved symptoms (e.g., musculoskeletal pain). As previously mentioned, it is extremely rare to experience residual symptoms from mTBI more than 12 months after the injury. In cases in which persistent symptoms cannot be explained by a general medical condition or other psychiatric disorder, a somatoform disorder may be suspected, and referral to a psychologist or psychiatrist for further evaluation and treatment is recommended.

As mentioned earlier, one of the most common predictors of delayed recovery from mTBI is ongoing litigation/pursuit of compensation [2, 12, 23]. Such circumstances should be explored during the patient's evaluation. The relationship between litigation and postconcussive symptoms remains poorly understood, and clinicians should not necessarily assume that all individuals who are actively involved in litigation are malingering [2].

Brief Case Vignette

At the time of her mild concussion at 28 years of age, Sarah had been working full-time as a waitress at a popular restaurant in Milwaukee. Her supervisor and coworkers described her as a hard worker, and regular patrons enjoyed her bubbly personality and attentive serving style. After leaving work one evening as the unhelmeted passenger of her boyfriend's motorcycle, she was involved in a motor vehicle collision. An automobile ran through a stop sign and collided with the motorcycle at an estimated 20–30 mph. Sarah fell from the motorcycle and sustained a brief loss of consciousness (<5 min) after she hit her head on the ground. Upon EMS arrival, she was alert but confused and complained of headache and dizziness. In the emergency department, a CT scan of her head was normal, and her Glasgow Coma Scale was 15. She continued to complain of headache and dizziness, however, and her physicians informed her that her symptoms were a normal reaction to mTBI. Furthermore, she was assured that her symptoms would likely remit within days to weeks, but that she should limit exertional activities until her symptoms diminished. She was discharged home with a plan to follow-up in the outpatient mTBI multidisciplinary clinic at the hospital in 2 weeks.

Sarah subsequently took sick leave from work for the following week due to mild headaches, fatigue, and occasional lightheadedness. Upon her return to work 1 week later, she reported no functional difficulties, although her employer and coworkers had noticed that she had seemed less energetic and mildly distractible. In the mTBI clinic appointment the following week, Sarah described daily light headaches and fatigue, and her boyfriend described mild, but improving, irritability. Sarah's physician again assured her that her symptoms were normal and would be expected to continue to improve as time progressed. She was informed that at this phase in her recovery, she was mentally working much harder to do routine tasks and she should expect to get mentally tired more easily. She was informed that her headaches might return to some degree if she mentally overtaxed herself. She indicated that she felt reassured. She was provided with con-

Table 1. Summary of intervention strategies for each stage of recovery from mTBI

Acute recovery period (0–7 days) 1. Educate patient about common symptoms and natural recovery course 2. Reassure patient about good outcome without permanent brain damage 3. Limit activity levels 4. Adjust self-expectations for performance 5. Take precautions to reduce risk of reinjury (e.g., do not drive or consume alcohol) 6. Gradual resumptions of work, school, and lifestyle activities as symptoms permit 7. Provide patient with contact information and assure your availability
Subacute recovery period (1 week to 3 months) 1. Continue education and expectation of good outcome from mTBI 2. Resurvey PCS symptoms and initiate symptom-specific evaluation and treatment 3. Introduce notion that symptoms may not be due to mTBI but rather to other injuries 4. Continue efforts toward gradual resumption of normal activity levels 5. Assure patient of your availability
Chronic recovery period (>3 months after injury) 1. Continue education and expectation of good outcome from mTBI 2. Monitor PCS symptoms and continue/initiate symptom-specific treatment as needed 3. Educate patient about possible mechanisms of symptoms other than mTBI 4. Refer to specialists as needed to optimize treatment of persistent symptoms 5. Counsel patient about lifestyle changes to optimize adjustment

tact information for her physician in the event that her symptoms did not improve, and she was again encouraged to take frequent rest breaks to assist with her fatigue and concentration difficulties. Three weeks after her injury, Sarah's symptoms remitted, and her supervisor and boyfriend noted that she had returned to her baseline with regards to work abilities and emotional functioning.

Conclusion

While PCS after mTBI resolves within a few weeks of injury for most patients, some patients have a more prolonged or otherwise adverse recovery course. This report offers best practice strategies for nonpharmacological treatment of PCS during the acute, subacute, and chronic stages of recovery following mTBI (table 1). Core treatment strategies emphasize (1) education about mTBI, PCS, and the natural recovery course, (2) reassurance of a good outcome, (3) reduction in activity level and refraining from hazardous behavior during the acute phase, (4) gradual return to lifestyle activities as symptoms permit, (5) careful monitoring and early intervention for adverse emotional responses, (6) symptom-specific treatment when needed, and (7) ready access to providers during acute and subacute recovery periods.

References

1 Faul M: Traumatic brain injury in the United States emergency department visits, hospitalizations, and deaths, 2002–2006. Atlanta, US Department of Health and Human Services, Centers for Disease Control and Prevention, National Center for Injury Prevention and Control, 2010. http://www.cdc.gov/traumaticbraininjury/pdf/blue_book.pdf.

2 Carroll LJ, Cassidy D, Peloso PM, Borg J, von Holst H, Holm L, et al: Prognosis for mild traumatic brain injury: results of the WHO Collaborating Centre Task Force on Mild Traumatic Brain Injury. J Rehabil Med 2004;(suppl 43):84–105.

3 American Psychiatric Association: Diagnostic and Statistical Manual of Mental Disorders: DSM-IV-TR, ed 4. Washington, American Psychiatric Association, 2000.

4 Iverson GL, Lange RT, Gaetz MB, Zasler ND: Mild traumatic brain injury; in Zasler ND, Katz DI, Zafonte RD (eds): Brain Injury Medicine. New York, Demos Medical Publishing LLC, 2013, pp 434–469.

5 Rohling ML, Larrabee GJ, Millis SR: The 'miserable minority' following mild traumatic brain injury: who are they and do meta-analyses hide them? Clin Neuropsychol 2012;26:197–213.

6 Ruff RM, Camenzuli L, Mueller J: Miserable minority: emotional risk factors that influence the outcome of a mild traumatic brain injury. Brain Inj 1996;10:551–565.

7 Alexander MP: Mild traumatic brain injury: pathophysiology, natural history, and clinical management. Neurology 1995;45:1253–1260.

8 McCrea M: Mild traumatic brain injury and postconcussion syndrome: the new evidence base for diagnosis and treatment. New York, Oxford University Press, 2008.

9 Meares S, Shores EA, Taylor AJ, Batchelor J, Bryant RA, Baguley IJ, et al: The prospective course of postconcussion syndrome: the role of mild traumatic brain injury. Neuropsychology 2011;25:454–465.

10 Ponsford J, Cameron P, Fitzgerald M, Grant M, Mikocka-Walus A, Schönberger M: Predictors of postconcussive symptoms 3 months after mild traumatic brain injury. Neuropsychology 2012;26:304–313.

11 Ponsford J: Treatment of mTBI; in Vasterling JJ, Bryant RA, Keane T (eds): PTSD and Mild Traumatic Brain Injury. New York, Guilford Press, 2012.

12 Kashluba S, Paniak C, Casey JE: Persistent symptoms associated with factors identified by the WHO Task Force on Mild Traumatic Brain Injury. Clin Neuropsychol 2008;22:195–208.

13 Lees-Haley PR, Brown RS: Neuropsychological complaint base rates of 170 personal injury claimants. Arch Clin Neuropsychol 1993;8:203–209.

14 Wang Y, Chan RC, Deng Y: Examination of postconcussion-like symptoms in healthy university students: relationships to subjective and objective neuropsychological function performance. Arch Clin Neuropsychol 2006;21:339–347.

15 Potter S, Brown RG: Cognitive behavioural therapy and persistent post-concussional symptoms: integrating conceptual issues and practical aspects in treatment. Neuropsychol Rehab 2012;22:1–25.

16 Wood RL: Understanding the 'miserable minority': a diasthesis-stress paradigm for post-concussional syndrome. Brain Inj 2004;18:1135–1153.

17 Mittenberg W, Tremont G, Zielinski RE, Fichera S, Rayls KR: Cognitive-behavioral prevention of postconcussion syndrome. Arch Clin Neuropsychol 1996;11:139–145.

18 Centers for Disease Control and Prevention: Injury Prevention and Control: TBI. http://www.cdc.gov/concussion/feel_better.html (accessed September 3, 2013).

19 Veterans Affairs/Department of Defense: Clinical Practice Guidelines: Management of Concussion/Mild Traumatic Brain Injury. 2009. v.1.0.http://www.healthquality.va.gov/mtbi/concussion_mtbi_full_1_0.pdf (accessed September 3, 2013).

20 Paniak C, Toller-Lobe G, Reynolds S, Melnyk A, Nagy J: A randomized trial of two treatments for mild traumatic brain injury: 1 year follow-up. Brain Inj 2000;14:219–226.

21 Defense and Veterans Brain Injury Center: TBI Symptom Management: Healthy Sleep. http://www.dvbic.org/material/tbi-symptom-management-healthy-sleep (accessed September 3, 2013).

22 Beck AT: Cognitive Therapy of Depression. New York, Guilford Press, 1979.

23 Paniak C, Reynolds S, Toller-Lobe G, Melnyk A, Nagy J, Schmidt D: A longitudinal study of the relationship between financial compensation and symptoms after treated mild traumatic brain injury. J Clin Exp Neuropsychol 2002;24:187–193.

Thomas A. Hammeke, PhD, ABPP-Cn
Acute Mental Health, Bldg 111, Zablocki VA Medical Center
5000 West National Avenue
Milwaukee, WI 53295 (USA)
E-Mail thammeke@mcw.edu

Niranjan A, Lunsford LD (eds): Concussion. Prog Neurol Surg. Basel, Karger, 2014, vol 28, pp 161–170
DOI: 10.1159/000358777

Concussion in Ice Hockey

Christopher M. Bonfield · Daniel A. Wecht · L. Dade Lunsford

Department of Neurological Surgery, Center for Sports Medicine, University of Pittsburgh Medical Center, Pittsburgh, Pa., USA

Abstract

Ice hockey is an aggressive and fast-paced sport which has a high risk of injury, concussions in particular. Although serious head injury has been recognized for nearly 50 years, an increase in mainstream media attention in recent years has led to unprecedented public awareness. As a result, the National Hockey League (NHL) and other professional leagues around the world have initiated concussion protocols in order to better prevent, recognize, and treat concussions. With over 1,000,000 youth hockey participants in Canada and the USA combined, concussion is an issue that reaches beyond the professional level. In this report we review the incidence, evaluation, treatment, return-to-play protocol, and prevention efforts related to concussion in ice hockey.

© 2014 S. Karger AG, Basel

Ice hockey, at all levels, is a high-risk sport for injury, and specifically concussion. The game is played at a high rate of speed on an ice rink encircled by rigid boards. Players are larger and faster than before, can reach speeds of over 30 miles per hour [1], and come in contact with hard surfaces such as boards, glass, ice, goal posts, sticks, pucks, and other players. These collisions cause severe changes in speeds and result in acceleration/deceleration injuries. There is no debate on why it is classified as a collision sport [2].

Furthermore, hockey is an aggressive sport that involves regular body-to-body contact, and the only sport outside of boxing and mixed martial arts to allow fighting. Hockey players have the reputation of being some of the toughest athletes and are seen as 'warriors' or 'soldiers' when playing through pain or injury. This leads to a potential problem of underreporting symptoms by the players and coaches looking past injuries to give their team a better chance to win [3]. Unlike other sports, National Hockey League (NHL) clubs are not required to disclose the specific nature of a player's injury. In certain cases, concussions may be underrecognized and determined to be an 'upper body injury'.

Although serious head injury has been recognized for nearly 50 years [4], an increase in mainstream media attention in recent years [5] has led to unprecedented public awareness. NHL stars like Sidney Crosby and Chris Pronger have been sidelined for extended periods of time. Many careers, including those of Paul Kariya, Pat LaFontaine, Eric Lindros, Keith Primeau, and most recently Marc Savard, have been prematurely ended by multiple concussions. The unanticipated apparent suicides of three NHL 'enforcers' (Derek Boogaard, Rick Rypien, and Wade Belak) between May and September of 2011 again brought the issue of head injury in sports to the forefront, and raised questions about long-lasting effects of repeated trauma to the head [6]. An increase of public concern over postconcussive syndrome, second-impact syndrome, and chronic traumatic encephalopathy has also raised awareness of and research in sport-related concussion.

As a result, the NHL and other leagues around the world have initiated concussion protocols in order to better prevent, recognize, and treat concussions. Gary Bettman, the current NHL commissioner, has stated, 'We (the NHL) are the first league that has had a protocol for the diagnosis and return-to-play decisions. We are the first sports league to do baseline testing with respect to concussions and this is just another in a series of steps' [7]. The NHL Protocol for Concussion Evaluation and Management was created in 1997, and a revised program was enacted in 2011 [8]. With this new awareness, the attitude towards concussion is changing.

Although the professional hockey leagues have received the most attention, over 1,000,000 male and female youths participate in hockey programs in Canada and the USA [9]. Langlois et al. [10] has estimated that as many as 1.6–3.8 million sport-related concussions happen in the USA annually. As such, this is a much greater concern beyond the athletes who participate at the professional level. In this report we review the incidence, evaluation, treatment, return-to-play protocol, and prevention efforts related to concussion in ice hockey.

Incidence

Calculation of the incidence of concussion in hockey is more difficult because of both the potential for underreporting and the lack of a standard reporting rate unit. Concussions per year, concussions per athlete exposures (AE; one athlete participating in one game, in which they are exposed to the possibility of athletic injury), concussions per game player-hours, and concussion per players per season have all been used in reporting concussion incidence in the literature.

In 2011–2012, the NHL reported approximately 90 players missed games due to concussion [11]. This is consistent with a mean of 80 concussions per year, 1.8 per 1,000 game player-hours, and 5.8% of players diagnosed from 1997 to 2004 [12]. Another report illustrated a slight decline in concussions from 1997 to 2008 with the most recent incidence of 1.26 concussions per 1,000 AE [13]. Incidence in the Swedish Elite League is similar with 5% of players per year experiencing a concussion [14].

Concussion rates vary depending on the level of play, players' age, and reporting methodology. In the USA National Collegiate Athletic Association (NCAA) programs, hockey has higher rates of concussion compared to other sports (0.41 per 1,000 AE for men and 0.91 per 1,000 AE for women) [15]. Another report lists the male concussion rate as 0.72 per 1,000 AE for men and 0.82 per 1,000 AE for women [16]. However, other published studies show a higher incidence in the same population at 3.1 per 1,000 AE, with concussion being the most common injury (18.6%) [17]. University hockey in New Zealand has been reported to have an incidence of 1.7 per 1,000 AE [18]. Echlin et al. [19] found a much larger incidence in Canada varsity hockey at 7.5 per 1,000 AE in men and 14.93 per 1,000 AE in women. USA high school male hockey has illustrated a much lower incidence at 0.54 per 1,000 AE [20]. Data related to the incidence of concussion in younger age groups is sparse.

A collision is nearly always the cause of concussion in hockey. Youth leagues that permit body-checking have an increased incidence of concussions. This is most clearly illustrated in leagues that have introduced body-checking into younger age groups [2, 21–24]. However, a substantial proportion of concussions occur in 'accidental contact' situations, and in youth or female leagues that do not allow body-checking. The NHL defines an accidental concussion as a hit from a teammate, a trip or fall (not caused by an opponent), being struck by a puck, or an inadvertent collision with an opponent [25]. They report that in 2010–2011, 26% of concussions were accidental (double from the year prior), resulting in 31% of concussion-related man-games lost (fivefold increase from 2009–2010). In the same year, 44% of concussions were from legal hits, 17% from illegal hits (41% in 2009–2010), and 8% from fights. Similar causative relationships have been seen in college and youth leagues as well. Nearly half of concussions in NCAA women's hockey are caused by player contact, despite no body-checking permitted [16]. Also, it was found that female concussion rates are similar to men in Canada [26]. USA youth hockey reports more concussions from unintentional collisions compared to intentional hitting, although more concussions overall were seen in leagues with body-checking [22]. In Canadian youth hockey, the most common cause of concussion was collisions with ice or boards [27].

Numerous other potential risk factors for concussion have also been studied. The vast majority (approx. 80%) of concussions occur in game situations compared to a practice environment [14–17, 20, 27]. This makes sense, as the level of aggressive play is heightened in games and against opponents. At all levels of play, studies report that forwards, especially centers, sustain proportionally more concussions than defensemen. Goalies have the least incidence [12, 13, 17, 27]. Fatigue during the game may impact susceptibility to concussions, as a NHL player's average ice time per game was found to be a significant predictor of concussion; the total ice time for the season and number of games played was not [28]. In Canadian youth hockey, data indicate that teams with more wins tend to have fewer concussions. There also appeared to be no relationship between total penalty minutes and concussions [29]. Finally, baseline historical symptoms may be a risk factor as well. In Canadian youth hockey, players who report preinjury headaches or neck pain are at increased risk for concussion [30].

Evaluation

Since signs and symptoms of potential concussion vary, both team management and players themselves need to be vigilant. Symptoms can include loss of consciousness, motor incoordination or balance problems (stumbling, slow/labored movements, etc.), a blank or vacant look, disorientation or confusion (inability to respond appropriately to questions), loss of memory, slow to get up after a hit to the head, disorientation, or clutching of the head after a hit. It is important to realize that a loss of consciousness is not required for a concussion to occur. Cognitive clouding, headache, and dizziness are the most common initial symptoms. Between 11 and 50% of players eventually diagnosed with concussion had delayed symptom onset [12, 31].

According to the NHL revised concussion protocol enacted in 2011, players suspected of having a concussion must now be removed from the game and taken to a quiet place for evaluation by a team physician. Prior to this, an examination could be completed on the bench. For the initial evaluation, the NHL and International Ice Hockey Federation (IIHF) both utilize the Sport Concussion Assessment Tool (SCAT). It is now in its third version [32], after its initial introduction in in 2005 [33]. SCAT3 presents a series of questions, and responses are given scores. It includes the Glasgow Coma Score (GCS), Standardized Assessment of Concussion (SAC) [34], Maddocks questions [35], and the Balance Error Scoring System (BESS) [36]. It also encompasses symptom evaluation, cognitive assessment and memory, neck examination, and coordination examination. SCAT3 is recognized as a standardized method of evaluating injured athletes (age >13 years) for concussion. Overall, any player diagnosed with a concussion should be removed from competition, monitored for deterioration, and not allowed to reenter the game.

Evaluators must be aware of indicators of more serious brain injury and the need for emergency management. These include GCS less than 15, deteriorating mental status, potential spine injury, progressive/worsening symptoms, or new neurologic signs. In these cases, the patient should be urgently transferred to a hospital and further imaging obtained (e.g. a CT scan to evaluate for skull fracture or intracranial hemorrhage). Approximately 5% of NHL concussions required further evaluation in a hospital [12].

Providers must also understand the possibility of a concomitant spine injury. Prior to off-ice evaluation, the player should not be allowed to sit up until it is determined that there is no neck pain, no numbness or tingling, normal muscle strength, and normal sensation to light touch.

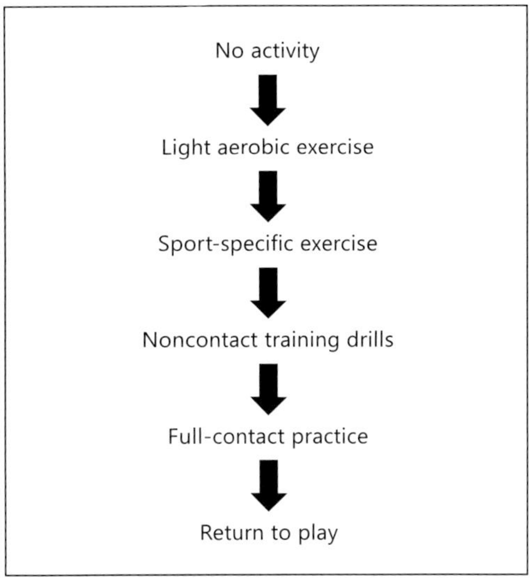

Fig. 1. Steps for return to play.

The concussed player may be observed if they are deemed stable without signs of serious complications. However, they must continue to be monitored for signs of deterioration over the next few days after the concussion. Worrisome signs and symptoms that require medical attending include worsening headache, excessive drowsiness, inability to recognize people or places, repeated vomiting, confusion, erratic behavior, increased irritability, seizures, reports of weakness or numbness in arms or legs, unsteadiness, and slurring of speech.

Return to Play

The First International Conference on Concussion in Sport in 2001 was the first to advocate a stepwise process for return to play [37]. The steps progress as follows: (1) no activity, (2) light aerobic exercise, (3) sport-specific exercise, (4) noncontact training drills, (5) full-contact practice, and (6) return to play (fig. 1). In the stepwise progression, the athlete should continue to proceed to the next level if asymptomatic at the current level. It is stated that each step should take at least 24 h so that an athlete would need at least 1 week to proceed through the full rehabilitation protocol once they are asymptomatic at rest and with provocative exercise. If any postconcussion symptoms occur while in the stepwise program, then the athlete should drop back to the previous asymptomatic level and try to progress again after another 24-hour period of rest has passed [32].

It is important to note that patients who are asymptomatic and have returned to their neuropsychological testing baseline at rest may still show neuropsychological decline after moderate exertion [38].

Table 1. Options for further treatment of concussion after an initial rest period

Therapy	Medication	Other
Physical therapy	Antidepressant	Hyperbaric oxygen
Vestibular therapy	Antimigraine	Meditation
Cognitive therapy		Biofeedback
		Massage

Further Treatment

While there has been a downward trend in concussion incidence, there has also been an upward trend in games missed per concussion [13]. From 1997 to 2004 in the NHL, 31% of players with concussions missed at least 10 days of activity. Patients with headaches, loss of consciousness, low energy or fatigue, or light sensitivity were at greater risk for longer recovery periods [12].

Care for patients with prolonged symptoms (>10 days) can be difficult. It requires a multidisciplinary approach in a coordinated center with special expertise. High-definition brain imaging using computed tomography or magnetic resonance imaging should be completed to rule out any underlying structural lesion, such as a cerebral contusion, Chiari malformation, or vascular malformation. Neuropsychological testing must be used to guide recovery. Immediate Measurement of Performance and Cognitive Testing (ImPACT) is often used to monitor recovery [39]. Its series of tests evaluate parameters including attention span, sustained and selective attention, reaction time, and several dimensions of memory. Persistent associated symptoms such as depression or anxiety may require additional medical management. Although other advanced imaging modalities are not routinely used, diffusion tensor imaging [40], functional magnetic resonance imaging, magnetic resonance spectroscopy [41], electroencephalography, and magnetoencephalography [42] have detected more subtle changes in selected patients with concussions. Investigations on the utility of genetic testing are also ongoing. After a short initial period of rest, more intense rehabilitation efforts including vestibular therapy, cognitive therapy, meditation, biofeedback, hyperbaric oxygen, and massage may be beneficial. Medications such as sertraline, amantadine, and antimigraine agents have provided benefit to some patients (table 1) [43].

Prevention

Equipment/Environment

Helmet use in the NHL was instituted for the 1979–1980 season, more than 50 years after head protection was first introduced. In 1929, the first leather facemask was worn by a by goalie. Jacques Plante used a facemask regularly for the Montreal Canadiens in 1959. Overall, NHL helmet use increased after Bill Masterson died in 1968 due to a head injury, but it was not made mandatory until 11 years later. Elsewhere, helmet use in Sweden began in the 1950s and became mandatory in 1963. In Canada, helmet use was mandated for youth hockey in 1965, a requirement that began shortly thereafter in the USA. After 2 deaths of amateur hockey players in Canada in the late 1960s, a call for new helmet technology led to the development of the Canadian Standards Association (CSA). The International Organization of Standardization (ISO) developed its first draft standards for helmets in 1987. Four official standards, including the Committee European Normalisation (CEN), ISO, CSA, and the American Society for Testing and Materials (ATSM), regulate helmet design and construction [44]. New technologies are currently being evaluated in order to make better, more protective helmets.

In all levels of youth hockey and many senior levels, full face shields are worn with the helmet. Most studies indicate that full face protection does not lessen the incidence of concussion compared to partial face protection or no face protection [45, 46]. However, Asplund et al. [47] reported that face protection could reduce concussion severity and result in an earlier return to play. Face protection did reduce nonconcussion head, face, and eye injuries. Similarly, the use of mouth guards did not reduce concussion in the NHL [48].

Equipment created for body protection has also been identified as an increased risk factor for head injury. Shoulder and elbow pads have increased in size and have incorporated harder material. Adjustments are attempting to be made to pad these hard surfaces, while still retaining adequate protection for the player [13].

The first hockey games were played outside on frozen ponds in the late 18th century. As the game moved indoors to a more enclosed space, the risk of collision and injury increased. European and Olympic hockey rinks are larger than those in the USA and Canada. Fewer collisions, head impacts, and injuries are seen in these rinks, and larger rinks may reduce the incidence of concussions [49].

Other preventative measures instituted by the NHL include the removal of seamless glass surrounding NHL rinks, additional assessment of ways to modify player equipment to make it safer, and a proposal that would hold teams, and perhaps coaches, responsible for the behavior of repeat offenders in the disciplinary process [7].

Rules/Suspensions

Rule changes have been implemented in all levels of hockey. In the NHL, rule 48 'renders illegal any lateral or blindside hit where the head is targeted and/or becomes the principle point of contact' [7]. Concurrently, suspensions are given and fines (over USD 2,400,000 in the 2011–2012 NHL season) [11] are levied to those players for illegal and dangerous hits. Concussions related to illegal hits have decreased in the NHL [25]. Despite this, there is still support for a no-tolerance ban to all hits to the head similar to the NCAA. Hits to the head in the NCAA result in a major penalty and an immediate game misconduct [50].

As mentioned previously, youth leagues with body-checking have increased risk of concussions. Past rule changes have reduced the age at which checking is allowed. As more data is reported, adjustments to increase the body-checking age have been made. As children begin to play sports at a younger age, they are at more risk for injury and concussion due to a longer playing career. Prevention of concussion must begin at the initial stages.

Education

Echlin [51] illustrated the differences and attitudes towards concussions between members of the team, including the coach, physician, athlete, trainer/first responder, athletic administration, and parents. In addition to attitudes, knowledge concerning rules, concussion recognition, and treatment varies. It has been reported that scattered youth hockey coaches allow players with concussion symptoms to reenter the game, depending on whether the coach thinks a 'minor' or 'major' concussion was sustained [52]. Programs, such as the ThinkFirst Canada have shown promising results with improvement in concussion knowledge, reduction in cross-checking, and major penalties for players who target players from behind [53]. DVDs and interactive computer modules have been used to educate players with positive results [54]. The Hockey Education Program (HEP), which includes Fair Play, Play It Cool (PIC), and other educational programs for coaches, parents, and athletes, has also been implemented and disseminated [1].

Conclusion

With mainstream media attention, many issues associated with concussion recognition have been brought to the forefront of the game. Standardized protocols have been put in place and rules have been created or modified. There is concern that banning certain hits will take the physical nature out of hockey. However, player safety must be of primary concern. Rules and equipment must continue to evolve, with steady improvement in better strategies for recognizing and treating concussions.

References

1 Smith AM, Stuart MJ, Greenwald RM, Benson BW, Dodick DW, Emery CA, Finnoff JT, Mihalik JP, Roberts WO, Sullivan CA, Meeuwisse WH: Proceedings from the ice hockey summit on concussion: a call to action. Clin J Sport Med 2011;21:281–287.

2 Safety in youth ice hockey: the effects of body checking. American Academy of Pediatrics. Committee on Sports Medicine and Fitness. Pediatrics 2000;105:657–658.

3 Williamson IJ, Goodman D: Converging evidence for the under-reporting of concussions in youth ice hockey. Br J Sports Med 2006;40:128–132.

4 Fekete JF: Severe brain injury and death following minor hockey accidents: the effectiveness of the 'safety helmets' of amateur hockey players. Can Med Assoc J 1968;99:1234–1239.

5 Garofalo P: For NHL players, concussions last a lifetime. April 22, 2013. http://www.usnews.com/opinion/blogs/pat-garofalo/2013/04/22/study-shows-nhl-concussions-last-a-lifetime (accessed May 20, 2013).

6 Branch J: Hockey players' deaths pose a tragic riddle. September 1, 2011. http://www.nytimes.com/2011/09/02/sports/hockey/deaths-of-three-nhl-players-raises-a-deadly-riddle.html?pagewanted=all (accessed May 20, 2013).
7 Roarke S: Bettman discusses concussions, player safety. March 14, 2011. http://www.nhl.com/ice/news.htm?id=556046 (accessed May 20, 2013).
8 Rosen D: New concussion protocol goes into effect tonight. March 16, 2011. http://www.nhl.com/ice/news.htm?id=556289 (accessed May 20, 2013).
9 Hemond C: Hockey concussion: is it child abuse? CMAJ 2012;184:861–862.
10 Langlois JA, Rutland-Brown W, Wald MM: The epidemiology and impact of traumatic brain injury: a brief overview. J Head Trauma Rehabil 2006;21:375–378.
11 Whamsby T: Final concussions and suspensions list. April 10, 2012. http://www.cbc.ca/sports/hockey/opinion/2012/04/concussions-and-suspensions-list.html (accessed May 20, 2013).
12 Benson BW, Meeuwisse WH, Rizos J, Kang J, Burke CJ: A prospective study of concussions among National Hockey League players during regular season games: the NHL-NHLPA Concussion Program. CMAJ 2011;183:905–911.
13 Wennberg RA, Tator CH: Concussion incidence and time lost from play in the NHL during the past ten years. Can J Neurol Sci 2008;35:647–651.
14 Tegner Y, Lorentzon R: Concussion among Swedish elite ice hockey players. Br J Sports Med 1996;30:251–255.
15 Hootman JM, Dick R, Agel J: Epidemiology of collegiate injuries for 15 sports: summary and recommendations for injury prevention initiatives. J Athl Train 2007;42:311–319.
16 Agel J, Harvey EJ: A 7-year review of men's and women's ice hockey injuries in the NCAA. Can J Surg 2010;53:319–323.
17 Flik K, Lyman S, Marx RG: American collegiate men's ice hockey: an analysis of injuries. Am J Sports Med 2005;33:183–187.
18 Rishiraj N, Lloyd-Smith R, Lorenz T, Niven B, Michel M: University men's ice hockey: rates and risk of injuries over 6-years. J Sports Med Phys Fitness 2009;49:159–166.
19 Echlin PS, Skopelja EN, Worsley R, Dadachanji SB, Lloyd-Smith DR, Taunton JA, Forwell LA, Johnson AM: A prospective study of physician-observed concussion during a varsity university ice hockey season: incidence and neuropsychological changes. Part 2 of 4. Neurosurg Focus 2012;33:1–11.
20 Marar M, McIlvain NM, Fields SK, Comstock RD: Epidemiology of concussions among United States high school athletes in 20 sports. Am J Sports Med 2012;40:747–755.
21 Cusimano MD, Taback NA, McFaull SR, Hodgins R, Bekele TM, Elfeki N; Canadian Research Team in Traumatic Brain Injury and Violence: Effect of bodychecking on rate of injuries among minor hockey players. Open Med 2011;5:e57–e64.
22 Darling SR, Schaubel DE, Baker JG, Leddy JJ, Bisson LJ, Willer B: Intentional versus unintentional contact as a mechanism of injury in youth ice hockey. Br J Sports Med 2011;45:492–497.
23 Marchie A, Cusimano MD: Bodychecking and concussions in ice hockey: should our youth pay the price? CMAJ 2003;169:124–128.
24 Emery CA, Hagel B, Decloe M, Carly M: Risk factors for injury and severe injury in youth ice hockey: a systematic review of the literature. Inj Prev 2010;16:113–118.
25 Roarke S: Study: time lost from illegal hits are down. March 14, 2011. http://www.nhl.com/ice/news.htm?id=555980 (accessed May 20, 2013).
26 Schick DM, Meeuwisse WH: Injury rates and profiles in female ice hockey players. Am J Sports Med 2003;31:47–52.
27 Goodman D, Gaetz M, Meichenbaum D: Concussions in hockey: there is cause for concern. Med Sci Sports Exerc 2001;33:2004–2009.
28 Stevens ST, Lassonde M, de Beaumont L, Keenan JP: In-game fatigue influences concussions in national hockey league players. Res Sports Med 2008;16:68–74.
29 Emery CA, Kang J, Schneider KJ, Meeuwisse WH: Risk of injury and concussion associated with team performance and penalty minutes in competitive youth ice hockey. Br J Sports Med 2011;45:1289–1293.
30 Schneider KJ, Meeuwisse WH, Kang J, Schneider GM, Emery CA: Preseason reports of neck pain, dizziness, and headache as risk factors for concussion in male youth ice hockey players. Clin J Sport Med 2013;23:267–272.
31 Duhaime AC, Beckwith JG, Maerlender AC, McAllister TW, Crisco JJ, Duma SM, Brolinson PG, Rowson S, Flashman LA, Chu JJ, Greenwald RM: Spectrum of acute clinical characteristics of diagnosed concussions in college athletes wearing instrumented helmets: clinical article. J Neurosurg 2012;117:1092–1099.
32 McCrory P, Meeuwisse WH, Aubry M, Cantu B, Dvorák J, Echemendia RJ, Engebretsen L, Johnston K, Kutcher JS, Raftery M, Sills A, Benson BW, Davis GA, Ellenbogen RG, Guskiewicz K, Herring SA, Iverson GL, Jordan BD, Kissick J, McCrea M, McIntosh AS, Maddocks D, Makdissi M, Purcell L, Putukian M, Schneider K, Tator CH, Turner M: Consensus statement on concussion in sport: the 4th International Conference on Concussion in Sport held in Zurich, November 2012. Br J Sports Med 2013;47:250–258.

33 McCrory P, Johnston K, Meeuwisse W, Aubry M, Cantu R, Dvorak J, Graf-Baumann T, Kelly J, Lovell M, Schamasch P: Summary and agreement statement of the 2nd International Conference on Concussion in Sport, Prague 2004. Br J Sports Med 2005; 39:196–204.
34 McCrea M: Standardized mental status testing on the sideline after sport-related concussion. J Athl Train 2001;36:274–279.
35 Maddocks DL, Dicker GD, Saling MM: The assessment of orientation following concussion in athletes. Clin J Sport Med 1995;5:32–35.
36 Guskiewicz KM: Assessment of postural stability following sport-related concussion. Curr Sports Med Rep 2003;2:24–30.
37 Aubry M, Cantu R, Dvorak J, Graf-Baumann T, Johnston K, Kelly J, Lovell M, McCrory P, Meeuwisse W, Schamasch P; Concussion in Sport Group: Summary and agreement statement of the First International Conference on Concussion in Sport, Vienna 2001. Recommendations for the improvement of safety and health of athletes who may suffer concussive injuries. Br J Sports Med 2002;36:6–10.
38 McGrath N, Dinn WM, Collins MW, Lovell MR, Elbin RJ, Kontos AP: Post-exertion neurocognitive test failure among student-athletes following concussion. Brain Inj 2013;27:103–113.
39 Maroon JC, Lovell MR, Norwig J, Podell K, Powell JW, Hartl R: Cerebral concussion in athletes: evaluation and neuropsychological testing. Neurosurgery 2000;47:659–669.
40 Koerte IK, Kaufmann D, Hartl E, Bouix S, Pasternak O, Kubicki M, Rauscher A, Li DK, Dadachanji SB, Taunton JA, Forwell LA, Johnson AM, Echlin PS, Shenton ME: A prospective study of physician-observed concussion during a varsity university hockey season: white matter integrity in ice hockey players. Part 3 of 4. Neurosurg Focus 2012;33:1–7.
41 Chamard E, Théoret H, Skopelja EN, Forwell LA, Johnson AM, Echlin PS: A prospective study of physician-observed concussion during a varsity university hockey season: metabolic changes in ice hockey players. Part 4 of 4. Neurosurg Focus 2012;33:1–7.
42 Tormenti M, Krieger D, Puccio AM, McNeil MR, Schneider W, Okonkwo DO: Magnetoencephalographic virtual recording: a novel diagnostic tool for concussion. Neurosurg Focus 2012;6:1–7.
43 Makdissi M, Cantu RC, Johnston KM, McCrory P, Meeuwisse WH: The difficult concussion patient: what is the best approach to investigation and management of persistent (>10 days) postconcussive symptoms? Br J Sports Med 2013;47:308–313.
44 Biasca N, Wirth S, Tegner Y: The avoidability of head and neck injuries in ice hockey: an historical review. Br J Sports Med 2002;36:410–427.
45 Stevens ST, Lassonde M, de Beaumont L, Keenan JP: The effect of visors on head and facial injury in National Hockey League players. J Sci Med Sport 2006; 9:238–242.
46 Benson BW, Rose MS, Meeuwisse WH: The impact of face shield use on concussions in ice hockey: a multivariate analysis. Br J Sports Med 2002;36:27–32.
47 Asplund C, Bettcher S, Borchers J: Facial protection and head injuries in ice hockey: a systematic review. Br J Sports Med 2009;43:993–999.
48 Benson BW, Hamilton GM, Meeuwisse WH, McCrory P, Dvorak J: Is protective equipment useful in preventing concussion? A systematic review of the literature. Br J Sports Med 2009;43:i56–i67.
49 Wennberg R: Effect of ice surface size on collision rates and head impacts at the World Junior Hockey Championships, 2002 to 2004. Clin J Sport Med 2005;15:67–72.
50 Peters C: NHL concussion crisis requires further rule changes. February 26, 2013. http://www.cbssports.com/nhl/blog/eye-on-hockey/21773717/nhl-concussion-crisis-requires-further-rule-changes (accessed May 20, 2013).
51 Echlin PS: A prospective study of physician-observed concussion during a varsity university ice hockey season. Part 1 of 4. Neurosurg Focus 2012;33: 1–7.
52 Bramley H, Kroft C, Polk D, Newberry T, Silvis M: Do youth hockey coaches allow players with a known concussion to participate in a game? Clin Pediatr (Phila) 2012;51:283–287.
53 Cook DJ, Cusimano MD, Tator CH, Chipman ML: Evaluation of the ThinkFirst Canada, Smart Hockey, brain and spinal cord injury prevention video. Inj Prev 2003;9:361–366.
54 Echlin PS, Johnson AM, Riverin S, Tator CH, Cantu RC, Cusimano MD, Taunton JE, Upshur RE, Hall CR, Forwell LA, Skopelja EN: A prospective study of concussion education in 2 junior ice hockey teams: implications for sports concussion education. Neurosurg Focus 2010;29:E6.

Christopher M. Bonfield, MD
Department of Neurological Surgery, Center for Sports Medicine
University of Pittsburgh Medical Center, 200 Lothrop Street Suite B-400
Pittsburgh, PA 15213 (USA)
E-Mail bonfieldcm@upmc.edu

Niranjan A, Lunsford LD (eds): Concussion. Prog Neurol Surg. Basel, Karger, 2014, vol 28, pp 171–183
DOI: 10.1159/000358778

Management of Concussion in the Professional Football Player

Elizabeth M. Pieroth[a] · Christopher Hanks[b]

[a]NorthShore University HealthSystem, Glenview, Ill., and [b]Chicago Bears Football Club, Chicago, Ill., USA

Abstract

There is no other sport that has come under greater scrutiny surrounding the incidence and treatment of concussion than football, and there is no other professional sports league that has experienced more intense focus of its handling of concussions than the National Football League (NFL). The NFL has received significant criticism of their management of concussion in players from both the popular press and the medical community. However, those working with active NFL players have changed their assessment and treatment of these injuries as the knowledge of concussions has evolved over time. We review the current approach to the management of concussions in the professional football player.
© 2014 S. Karger AG, Basel

Football has long been considered a dangerous sport. After the deaths of eighteen collegiate and high school football players in 1904, President Theodore Roosevelt, a strident fan of the game, gathered the head coaches of Harvard, Yale, and Princeton to the White House on October 9, 1905. He warned the teams to reduce the level of violence or risk the abolishment of collegiate football [1].

However, little changed and there were 19 deaths in the 1905 season. Another meeting of collegiate football leaders was conducted at the White House in the off-season with the goal to 'minimize the danger' without football becoming 'too ladylike'. An intercollegiate conference was formed, which would later develop into the NCAA, and approved changes that would be implemented in the 1906 season. Fatalities and injuries did decline, and additional safety measures were enacted after a 1909 conference attended by football officials from the most prestigious universities, including the then president of Princeton University, Woodrow Wilson [2]. Since that time, countless rule changes and advances in the quality of player equipment have been made, greatly improving the safety of the sport. However, football continues to have the highest number of traumatic brain injuries, including concussions, in youth sports [3] (table 1).

Over the past decade the media has taken a much closer look at how concussions have been handled by the National Football League (NFL). Public awareness was significantly

Table 1. Sport-specific injury rates[a] in practice, competition, and overall in the USA (2005–2006 school year): High School Sports-Related Injury Surveillance Study [20]

Sport	Rate		
	practice	competition	overall
Boys' football	2.54	12.09	4.36
Boys' wrestling	2.04	3.93	2.50
Boys' soccer	1.58	4.22	2.43
Girls' soccer	1.10	5.21	2.36
Girls' basketball	1.37	3.60	2.01
Boys' basketball	1.46	2.98	1.89
Girls' volleyball	1.48	1.92	1.64
Boys' baseball	0.87	1.77	1.19
Girls' softball	0.79	1.78	1.13
Total	1.69	4.63	2.44

[a] Per 1,000 athlete exposures (i.e. practices or competitions).

raised after a series of articles by Allen Schwarz was published in *The New York Times* [4–6]. Other publications, such as the 2011 piece in *The New Yorker* provocatively titled, 'Does football have a future: the NFL and the concussion crisis', brought further attention to this issue [7]. The question of how the NFL has managed concussions was even debated on Capitol Hill in October 2009 [8]. The recent settlement of USD 765,000,000 between the NFL and more than 4,000 retired NFL players has not silenced the critics of the sport [9]. However, there remains little consensus on the possible long-term sequelae of participation in football or other contact sports amongst researchers.

While the debate about concussions in football rages on, there are 1,602 active NFL players each year who require medical care for a variety of injuries, including concussions. A thorough review of the literature on concussions in football or within the NFL is outside the scope of this report. The focus of this report is detailing how the medical professions working with NFL players assess and manage concussions in their athletes. The first author (E.M.P.) has 16 years of experience as a sports neuropsychologist and has spent the last 10 years as the consulting neuropsychologist to the Chicago Bears. The second author (C.H.) has worked as a certified athletic trainer for 24 years, the last 14 years with the Chicago Bears.

A Brief History of the NFL Concussion Program

The NFL's Committee on Concussion was first announced in 2009 and developed in conjunction with team physicians, unaffiliated medical experts, and the NFL Players Association (NFLPA). The initial return-to-play guidelines initially presented in 2007 were expanded to include the requirement that any concussed player be fully asymptomatic at both rest and with exertion, have a normal neurological examination, normal neuropsychological testing, and be cleared by the team physician and the neurological consultant.

In March 2010, the NFL announced the Committee on Concussion would be renamed 'The NFL Head, Neck and Spine Medical Committee' (HNS). Two neurosurgeons, Hunt Batjer, MD, and Richard Ellenbogen, MD, were chosen as co-committee chairs. The HNS was designed to provide a platform for disseminating current research and providing education on concussions to the teams' medical personnel. The HNS is tasked with formulating and implementing the best practices in the management of concussions for players in the NFL.

The Current NFL Program

The existing NFL concussion protocol has a number of components: player education, preseason physicals and cognitive testing, identification of injuries during practice and game play, and treatment of the concussed athlete.

Prior to the Season

An important part of any concussion program is the education of athletes, which has been a long-standing focus with NFL players. All NFL players are provided with information about the signs/symptoms of concussion, as well as the management of these injuries. This includes informational seminars, educational literature, and posting of concussion posters in each NFL locker room (fig. 1). The NFL concussion posters were based on information available from the Centers for Disease Control and Prevention (CDC) and produced by agreement of the NFL, NFL Players Association, NFL Physicians Society, and NFL Athletic Trainers Society.

Preseason physicals are required by the Collective Bargaining Agreement (CBA) between the NFL and the NFL Players Association. In addition to standard medical testing (lab work, EKGs, X-rays), physicians also review each player's concussion history during their physical. Particular emphasis is placed on players who had been diagnosed with multiple concussions or sustained a concussion during the past season. Each player is also administered a baseline SCAT3 (Sport Concussion Assessment Tool) [10] to assess basic cognition and balance functioning.

Baseline neurocognitive testing (discussed in greater detail later in this report) is completed during this off-season period as well. The Chicago Bears and many other NFL teams utilize ImPACT (Immediate Post-Concussion Assessment and Cognitive Testing) [11] for their neuropsychological baseline assessments. All players are required to complete a baseline neurocognitive test before the start of training camp in July. There is variability between NFL teams in the frequency of retesting. The Chicago Bears require any player with a baseline assessment older

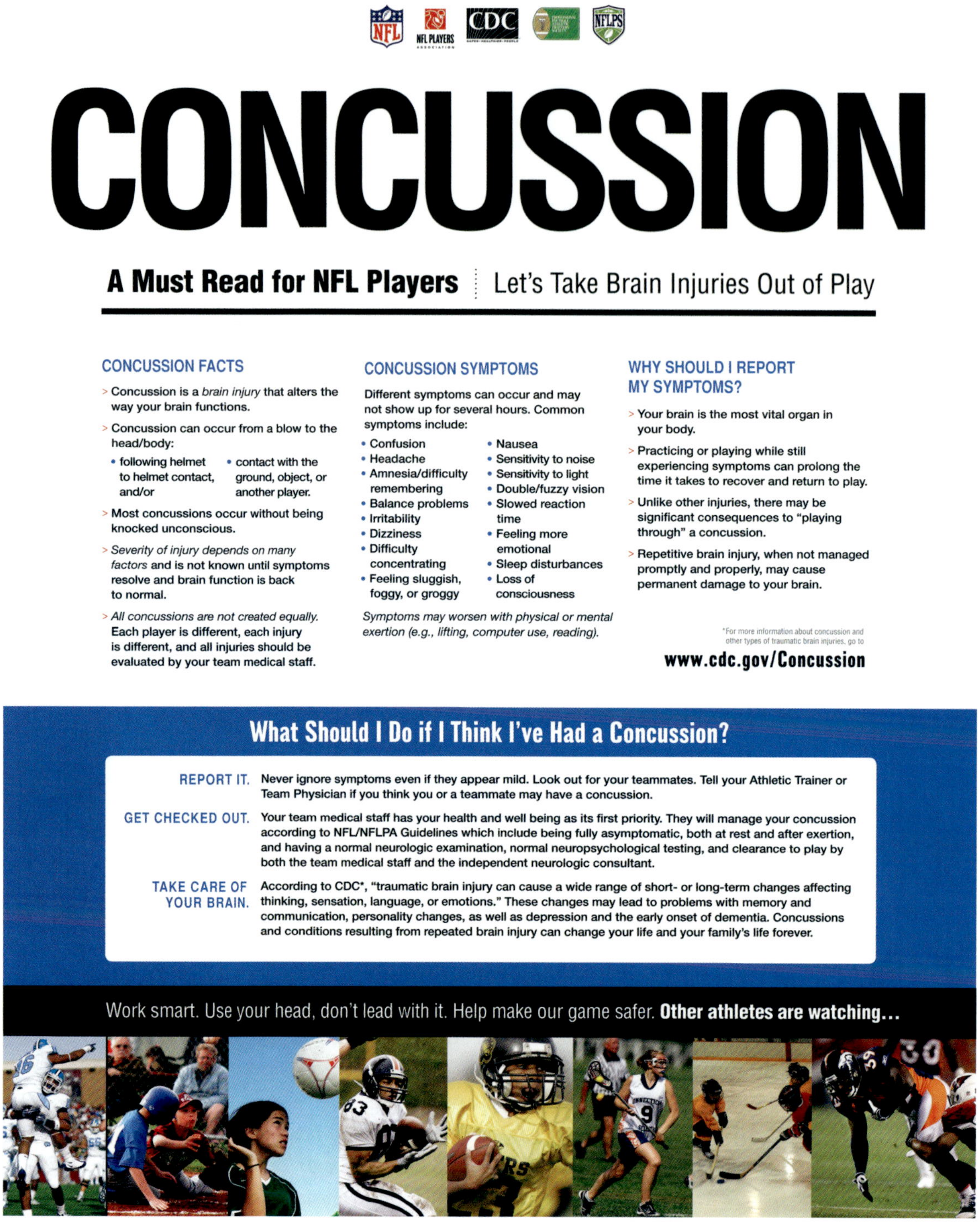

Fig. 1. Educational poster about sport-related concussion [18, http://www.cdc.gov/concussion/pdf/NFL_Player_Poster-a.pdf].

than 3 years to be readministered a baseline test. In addition, any player who sustained a concussion in the prior season will also complete a new baseline ImPACT.

Practice and Game Day

The underreporting of concussions by athletes has long been documented [12], and continues to be a challenge for the medical staff of any sport team. This is particularly difficult for the NFL on-field medical staff who have large numbers of athletes to care for and who may be unable to watch the behaviors of each player. To address this issue, the NFL enacted a new rule in the 2012–2013 season that required each game to have an athletic trainer, who was not affiliated with either team, monitoring the players from the press box to serve as a 'spotter' for both teams. This 'eye in the sky' is able to watch both sidelines, as well review specific plays where he/she feels there was enough contact to cause a concussion.

The position in the skybox also allows the unaffiliated athletic trainer to watch all players for on- or off-field behavior that may be indicative of a concussion. This includes a player who shows gait disturbance ('wobbly'), is slow to return to their position, or holds their hands to their head after contact suggesting pain. The unaffiliated athletic trainer may also simply advise the on-field medical staff that a player took a direct contact to the head and should be examined, even if no outward behaviors are observed.

The unaffiliated athletic trainer has the ability to radio down to the sidelines to speak with a team physician or head athletic trainer to alert them of a possible injury. The medical staff is then able to review the play on a monitor stationed on the sidelines and assess the player in question. The intent of this system was to assist with concussion, but it has been used to review other injuries as well. However, this system is used only during game play and not during practice.

The HNS Committee also requires the use of a computerized sideline concussion assessment tool for NFL medical staff (fig. 2). This tool was created by X2 Biosystems [13] for use on tablets and is utilized during a game or practice if a concussion is suspected. As noted, each player is administered the SCAT3 test prior to the season and this information is entered into X2 Biosystems' database. If an athlete is being evaluated for a possible concussion, they can be reassessed on the sideline or training room and this information can be easily entered on a tablet device and then compared to the baseline data. NFL players can change teams, which can create difficulty in sharing medical data between teams. The X2 Biosystems program is tied in with the NFL head office so the baseline data can be automatically downloaded to the new team's database. This computerized system allows for improved record keeping as well.

After a player is diagnosed with a concussion, he is required to immediately be removed from the field for further evaluation in the locker room. This is referred to as the Madden Rule, which was adopted at the recommendation of former coach John Madden, and is followed by all NFL teams. This allows for further evaluation and constant

This tool does not constitute, and is not intended to constitute, a standard of medical care. It is a guide derived from the Standardized Concussion Assessment Tool 2 (SCAT2) (McCrory, et al, BJSM '09) and represents a standardized method of evaluating NFL players for concussion consistent with the reasonable, objective practice of the healthcare profession. This guide is not intended to be a substitute for the clinical judgment of the treating healthcare professional and should be interpreted based on the individual needs of the patient and the specific facts and circumstances presented.

NFL Sideline Concussion Assessment Tool: BASELINE TEST. Athlete completes blue sections. ATC/MD/DO completes sheet.

Athlete ____________ Position ____________ Team ____________ Athlete Initials _____

Date & Time of Baseline Test: Date _____ Time ____am / pm Evaluator ____________ ATC / MD / DO /Other

RISK FACTORS:

Concussion History

Have you EVER had a concussion, had your "bell rung", or had any of the symptoms below as a result of a head injury? Y N

If yes, previous number 0 1 2 3 4 5 6+

What type of symptoms did you have? ____________

How long were you out of activity? ____________

Have you ever lost consciousness as a result of a head injury? Y N If yes, how long? ____________

Have you ever been hospitalized as a result of a head injury? Y N Details ____________

Have you ever had any imaging tests of your brain (CT, MRI, DTI, other)? Y N Details ____________

Date of most recent concussion? ________

Additional Risk Factors: Personal History

Have you ever been diagnosed with:

- ☐ Headache or migraines?
- ☐ Learning disability / dyslexia?
- ☐ ADD / ADHD?
- ☐ Depression, anxiety or other psychiatric disorder?
- ☐ Seizure disorder?

Family History

Has anyone in your family ever been diagnosed with:

- ☐ Headache or migraines?
- ☐ Learning disability / dyslexia
- ☐ ADD / ADHD
- ☐ Depression, anxiety or other psychiatric disorder?
- ☐ Seizure disorder?

Are you on any medications? If yes please list ____________

How do you feel? The athlete should score themselves on the following symptoms, based on how they feel at the time.
(i.e. 0 = not present, 1 = mild, 3 = moderate, 6 = severe)

Symptom	Score	Symptom	Score
Headache / head pressure	0 1 2 3 4 5 6	Feeling slowed down	0 1 2 3 4 5 6
Nausea / vomiting	0 1 2 3 4 5 6	Sensitivity to noise	0 1 2 3 4 5 6
Neck pain	0 1 2 3 4 5 6	Sensitivity to light	0 1 2 3 4 5 6
Drowsiness	0 1 2 3 4 5 6	Visual problems /blurred vision	0 1 2 3 4 5 6
Balance problems	0 1 2 3 4 5 6	Sleeping more than usual	0 1 2 3 4 5 6
Dizziness	0 1 2 3 4 5 6	Sleeping less than usual	0 1 2 3 4 5 6
Fatigue / low energy	0 1 2 3 4 5 6	Trouble falling asleep	0 1 2 3 4 5 6
Confusion	0 1 2 3 4 5 6	Sadness	0 1 2 3 4 5 6
"Don't feel right"	0 1 2 3 4 5 6	Nervous or anxious	0 1 2 3 4 5 6
Feeling "in a fog"	0 1 2 3 4 5 6	Feeling more emotional	0 1 2 3 4 5 6
Difficulty remembering	0 1 2 3 4 5 6	Irritability	0 1 2 3 4 5 6
Difficulty concentrating	0 1 2 3 4 5 6	Numbness or tingling	0 1 2 3 4 5 6

Total # Symptoms: of 24 = ____ Symptom Severity Score: (max 24 symptoms X max 6 rating) of 144 = ____

Athlete should initial in upper right hand corner that information provided above is accurate to the best of their knowledge

BELOW IS FOR ATC / MD / DO / OTHER PROVIDER USE ONLY

Select Physical Signs or Symptoms: Screen for Cervical Spine and/or More Serious Brain Trauma

Any reported neck pain, c-spine tenderness or decreased range of motion? Y N

Pupil reaction abnormal or pupils unequal ? Y N

Extra-ocular movements abnormal and/or cause double vision? Y N

Asymmetry or abnormalities on screening motor or sensory exam? Y N

Other ____________

Fig. 2. NFL sideline concussion assessment tool [19].

NFL Sideline Concussion Assessment Tool: BASELINE TEST (continued)

ORIENTATION / SAC	**of 5 = ____**	
What month is it?	0	1
What is the date today?	0	1
What is the day of the week?	0	1
What year is it?	0	1
What time is it right now? (within an hour)	0	1

SAC / Word Recall: Read list of 5 words 1 per second, ask athlete to repeat list, in any order. (Use of specific lists below optional) For Trial 2 & 3, read the same list of words again and have athlete repeat them back, in any order. One point for each word remembered. You must conduct all 3 trials regardless of their success on trial 1. **Do not tell athlete that delayed recall will be tested**

List 1	**Immediate Recall Trials #1**	**#2**	**#3**	**Alternative Lists**		**Delayed recall (perform at end of all sideline testing, at least > 5 minutes)**
elbow	______	______	______	candle	baby	______
apple	______	______	______	paper	monkey	______
carpet	______	______	______	sugar	perfume	______
saddle	______	______	______	sandwich	sunset	______
bubble	______	______	______	wagon	iron	______

Total of all three immediate word recalls: out of 15 = _____

Total delayed recall: out of 5 = _____

SAC / Concentration: Read string of numbers, ask athlete to repeat backwards. (Use of specific numbers below optional). If correct go to the next string length. If incorrect, read second string (same length) 1 point for each string length correct. Stop after incorrect on both trials. Read digits at rate of 1 digit /sec

Digits Backward:			**Alternative digit lists**	
4-9-3	0	1	6-2-9	5-2-6
3-8-1-4	0	1	3-2-7-9	1-7-9-5
6-2-9-7-1	0	1	1-5-2-8-6	3-8-5-2-7
7-1-8-4-6-2	0	1	5-3-9-1-4-8	8-3-1-9-6-4

SAC / Concentration cont. Months in reverse order

Dec - Nov - Oct - Sept - Aug - Jul - Jun - May - Apr - Mar - Feb - Jan

1 point for months in reverse correctly (< 30 sec) = ____

1 point for each sequence correct of 4 = _____

Total of SAC Concentration of 5 = _____

Modified BESS: This is calculated by adding 1 error point for each error during the three 20-sec tests. The maximum total # of errors for any single condition is 10. The higher the score, the worse is the player's balance.

Balance testing – types of errors

1. Hands lifted off iliac crest
2. Opening eyes
3. Step, stumble, or fall
4. Moving hip into > 30 degrees abduction
5. Lifting forefoot or heel
6. Remaining out of test position > 5 sec

Which foot tested (non-dominant foot) ☐ L ☐ R

Double leg stance (feet together)	# errors ___
Single leg stance (non dominant foot)	# errors ___
Tandem stance (non dominant foot at back)	# errors ___

BALANCE SCORE: (summed # of errors) = ____

SCORING:

All SAC scores (summed orange boxes)	= ___ of 30
BALANCE Score: (summed BESS Errors)	= ___
Symptom Score: (# symptoms reported)	= ___ of 24

ADDITIONAL COMMENTS: ____________________

____

____

____

____

____

Fig. 2. Continued.

supervision in a quiet setting for a player suffering from a concussion. It also provides privacy for a player who might be exhibiting the signs of a concussion, as all games are televised and the cameras frequently focus on injured players on the sidelines.

For the 2013–2014 season, the NFL, on the recommendation of the HNS Committee and NFL Players Union, also required that an unaffiliated neurotrauma consultant be stationed on each sideline during games to provide a second opinion in the assessment and treatment of any traumatic brain injury or spine trauma. These neurosurgeons are independent of the teams and are able to provide impartial assistance if deemed necessary by the team physician. The unaffiliated neurotrauma consultants are also affiliated with local hospitals and are able to take over emergent care if a severely injured player requires transport from the field to the hospital. The unaffiliated neurotrauma consultant is not utilized during NFL practices.

After Injury

Each NFL team is required to have both a consulting neurologist and neuropsychologist. The NFL consulting neuropsychologists are clinicians who are experienced in the assessment and management of concussive injuries in athletes. They are not employees of the team, but act as independent consultants to the team's medical staff. The degree of involvement by the consulting neuropsychologist is not mandated by the NFL concussion protocol, but rather determined by each individual team. However, all NFL teams must utilize an unaffiliated neuropsychologist to administer and interpret postinjury cognitive tests with athletes who have been diagnosed with a concussion. The neuropsychologists provide an opinion regarding any evidence of residual cognitive impairment or psychological issues related to the injury, but does not make the final return-to-play decision. This is the responsibility of the team physician after consulting with both the independent neuropsychologist and neurologist.

The consulting neuropsychologist may become involved in the care of concussed athlete at various points in the recovery process, depending on the team's policy. The Chicago Bears, along with many other NFL teams, involve the neuropsychologist as soon as the injury has been diagnosed by the game-day staff. The neuropsychologist is advised of the mechanism of injury, the initial symptom presentation, any increase or resolution of symptoms during the initial monitoring of the injury, and general medical history of the player. Consulting neuropsychologists are typically not included as sideline staff, as the athletic trainers and team physicians are the most appropriate healthcare providers to diagnose and manage the concussed athlete at the time of injury. Any recommendation for further medical examination, such as neuroimaging or transport to a local emergency department, is outside the training of a neuropsychologist.

The timing of the initial appointment by the neuropsychologist is dependent on team policy as well. The Chicago Bears prefer to have the neuropsychologist provide an initial assessment within the first 1–2 days after the injury. This appointment does not typically involve cognitive testing, as the player is likely still symptomatic at that time. The appointment is focused on obtaining a thorough understanding of the injury, the current symptom profile, gathering of additional medical and psychological history, and providing education about concussion to the player. This opportunity for education to the athlete is one of the most important contributions by team neuropsychologists.

An NFL neuropsychological consultant is chosen because of his/her unique experience with concussed athletes and their thorough understanding of the current state of the science of concussions. Additionally, the neuropsychologist has the unique training to address psychological factors that may be impacting recovery. This may be a history of preexisting of psychiatric disorders, such as depression or anxiety, or may include the athlete's emotional reaction to the injury.

If the athlete continues to have persistent physical or cognitive symptoms of concussion, the neuropsychologist will review other possible causes of these symptoms (e.g. cervical injuries or persistent vestibular dysfunction). Recommendations for additional treatments, such as physical therapy, are then made in conjunction with the team's medical staff.

Once an athlete reports being fully asymptomatic, including not taking any medication for headaches, he is referred to the neuropsychologist for a cognitive assessment. The HNS Committee mandates that all postinjury neurocognitive test data be interpreted by the consulting neuropsychologist. The choice of tests administered by the neuropsychologist is not mandated by the NFL, but determined by the consulting neuropsychologist. For most NFL neuropsychologists, this includes administration of the ImPACT computerized test battery and an additional battery of traditional paper-and-pencil cognitive tests. Some NFL consulting neuropsychologists use only ImPACT after an injury, while others utilize only paper-and-pencil tests. Most NFL teams administer ImPACT to athletes prior to the season to obtain a baseline assessment of their functioning. A few teams also include paper-and-pencil tests in the baseline evaluations [McCrae, pers. commun., 2013].

Regardless of the chosen method of assessment, all NFL players diagnosed with a concussion are subjected to an evaluation of their cognitive and emotional functioning prior to being referred for a neurological consultation. All concussed athletes must report no subjective symptoms of concussion, not have any evidence of balance disturbance, and demonstrate intact neurocognitive functioning. Recovery of cognition after a concussion may be determined by comparison of baseline and preinjury cognitive test data if it has been determined that the baseline data is valid and reflective of the athlete's optimal cognitive abilities. The neuropsychological consultant must also review baseline data to ensure that the athlete did not purposefully reduce their baseline scores in order to increase the likelihood of a quicker return to play after an injury. If no baseline data is available or the data is not valid, the athlete's scores can be compared to normative data. The experienced clinician considers the patient's premorbid abilities to ensure proper comparison when utilizing normative data.

Once the team physician and neuropsychologist consultant are in agreement that the player has adequately recovered, the player will begin the exertional return-to-play protocol. The first step is light aerobic activity, such as a stationary bike or walking on a treadmill. The players are monitored for any return of their symptoms. In the absence of symptoms, the workload is increased to include weightlifting and moderate aerobic activity. The next step, if the athlete remains symptom-free, is to functional activity that is specific to that player's position. This may involve running and turning to catch passes for a wide receiver or sled drills for an offensive or defensive lineman. After that is practice in a noncontact environment, including all functional movements that are required for their position. If the player has any return of his symptoms, they are returned to the previous stage of the exertional protocol. Other possible physical or psychological causes of the return of their symptoms are reviewed as well.

Once the athlete has completed the above steps in the exertional program, they are again seen by team physician (and occasionally the consulting neuropsychologist) for a final assessment. The NFL then requires one final step before the player is fully cleared. He must also be evaluated and cleared by an independent neurologist that has been approved by the HNS Committee. When the team physician, neuropsychologist consultant, and the neurologist consultant have provided clearance and the player feels comfortable returning, he is allowed to participate in contact practice. He is continually monitored for any return of his symptoms. If he remains symptom-free, the athlete is cleared for return to unrestricted activity.

From a NFL Athletic Trainer Perspective (C.H.)

The NFL has become a league with highly motivated and competitive athletes. Although we continue to provide education on concussions to the players, there are still a few that will attempt to hide the injury from their team's medical staff. Therefore, the athletic trainers and physicians are constantly monitoring the players on the sidelines. We always talk to a player immediately after he comes off the field after taking a big hit or head-to-head contact, but we also continue to observe and monitor them.

From the stands it may appear that the sideline is a chaotic place, but it is organized chaos. Each player has a place where they sit. They each have rituals and routines that they go through. These players are creatures of habit. This is why having a medical staff that is familiar with each player is so important. The team's staff knows where each player is supposed to be, how they typically behave, and (most importantly) their personality. When I observe something out of the ordinary, I immediately go talk to the player. This will allow me to get a better idea if they are behaving differently or assess if they may be attempting to hide concussion symptoms. I have seen players hide from the medical staff by moving from one end of the bench to the other to avoid being face-to-face with us. I once noticed a player who was sitting at the end of the opposite bench of where he should be. When I went to see him, he was crying and could not explain why he was crying or why he was there. Without a trained medical professional on the sidelines looking for aberrant behavior, that athlete may have hidden his injury and returned to the game.

From a Sports Neuropsychologist's Perspective (E.M.P.)

The utilization of neuropsychologists in the care of concussed athletes has grown substantially. This includes our work with youth, high school, collegiate, and professional athletes. Research has demonstrated the role of cognitive assessment in the management of concussion [14–16]. However, this discussion has focused almost exclusively on cognitive testing. The sports neuropsychologist provides other aspects of care to the concussed athlete, in addition to the administration and interpretation of cognitive tests.

The review of the athlete's symptoms (the initial symptoms at the time of the injury or current symptom profile at the time of examination) can be different than what was reported to the team's medical staff. The neuropsychologist may ask the questions in a manner that elicits a different picture of their symptoms, or the athlete may simply respond more honestly to a non-team-affiliated healthcare provider. In my experience, the athlete typically reports a very positive relationship with the team's athletic training staff, but may be apprehensive about reporting lingering symptoms because they do not want to let the team down.

An experienced sports neuropsychologist also spends a great deal of time educating athletes on the pathophysiology of concussions and the typical recovery pattern. This is provided in terms that can be understood by a nonmedical professional. The current state of the science regarding the role of sports equipment in the prevention or reduction of concussions is also typically reviewed with the athlete. The professional football player, in particular, frequently has questions about the role of concussions and repetitive contact to the head in long-term cognitive decline and emotional disorders. There can be a great deal of anxiety surrounding these issues, especially if their loved ones have also expressed these concerns. The neuropsychologist consultant must be able to present this information to the athlete (and occasionally their family members) in an unbiased manner. It is vital that the athlete feels confident that the neuropsychologist is acting in their best behalf, not as an agent of the team or the NFL. These frank discussions are often the most rewarding for me in my work as a team consultant. Taking the time to answer their questions about concussions often provides the best reduction of the player's anxiety surrounding these injuries. However, occasionally problems with depression or anxiety after an injury also need to be addressed by the neuropsychologist. This is of particular concern if the athlete has a preexisting psychiatric history.

In a related note, it is important that the consulting neuropsychologist spend time with the team members when clinically appropriate so the athletes have some familiarity with them. However, it is even more imperative that the consultant retains his/her objectivity in assessing professional athletes. The excitement of working with professional sports teams, especially if the neuropsychologist is a fan of the sport or their team, can be quite alluring. It is vital that the consultant be able to withstand outside influence to return an athlete to the field of play before he is fully recovered. The return-to-play decision is made on the basis of evidence of recovery and what is in the best interest of the player, not the status of their season. In my work with four different professional teams in Chicago, I have no contact with the coaching staff. All communications about the player's injury is with the head athletic trainer and head team physician (for a more thorough examination of the role of neuropsychologists in concussion management in a recent book report [17]).

Further Directions

While research on the possible short- and long-term effects of concussions and repetitive contact to the head is ongoing, continual review of the protocol for managing concussions in professional football players is required. To date there have not been any published data examining whether the education provided to NFL players is effective. Do the athletes have an adequate understanding of the signs and symptoms of concussion? Does the information provided to them increase the likelihood that they will appreciate when they or one of their teammates have suffered a concussion? Has the education on concussion resulted in an increase in reporting of concussive injuries? Are there more effective ways to communicate this information to NFL players?

Additionally, the effectiveness of the current NFL program needs to be empirically studied. Does each component of the current program contribute to better identification of concussions and the subsequent management of these injuries? Does each member of the medical staff have the appropriate training and experience in concussions, and are they remaining up-to-date in their knowledge of the ever-evolving research on this injury? Are the measures being used on the sidelines and during the baseline/postinjury testing both reliable and valid for assessing concussions? Is there consistency in how these injuries are being managed between NFL teams? Should unaffiliated athletic trainer 'spotters' and unaffiliated neurotrauma consultants be made available at NFL practices? These are all unanswered questions that should be studied.

Conclusions

Football has a long and storied history, and professional and collegiate football remains the most popular sport in this country. The sport of football, and the NFL in particular, has come under great scrutiny regarding the handling of concussions in the past decade. Attention from the popular press, the medical community, and even Congress has placed a direct spotlight on how concussive injuries are managed in the NFL. This has resulted in the development of a complex system for identifying and treating concussed athletes. The current NFL protocol utilizes a number of highly trained medical professionals from the point of the initial injury to when the athlete has demonstrated recovery. This protocol will continue to evolve as research on the biomechanics of the injury, the use of sports equipment, and the effectiveness of our various methods of assessment and treatment improves our knowledge of the best practice methods. Additional research should address the effectiveness of each of the components of the current NFL model.

References

1 Smith R: Harvard and Columbia and a reconsideration of the 1905–06 football crisis. J Sports Hist 1981; 8:5–19.
2 Watterson JS: Political football: Theodore Roosevelt, Woodrow Wilson and the gridiron reform movement. Pres Stud Q 1995;25:555–564.
3 http://www.cdc.gov/mmwr/preview/mmwrhtml/mm5538a1.htm.
4 Schwarz A: Expert ties ex-player's suicide to brain damage. New York Times, January 18, 2007.
5 Schwarz A: Concussions tied to depression in ex-NFL players. New York Times, May 31, 2007.
6 Schwarz A: Dementia risk seen in players in NFL study. New York Times, September 29, 2009.
7 McGrath B: Does football have a future: the NFL and the concussion crisis. The New Yorker, January 31, 2011.
8 House of Representatives: Hearings before the Committee on the Judiciary: One Hundred Eleventh Congress, first and second sessions. October 28, 2009 and January 4, 2010.
9 NFL, ex-players agree to $765M settlement in concussions suit. August 29, 2013. http://www.nfl.com/news/story/0ap1000000235494/article/nfl-explayers-agree-to-765m-settlement-in-concussions-suit.
10 Concussion in Sport Group: SCAT3. Br J Sports Med 2013;47:259–262.
11 Lovell MR, Collins MW, Podell K, Powell K, Maroon J, et al: ImPACT: Immediate Post-Concussion Assessment and Cognitive Testing. Pittsburgh, NeuroHealth Systems, 2000.
12 McCrea M, Hammeke T, Olsen G, Leo P, Guskiewicz K: Unreported concussion in high school football players: implications for prevention. Clin J Sports Med 2004;14:13–17.
13 http://www.x2biosystems.com.
14 Broglio SP, Sosnoff JJ, Ferrara MS: The relationship of athlete-reported concussion symptoms and objective measures of neurocognitive function and postural control. Clin J Sports Med 2009;19:377–382.
15 Collie A, Madkissi M, Maruff P, Bennell K, McCrory P: Cognition in the days following concussion: comparison of symptomatic versus asymptomatic athletes. J Neurol Neurosurg Psychiatry 2006;77:241–245.
16 Fazio VC, Lovell MR, Pardini JE, Collins MW: The relation between post concussion symptoms and neurocognitive performance in concussed athletes. NeuroRehabilitation 2007;22:207–216.
17 Pieroth EM: The Role of the Neuropsychologist in Concussion Management; in Petraglia A, Bailes J, Day A (eds): Champaign, Human Kinetics Publishers, 2012 (in press).
18 http://web.mail.comcast.net/service/home/~/NFL_Player_Poster-a.pdf?auth = co&loc = en_US&id = 751647&part = 1
19 http://www.nflevolution.com/wordpress/wp-content/uploads/2012/08/nfl-sideline-tool-baseline.pdf.
20 Sports-related injuries among high school athletes -- United States, 2005–06 school year. http://www.cdc.gov/mmwr/preview/mmwrhtml/mm5538a1.htm#fig2.

Elizabeth M. Pieroth, PsyD, ABPP
NorthShore University HealthSystem
2180 Pfingsten Rd., Suite 2000
Glenview, IL 60026 (USA)
E-Mail epieroth@northshore.org

Niranjan A, Lunsford LD (eds): Concussion. Prog Neurol Surg. Basel, Karger, 2014, vol 28, pp 184–194
DOI: 10.1159/000358779

Developing an Interdisciplinary Community-Based Sports Concussion Management Program

Anthony LoGalbo[a, b] · Christine M. Salinas[b, c] · Michael Dougherty[b] · Mel Field[b, d]

[a]Medical Psychology Associates, Winter Park, Fla., and [b]Florida Hospital Sports Concussion Program, [c]Comprehensive Epilepsy Center, Florida Hospital for Children, and [d]Orlando Neurosurgery, Orlando, Fla., USA

Abstract

The increasing incidence and associated consequences of sport-related concussion have been at the forefront of public health concerns in recent years, prompting the need for safe and effective management guidelines and availability of appropriately trained healthcare providers. In this report we provide practical and user-friendly information regarding several important factors to consider when developing a sports concussion program, including how to select relevant team members, assess community needs and available resources, provide concussion education, secure and nurture partnerships with athletic programs, implement management strategies that align with current practice standards, and cater to athletes' unique needs in terms of program accessibility. It is hoped that the knowledge shared and proposed recommendations will be beneficial for guiding both newly developing and established concussion programs alike. © 2014 S. Karger AG, Basel

Over the past decade, there has been mounting evidence regarding the epidemiology and consequences of concussion to support that athletes of any age, gender, or sport may have equivalent or greater risk than the traditionally studied male football players [1–5]. Improved knowledge and awareness regarding the neurometabolic changes associated with concussion [6], and the effects of multiple injuries [7], along with highly publicized athlete retirements and cases that instill fear about potentially dangerous outcomes (including the controversial second impact syndrome and chronic traumatic encephalopathy) have placed concussion in the limelight as a public health issue. This has led to a series of international sports concussion consensus meetings [8, 9] and improved safety for the majority of athletes.

Prior to the mid-1990s, the cornerstone of concussion management included concussion grading scales. Although simple to use, they were not empirically validated and have subsequently been found to have many flaws, placing some athletes at risk for further injury while others are withheld from play in spite of full recovery. It is well known that athletes frequently underreport symptoms in order to avoid removal from athletic competition; therefore, the mantra 'when in doubt, sit them out' reflects the recent shift toward a more conservative management approach [10]. The recognized need for an individualized approach with an emphasis on demographic variables, neuropsychological status, balance, extended rest, and graded exertional protocols [8, 9] has resulted in an increasing demand for the establishment of concussion management programs at all levels of sports around the country.

Increased vigilance has also led to improved protective sport equipment, state regulation regarding helmet use, and concussion legislation in all states except for Mississippi (incited by the Zackery Lystedt Law of 2009) in hopes of protecting student-athletes from returning to play too soon and requiring athletes to seek medical attention by healthcare personnel. Unfortunately, despite this positive momentum, few states have infrastructure for access, provide aide for development, or mandate that insurance plans (including those that are state-run) cover services required for comprehensive concussion care. As healthcare providers, the onus of responsibility has fallen on us to ensure the proper care of this population. Few resources detail how to implement a successful community-based concussion program that satisfies individual state mandates and ensures buy-in by local and regional schools, parents, coaches, and athletes. In this report we will review multiple factors that need to be considered when creating a sports-concussion program, and provide management strategies that align with current practice standards.

Key Components to Program Establishment

Select an 'A' Team

Starting a concussion program requires much time and effort, often beyond the realm of an individual's capacity. Therefore, establishing a team of individuals from multiple disciplines with a strong passion and competence in this area is paramount. Each contributes an important role in the process of diagnosis and management of concussion, and ultimately return-to-play decisions. Team members typically include neuropsychologists, neurologists, neurosurgeons, sports medicine specialists, athletic trainers, and physical therapists. At a minimum, a core triad of a physician, neuropsychologist, and athletic trainer is highly recommended. The program's setting (e.g. university-based, private hospital, or independent organization) will have an enormous influence on the roles each of these team members will play in developing and implementing the program, and available resources for the program in terms of financial and administrative support. In university- and hospital-based programs, strong physician and organizational leadership support can be influential in getting the program up and running: from providing financial support and a physical location to house the program, to allocating resources for marketing and community outreach efforts. Independent organizations, on the other hand, may depend on philanthropic support from local foundations, charities, or athletic associations.

Identify and Address Community Needs

Developing a vision, including the main purpose and goals, is vital during the initial stages of program development. Part of this process includes assessing community needs to establish your target athlete populations. For example, will the program focus on middle or high school athletes? Are there enough professional and/or collegiate athletic organizations in the community that have a need for such a program? Are youth recreational and club leagues accessible and interested in participating? Are there other sports or entertainment performers in the area which may be vulnerable to concussions (e.g. skiing/snowboarding and stunting/acrobatics)? Will the focus be on securing physician or professional referrals, such as from pediatricians or emergency room and urgent care visits? Do other concussion management programs already exist in the community? If so, how can the program be unique? Communities will have different needs, depending on various factors, such as whether the area is urban or rural, what the popular sports are in the area, and importantly, how invested athletic programs are in incorporating concussion management into their system. We recommend exploring the number of high schools with athletic programs and club and recreational leagues in the area. Developing relationships with local hospitals, universities, and sports medicine organizations (often orthopedic in nature) can be helpful to pool resources and facilitate referral sources. Newly developed concussion programs might initially consider selecting just a few schools or athletic organizations to ensure quality management practices.

Build a Local Network

To get athletic programs 'on board', it is vital to establish and maintain ongoing communication with school districts, school administrators, athletic directors, club organization officials, team physicians, athletic trainers, coaches, and even athletes and their families, especially when dealing with youth. Obtaining support from organizational leadership typically helps with program implementation and expansion. For example, making an arrangement to conduct baseline and postconcussive testing with an athletic trainer for specific team sports is a good step forward; however, having an athletic department mandate evaluation of all athletes is a huge leap. We encourage newly developed programs to create a template to guide schools in their institutional policies regarding concussion management. The most powerful method is to gain support from a local school district through development of concussion management policies. Notably, parents of established athletes are often the biggest advocates for the program and represent an important voice in the community. Parents frequently spread the message to other families or may be linked with a school's booster club, which can create positive momentum toward changing a concussion management policy. Their experience and passion may expand your local audience, help provide more resources, and ensure a school's policy is implemented.

Raise Awareness in the Athletic Community

Concussion education that emphasizes signs and symptoms, common injury mechanisms, evaluation procedures, recovery expectations, and management protocols should be developed for coaches, parents, athletes, officials, and healthcare providers. Within the context of youth, the likelihood that a healthcare professional will be accessible and/or familiar with guidelines for identification, treatment, and management of concussions is low. Therefore, education should ideally begin with individuals that are on the first line of preventing or detecting a concussion (e.g. parents, coaches, athletic trainers, and athletes themselves). Providing knowledge of subtle signs dispels misconceptions, leading to accurate injury identification. Education regarding concussion prevalence and risk in various sports, including those less commonly recognized (such as girls' soccer, lacrosse, or cheerleading) is vital to ensuring all athletes' safety. Ask athletic programs to identify their approach to managing concussions and areas that could be improved upon in the future. Educate them about how your concussion program may help relieve excess burden, facilitate athletes' recovery, and ensure safe return to athletic play. Provide training to athletic trainers and coaches so that they can perform accurate sideline evaluations to assist with early injury detection and emphasize athlete removal from play when there is a doubt of injury and until the athlete can be evaluated by a healthcare professional competent in concussion management. Implementation of management guidelines is a high priority, both initially and throughout each sport season. Organizational leadership benefits from education about concussion so that they understand the risks and allocate funding toward acquiring qualified personnel to monitor athletic activities and implement management protocols. The 'Heads Up: Concussion' toolkits are free resources provided by the Centers for Disease Control and Prevention (CDC; http://www.cdc.gov/concussion/headsup/) that are useful in disseminating concussion-related information to parents, players, coaches, physicians, and schools.

Educate Healthcare Professionals

Create opportunities to meet with local physicians, nurses, urgent care facilities, and emergency departments to inform them of the current standards of care for diagnosis and management of concussion, and tell them about the comprehensive services your program can provide for athletes. Create a "lunch-n'-learn", set up a physician dinner with lectures, participate in medical department meetings, be visible at athletic games, and initiate conversation with team physicians on the sideline. Provide continuing education unit lectures and figure this into the program's budget. Costs may include money to become a continuing education unit provider for certified athletic trainers (ATCs) or other disciplines, postage, and media (or you can opt for electronic distribution and 'go green'). Choosing a targeted audience such as your local ATC partners, athletic directors, coaches, and team physicians can reduce costs and ensure optimal participation. With more resources, a program may be able to establish a statewide or national miniconference.

Support School Partners
An athletic trainer and athletic program solidify schools as referral sources when concussions occur; therefore, a close working relationship with both is key to a program's success. Provide support in many ways from increasing manpower to proctoring baseline testing and assisting with sideline evaluations. This approach ensures that testing is done properly with adequate oversight, minimizing the frequency of invalid testing. Your staff will often serve as a liaison between the athletic trainer, coach, and/or parent. It is helpful to check daily if testing has been performed at a school as routine practice. Tracking concussed athletes relieves excessive burden on school personnel since they may support 10 or more contact sports annually. Educate staff regarding the necessary course of action when a concussion occurs. Advise school athletic staff if an appointment is necessary, whom would be best to schedule, and make sure information pertaining to injury characteristics, symptomatology, associated consequences (including cognitive changes that may impact academic functions), risk factors for prolonged recovery, and compliance with recommendations is gathered. Inform ATCs if a concussed athlete has not followed up to avoid premature return to athletic play.

Market Your Program
Develop a program logo, professional brochure, field cards (fig. 1), a banner, and a program website. Free promotion can be conducted through social media and blogs, patient testimonials, and word of mouth. Investing in the educational aspects of the program, partnering with local schools and teams, and providing excellent patient experience can be more influential to the program's success than paying for expensive radio spots, television ads, or a billboard. Conducting internal research regarding concussion incidence and recovery can be powerful data to share with your local community and helps raise awareness about particularly vulnerable groups. Tracking trends can help anticipate patient volume for planning costs and expenditures, time and resource allocation, and potential growth.

Developing and Implementing Management Practices for Concussed Athletes

A successful program should be equipped to support athletic programs as well as evaluate and manage sport-related concussion in accordance with the consensus of the scientific community [8, 9]. The typical protocol includes preseason baseline computerized neurocognitive assessments for all athletes, sideline assessment when a suspected concussion has occurred and determination of appropriateness for immediate urgent care, postinjury neurocognitive assessment, reassessment of symptoms and cognitive functions as necessary throughout the recovery process, and facilitation of a safe return to play. Supplemental balance, vestibular, ocular-motor, and visual assessments may be included. The general consensus regarding determination of an athlete's recovery is based on at least three factors: resolution of postconcussive symptoms while at

Florida Hospital
SPORTSMEDICINE
AND REHABILITATION

CONCUSSION MANAGEMENT PROTOCOL

Go home and rest. You may move around and engage in everyday activities, but do not exert yourself, physically or mentally. Report to your team athletic trainer, coach, physician, or medical professional as arranged or scheduled.

SEEK MEDICAL ATTENTION IMMEDIATELY IF YOU EXPERIENCE THE FOLLOWING SYMPTOMS:

- Abnormal pupils
  Difference in size left to right
- Arm/leg weakness (unilateral)
- Headache that is severe or gets worse
- Difficulty speaking and/or slurred speech
- Changes in gait or balance
  Difficulty walking
  Unsteady on your feet
  Dizziness or vertigo
- Changes in level of consciousness
  Difficult to awaken
  "Black out"
  Loss of consciousness
- Memory loss
  Unable to recognize familiar people, places or things
- Behavior changes
  Irritable/restless
- Mental confusion
- Repeated vomiting
- Seizure activity
- Fever or stiff neck
- Urine or bowel incontinence

PAIN RELIEF

Do not take aspirin or any medication containing aspirin unless specifically directed to do so by your physician. It is safe to take acetaminophen for headache/pain.

Return to Participation

You cannot return to participation until you are medically cleared, are symptom-free at rest, have normal neurocognitive scores AND no return of symptoms with controlled exertion.

Why is this so important?

- You can increase your risk for another concussion if you return to participation before recovering from your current concussion. Slower reaction time, along with decreased balance, coordination and concentration, set the stage for reinjury.
- If you have another concussion before recovering from this one, you can havepermanent brain injury or death from "second-impact syndrome."

SLEEPING

During the first night after a concussion, someone should wake the patient every hour to check on him/her. If they are harder to wake than usual, confused, unable to speak normally, or walk steadily, someone should take him/her to the hospital immediately.

DRINKING

Do not drink alcohol or take sleeping pills until you receive medical clearance to do so.

DRIVING

Do not operate a motorized vehicle until you receive medical clearance to do so.

Return To School Or Work.

If your symptoms last longer than three days, you will need to get specific advice from the concussion specialists about how to return to school/work successfully.

For more information or to schedule an appointment, call (407) 303-8012 or visit
www.FHSportsMed.com/Concussion.

Fig. 1. An example of a Concussion Guide Field Card given to all athletic trainers and team physicians.

rest, neurocognitive testing performance returning to an established baseline or otherwise within expectation, and completion of a stepwise physical exertional testing protocol while remaining asymptomatic. Legislative and organizational policies may specify whether additional steps are required and who is capable of providing medical clearance (e.g. any 'healthcare provider with experience and training in concussion management', or a physician MD/DO only); therefore, it is imperative to be knowledgeable about policies in your state to ensure your program satisfies these criteria and implements strategies that support a successful reentry to sports, school, or work.

Baseline Testing

A program member (frequently an ATC) should go to the school or athletic organization to assist with baseline testing, and this should be done before a sport season begins. Parental consent may be needed for performing such testing with youth, and this can be incorporated into documentation parents complete to allow their child's athletic participation. Selecting 1–2 days per sport during preseason workouts and conditioning often works best for administration of baseline assessments. School computer labs can be used to streamline the process and test multiple athletes simultaneously, although caution needs to be exercised to ensure an optimal test-taking environment and valid test results. Computerized neurocognitive measures have embedded validity indicators; however, we recommend that a neuropsychologist review tests that have been flagged as 'invalid' to deem whether repeat testing is appropriate.

Sideline Evaluation

When a concussion is suspected, it is important to perform a brief yet multifaceted sideline assessment as soon as possible (e.g. SCAT3). This will typically be performed by an ATC, if available; however, other athletic staff could also be trained to perform this assessment. A predetermined set of critical signs and symptoms (e.g. decreased consciousness or arousal, emesis, increasing symptom severity, focal neurological deficits, behavioral changes), if observed, should trigger an immediate referral to the emergency department. Otherwise, the athlete should be closely monitored for acute symptom onset and a parent should be informed of the injury if the athlete is a minor. Detailed information regarding concussive injuries should be provided to caregivers including warning signs that may indicate a worsening condition, along with recommendations for an acute follow-up plan, including removal from play until being evaluated by an appropriate healthcare professional (fig. 2).

Postconcussive Neuropsychological Evaluation

Athletes typically undergo an initial postinjury neurocognitive assessment that may include both computerized and traditional paper and pencil measures within 24–72 h. Face-to-face neuropsychological consultation to review test results in the context of the athlete's medical and psychosocial history and to generate treatment recommendations (e.g. including extended cognitive and physical rest) for symptom manage-

Florida Hospital
SPORTSMEDICINE
AND REHABILITATION

CONCUSSION PROGRAM INFORMATION AND SCHEDULING
(407) 303-8012 www.FHSportsMed.com/Concussion

SIGNS AND SYMPTOMS MAY WORSEN WITH EXERTION.

- Always assume the possibility of neck or brain injury if the patient is unconscious. Take appropriate steps for neck injury.
- You DO NOT have to lose consciousness to have sustained a concussion.
- The patient should not return to Participation if he/she shows any signs or symptoms of concussion. Patient should be cleared medically prior to returning to participation.
- Re-assess the patient's condition every five minutes. If the condition or symptoms get worse, seek immediate medical attention.

SYMPTOMS REPORTED

- Headache
- Nausea/vomiting
- Balance problems or dizziness
- Double or fuzzy vision
- Sensitivity to light or noise
- Feeling sluggish, foggy or groggy
- Change in sleep pattern
- Concentration or memory problems
- Confusion
- Tinnitus (ringing in the ears)
- Personality change
- Irritability (late-onset symptom)
- Sleep disturbance (late-onset symptom)

SIGNS OBSERVED

- Appears to be dazed or stunned
- Confused in general or about assignment
- Forgets team moves or plays
- Unsure of game, score or opponent
- Moves clumsily
- Answers questions slowly
- Loses consciousness (even briefly)
- Shows behavior or personality / change
- Forgets events prior to impact (retrograde)
- Forgets events after impact (anterograde)
- Seizures
- Pupils appear different in size

THE PATIENT MUST NOT RETURN TO PARTICIPATION UNTIL THEY ARE EVALUATED BY A CONCUSSION SPECIALIST. *"WHEN IN DOUBT, SIT THEM OUT."*

To report a concussion to the Florida Hospital Concussion Team, call (407) 303-8012.

Fig. 2. An example of a fold-up pocket-sized Concussion Care Card given to concussed athletes and their caregivers at the time a concussion occurs.

ment is helpful during the acute phase of recovery. Providing detailed recommendations regarding classroom or work accommodations can inform others about the injury and specific guidelines to facilitate recovery, which may help minimize an adverse impact on the athlete's academic or work performance. Implementation of a 504 or Individualized Education Plan may be needed for youth. The Acute Concussion Evaluation (ACE) care plan is a freely accessible resource on the CDC website: www.cdc.gov/concussion/HeadsUp/physicians_tool_kit.html [11].

Monitoring and Managing the Injured Athlete

Frequent communication between the concussion program and athletic staff (as well as parents) regarding an athlete's status is imperative during the recovery process, as symptoms may fluctuate and may be highly dependent on compliance with activity restrictions (i.e. he/she may have a hard time resisting social media, computers, videogames, and physical exercise). Adjustments to recovery guidelines and accommodations are needed as the athlete gradually recovers or in the event of a prolonged course. Repeat computerized neurocognitive assessment is performed once the athlete is asymptomatic at rest, commonly at least 2 consecutive days. Caution is advised in administering serial assessments within a short time span, especially while the athlete remains symptomatic as this may exacerbate symptoms and lead to practice effects, skewing conclusions which may be drawn from the data. Reassessments may be performed at various locations with neuropsychologists solely providing test interpretation. Notably, many factors need to be considered when comparing baseline and postinjury data, including but not limited to an athlete's prior history of concussion or other neurological conditions (e.g. seizures, migraine syndromes), learning disability, and attention-deficit/hyperactivity disorder. Because of neuropsychologists' expertise in understanding brain-behavior relationships and competence with standardized neuropsychological assessment, they are in the 'best position' to analyze baseline and postinjury testing data [9], especially in the context of these comorbid conditions. Some athletes also experience a protracted recovery that lasts beyond several weeks. In these cases, comprehensive neuropsychological evaluations are warranted to better understand the athlete's cognitive and psychological status, along with other demographic, situational, and familial factors that may be contributory. Referrals to neurologists, physiatrists, physical therapists, psychiatrists, and psychologists may be necessary.

Exertional Testing

After an athlete's postinjury test results are considered to be within expectation, the athlete then undergoes physical exertional testing, which is usually performed under the supervision of an athletic trainer or coach. While initial steps can be employed through the concussion program (e.g. engaging the athlete in gradually more intense aerobic activities), subsequent steps may be effectively completed with the athletic program (e.g. participating first in noncontact drills and then participating in contact practices before competing in a game).

Concussion Program Accessibility: Catering to Athletes' Unique Needs

The concussion management practice model is unique in that athletic events occur daily and present a risk for injury, requiring acute evaluation and education regarding symptom management. To make matters more complex, there can be high stakes involved; therefore, athletes themselves, coaches, and even parents may want him/her to return to play as soon as possible. Hence, prompt availability of clinicians to perform assessments and make recommendations is vital to a concussion management program's effectiveness. The following are some suggestions to improve flexibility and efficiency in this setting.

We recommend blocking specific time in clinicians' schedules for concussion patients, perhaps on a weekly or biweekly basis depending on the anticipated need. Patient volume can be difficult to predict across the school year and from one sport season to the next, even in already established concussion programs. While making appointments in advance is preferred in most clinical settings, with respect to concussions, there is often a need to adopt an urgent care-like model allowing for 'walk-ins'. The majority of concussed athletes will seek an evaluation as soon as possible. They are often directed to the program by an athletic trainer for an initial assessment after sustaining an injury the night before, or upon presenting to school, urgent care, or their primary care provider with postconcussive symptoms the morning after an injury occurred. Clinician availability within a day or two following an injury or initial point of contact with the athlete is crucial for all the aforementioned reasons in this report. It is ideal to allocate specific time earlier in the week for injuries that occurred over the weekend and later in the week for events that occurred midweek (i.e. our program has successfully implemented a Tuesday and Thursday walk-in morning clinic with additional flexibility set aside during the week).

Another unique aspect to a concussion clinic model, especially for neuropsychologists, is the need to see multiple patients in a relatively shorter period of time. For example, the initial sports concussion consultation may last 30 min. Having a multidisciplinary team in place is beneficial to facilitating clinic flow. An athletic trainer or other team member can check in newly arriving athletes and set them up with computerized testing, while the neuropsychologist and physician meet with athletes who have completed testing. A neuropsychology trainee may also assist with traditional neuropsychological testing. A mechanism needs to be in place for communicating results back to referral sources. The program's athletic trainers can communicate with the athletic program directly by phone or email, and progress notes along with recommendations can be sent to referring physicians. It is important for the concussion program to delegate responsibilities among team members to ensure follow-through and efficiency.

There are many additional key concepts regarding program accessibility to consider. The physical and geographic location of the concussion clinic should ideally be easily accessible and within reasonable proximity to the athletic organizations which it is supporting. The space should be large enough to accommodate all program team members and also allow for anticipated patient volume during clinic hours. Financial considerations regarding how to manage athletes who are underinsured or who have insurance that is not typically accepted by the providers is critical. Providing occasional pro bono services can accommodate an individual athlete's needs and often facilitates establishing and maintaining consistent participation with specific schools, school districts, and nonacademic athletic organizations. However, informing athletic staff that the program only serves athletes with certain insurance requirements may lead to a drop off in commitment to the program and referrals. Grant funding, philanthropic support, and/or sliding fee scales are helpful to ensure sustainability.

In summary, the large accumulation of evidence pertaining to sport-related concussion and its associated consequences has led to the establishment of legislative, athletic organization, and international guidelines to appropriately diagnose and manage injured athletes. Athletic participation has reached an all-time high in younger ages, often resulting in concussions sustained during play and, with increased vigilance and monitoring, better injury detection. All of these factors in combination have created an unprecedented demand for healthcare professionals that are qualified to provide competent services to concussed athletes. The development of interdisciplinary and multimodal concussion management programs, particularly at the high school level, may help address this public health concern. Interdisciplinary management programs also lend themselves well to research, which can lead to improvements regarding empirically validated approaches to the diagnosis and treatment of athletes in the future, particularly youth, who still represent relatively new unchartered territory.

References

1 Covassin T, Elbin RJ: The female athlete: the role of gender in the assessment and management of sport-related concussion. Clin J Sport Med 2011;30:125–131.

2 Gessel LM, Fields SK, Collins CL, Dick RW, Comstock RD: Concussions among United States high school and collegiate athletes. J Athl Train 2007;42: 495–503.

3 McClincy MP, Lovell MR, Pardini J, Collins MW, Spore MK: Recovery from sports concussion in high school and collegiate athletes. Brain Inj 2006;20:33–39.

4 McCrea M, Guskiewicz KM, Marshall SW, Barr W, Randolph C, Cantu RC, et al: Acute effects and recovery time following concussion in collegiate football players: the NCAA Concussion Study. JAMA 2003;290:2556–2563.

5 Field M, Collins MW, Lovell MR, Maroon J: Does age play a role in recovery from sports-related concussion? A comparison of high school and collegiate athletes. J Pediatr 2003;142:546–553.

6 Giza CC, Hovda DA: Neurometabolic cascade of concussion. J Athl Train 2001;36:228–235.

7 Guskiewicz KM, McCrea M, Marshall SW, Cantu RC, Randolph C, Barr W, et al: Cumulative effects associated with recurrent concussion in collegiate football players: the NCAA Concussion Study. JAMA 2003;290:2549–2555.

8 McCrory P, Meeuwisse WH, Aubry M, Cantu RC, Dvorak J, Echemendia RJ, et al: Consensus statement on concussion in sport: the 4th International Conference on Concussion in Sport, Zurich, November 2012. Br J Sports Med 2013;47:250–258.

9 McCrory P, Meeuwisse W, Johnston K, Dvorak J, Aubry M, Molloy M, Cantu R: Consensus statement on concussion in sport: 3rd International Conference on Concussion in Sport held in Zurich, November 2008. Clin J Sport Med 2009;19:185–200.

10 Aubry M, Cantu R, Dvorak J, Graf-Baumann T, Johnston KM, James K, et al: Summary and agreement statement of the 1st International Symposium on Concussion in Sport, Vienna 2001. Clin J Sport Med 2002;12:6–11.

11 Gioia G, Collins M: Acute Concussion Evaluation (ACE) Care Plan. 2006. Accessed at http://www.cdc.gov/concussion/HeadsUp/physicians_tool_kit.html. August 31, 2013.

Anthony LoGalbo, PhD
Medical Psychology Associates
1685 Lee Road, Suite 200
Winter Park, FL 32789 (USA)
E-Mail anthony.logalbo@flhosp.org

Niranjan A, Lunsford LD (eds): Concussion. Prog Neurol Surg. Basel, Karger, 2014, vol 28, pp 195–212
DOI: 10.1159/000358780

The Multidisciplinary Concussion Management Program

David M. Panczykowski · Jamie E. Pardini

Department of Neurosurgery, University of Pittsburgh Medical Center, Pittsburgh, Pa., USA

Abstract

Over the past decade, research has increased scientific and public knowledge about the importance of identification and proper management of concussion. These concerns have prompted many state, regional, and private organizations to mandate the creation of, and strict adherence to, concussion management protocols, particularly with regard to sport-related concussion and subsequent return to play. Because of the individualized nature of the concussive injury and its recovery, a multidisciplinary approach provides comprehensive patient care that best addresses treatment and management of changing symptoms and their impact on multiple aspects of a patient's life and overall function. The current report will explore a model of multidisciplinary concussion management from program establishment and baseline testing to recovery from chronic postconcussion symptoms.

© 2014 S. Karger AG, Basel

Foundations of Multidisciplinary Management

Understand Relevant Laws and Mandates

When creating a concussion management program, it is important to first determine current law regarding concussion management. At present, 49 states and the District of Columbia have passed laws designed to protect student-athletes with concussion from premature return to play. Most state laws mandate three important components of concussion management: education, identification of injury, and return to play only with documented permission from an appropriately trained medical professional. The type of medical professional who can approve a return to play following concussion varies among states, all of which indicate MDs or DOs properly trained in concussion management, and some of which also allow properly trained neuropsychologists, athletic trainers, nurse practitioners, physician assistants, psychologists, chiropractors, and/or registered nurses to approve return to play. There are multiple websites that provide information about concussion management laws by state, including the Centers for Disease Control and Prevention (CDC; www.cdc.gov/concussion/policies.html). In addition, athletic organizations, schools, and school districts may have institution-specific rules for concussion management that may be more restrictive than the governing state laws. As explained in other reports within this volume, organizations like the National Football League, Major League Soccer, National Hockey League, National Collegiate Athletic Association (NCAA), National Federation of State High School Associations, etc. may have their own guidelines or rules that govern return to play following concussion. Medical practitioners establishing a concussion management program should be aware of all rules and regulations that may govern the return to play of potential injured patients in order to design an effective program that can be seen as a valuable community resource.

Join, or Vet, a Good Multidisciplinary Team

While a neurosurgeon may certainly be the cornerstone of a concussion management program, it is likely that concussion management will be a small portion of a busy neurosurgeon's practice. Thus, it is important to recruit or join a team of other professionals who are interested in and who are properly educated about the diagnosis and management of concussion. Valuable team members with whom you will regularly interact regarding patient care may include athletic trainers, neuropsychologists, primary care physicians, and team physicians. If the patient has a prolonged recovery, other professionals may also join the care team, including physiatry, neurology, physical therapy, vestibular therapy, visual therapy, and/or relevant academic officials. The potential role of these team members will be outlined in subsequent sections of this report. Concussion symptoms and their impact on daily function can change relatively quickly and thus require regular monitoring so treatment, activity level, and recommendations can be adjusted when appropriate.

Preinjury Preparations

Educate Everyone

Education about the common signs and symptoms of concussion, as well as the potential dangers of premature return to play, is a vital component of a successful concussion management program. Many states and organizations mandate education of coaches, involved medical practitioners, student-athletes, and/or parents of athletes, and some require parents and students to sign forms indicating they have received educational information about concussion. Regardless of policy, education is critical. Over the past decade, it has become more common for educated student-athletes or parents to be the first to identify that an athlete may be hiding a head injury and bring it to the attention of an appropriate medical professional. Excellent educational materials are available at no cost from the CDC, and many organizations have created institution- or sport-specific educational materials. Often, concussion education sessions are provided to student-athletes by athletic trainers or team physicians as part of required preseason activities, along with education about other common sport-related injuries, such as heat stroke and orthopedic injuries. Parents can be invited to attend these sessions or may receive the opportunity to attend talks during PTA (parent-teacher association) or other school meetings. States that require education of coaches, athletic trainers, and/or other medical professionals provide live or online access to approved courses or materials that meet the requirement for training.

Foster Communication and Compliance

Organizations with the most successful concussion management programs or systems are those that foster open communication between all involved members of the interdisciplinary management team and which have agreed upon the approach and procedures for injury management. Establishing rapport and a good working relationship with the schools and organizations with which you will often work will also improve the monitoring of an athlete's recovery and compliance with activity restrictions and treatment. One way to foster good compliance is to have an initial meeting of all professionals who may be involved with managing a concussed athlete, from baseline to return to play, in order to establish procedures and clarify roles (e.g. who will manage accommodations, exertion, cognitive evaluation, etc.). Those providers who will have the most direct contact with potentially injured athletes should also dedicate effort to promoting compliance among the athletes themselves by discussing the importance of immediately notifying a medical professional if a concussion is suspected, and creating a safe environment for a teammate to come forward if he/she suspects a peer is hiding or is unaware of an injury. As awareness about the potential dangers of improperly managed concussion has increased, we have increasingly treated injured athletes whose injury was first spotted by a teammate who noticed the athlete was acting differently in the huddle, locker room, or field.

Provide Baseline Testing

An important component of any concussion management program is acquisition of valid information about the baseline functioning of those at risk for sustaining concussion. It has become common practice to provide baseline testing of an athlete's cognitive function, symptom report, and balance prior to the start of a contact sport season. Other reports in this series provide detailed information about cognitive testing platforms and management of concussion based upon level of sport. Many baseline testing protocols encourage or require acquisition of a baseline symptom report in addition to cognitive and balance testing. Having access to preinjury symptom reporting is helpful when an athlete does sustain a concussion to better understand the patient's usual experience of commonly experienced symptoms that overlap with concussion, such as migraine, attention problems, and mood difficulties. In addition, completing a baseline symptom checklist can reinforce other educational efforts that address common signs and symptoms of concussion. Reviewing baseline symptom reports and cognitive testing can occasionally lead to identification of an athlete hiding an unresolved injury.

Postinjury Management: Initial Evaluation and Diagnosis

The primary objectives in the evaluation of anyone suspected of suffering a traumatic brain injury (TBI) are to (1) diagnose acute intracranial, spinal, or other injury, (2) determine existence of an antecedent/precipitating medical event, and (3) determine appropriate disposition and referral from the acute care setting.

Concussion, a subset of TBI, is a biomechanically induced alteration of brain function that results in acute, short-lived impairment of neurologic function with spontaneous resolution. Although concussion may result in neuropathological changes, acute clinical symptoms are primarily a result of functional disturbance, not macroscopic structural injury. As well, concussion should be viewed as the acute phase of an injury in evolution; full symptom manifestation may occur over hours to days. In most cases, the onset of initial symptoms occurs immediately after the concussive event. However, some athletes may experience a delay of symptom onset [1]. In a study of NCAA football players, 11 of 94 athletes diagnosed with concussion experienced delayed symptom onset (mean = 14.4 min, SD = 15.5 min).

Different groups have produced varying criteria for clinical identification of concussion with subtle differences over a range of domains including clinical symptoms, physical signs, cognitive impairment, and neurobehavioral features (see table 1 for definitions of concussion and table 2 for common signs and symptoms). Criteria for identification typically include at least 1 of the following:

1 Any loss of consciousness (LOC)
2 Any loss of memory for events immediately before (retrograde amnesia) or after the accident (posttraumatic amnesia)
3 Any alteration in mental state (dazed, confused, mental fogginess, disoriented, irrational behavior, etc.)
4 Other transient neurologic abnormalities where the injury does not exceed any of the following: LOC >30 min, Glasgow Coma Scale (GCS) <13 persisting for >30 min, or posttraumatic amnesia >24 h

Clinical diagnosis is based on injury characteristics (LOC, posttraumatic amnesia, and/or confusion) evaluated through careful and deliberate history and neurologic examination. Although multiple definitions of concussion exist, commonly used

Table 1. Evolving definitions of concussion

American Congress of Rehabilitation Medicine (1993) [3]
A patient with mTBI is a person who has had a traumatically induced physiological disruption of brain function, as manifested by at least one of the following:
1. Any period of LOC
2. Any loss of memory for events immediately before or after the accident
3. Any alteration in mental state at the time of the accident (e.g. feeling dazed, disoriented, or confused)
4. Focal neurological deficit(s) that may or may not be transient, but where the severity of the injury does not exceed the following:
   - LOC of approx. 30 min or less
   - After 30 min, an initial GCS of 13–15
   - Posttraumatic amnesia not greater than 24 h

World Health Organization Collaborating Task Force on mTBI (2005) [21]
mTBI is an acute brain injury resulting from mechanical energy to the head from external physical forces. Operational criteria for clinical identification include: (i) 1 or more of the following: confusion or disorientation, LOC for 30 min or less, posttraumatic amnesia for less than 24 h, and/or other transient neurological abnormalities such as focal signs, seizure, and intracranial lesion not requiring surgery; (ii) GCS score of 13–15 30 min after injury or later upon presentation for healthcare. These manifestations of mTBI must not be due to drugs, alcohol, medications, caused by other injuries or treatment for other injuries (e.g. systemic injuries, facial injuries, or intubation), caused by other problems (e.g. psychological trauma, language barrier, or coexisting medical conditions), or caused by penetrating craniocerebral injury.

CDC (2007) [4]
'A mild traumatic brain injury (mTBI) or concussion is defined as a complex pathophysiologic process affecting the brain, induced by traumatic biomechanical forces secondary to direct or indirect forces to the head. mTBI is caused by a jolt to the head or body that disrupts the function of the brain. This disturbance of brain function is typically associated with normal structural neuroimaging findings (i.e., CT scan, MRI). mTBI results in a constellation of physical, cognitive, emotional, and sleep-related symptoms that may or may not involve a loss of consciousness (LOC). Duration of symptoms is highly variable and may last from several minutes to days, weeks, months, or longer in some cases.'

Concussion in Sport Group (2013) [3]
Concussion is a brain injury and is defined as a complex pathophysiological process affecting the brain, induced by biomechanical forces. Several common features that incorporate clinical, pathologic and biomechanical injury constructs that may be utilized in defining the nature of a concussive head injury include:
1. Concussion may be caused either by a direct blow to the head, face, neck or elsewhere on the body with an 'impulsive' force transmitted to the head
2. Concussion typically results in the rapid onset of short-lived impairment of neurological function that resolves spontaneously; however, in some cases, symptoms and signs may evolve over a number of minutes to hours
3. Concussion may result in neuropathological changes, but the acute clinical symptoms largely reflect a functional disturbance rather than a structural injury and, as such, no abnormality is seen on standard structural neuroimaging studies
4. Concussion results in a graded set of clinical symptoms that may or may not involve LOC; resolution of the clinical and cognitive symptoms typically follows a sequential course, but it is important to note that in some cases symptoms may be prolonged

Table 2. Common signs and symptoms of concussion

Signs and symptoms
Signs of injury
LOC
Retrograde amnesia (forgetting events that happened before the concussion)
Posttraumatic or anterograde amnesia (forgetting events happening after the concussion)
'Dazed' look
Confusion about injury events or details
Disorientation to person, place, or time
Emotional lability
Inappropriate emotions
Behavior or personality changes
Symptoms of injury
Headache
Dizziness
Lightheadedness
Balance problems
Fatigue
Visual changes (blurred vision, double vision, etc.)
Insomnia (trouble falling asleep, staying asleep, or early waking)
Hypersomnia
Drowsiness
Attention or concentration problems
Short-term memory problems
Difficulty with multitasking
Phonophobia (sensitivity to noise)
Photophobia (sensitivity to light)
Bradyphrenia (slowed thinking)
Mental 'fogginess'
Emotional changes (irritability, sadness, nervousness)
Vomiting

definitions include those published by the American Academy of Neurology [2], American Congress of Rehabilitation Medicine [3], and the Centers for Disease Control [4]. The CDC offers the following comprehensive definition (p. 2):

> A mild traumatic brain injury (mTBI) or concussion is defined as a complex pathophysiologic process affecting the brain, induced by traumatic biomechanical forces secondary to direct or indirect forces to the head. mTBI is caused by a jolt to the head or body that disrupts the function of the brain. This disturbance of brain function is typically associated with normal structural neuroimaging findings (i.e. CT scan, MRI). mTBI results in a constellation of physical, cognitive, emotional, and/or sleep-related symptoms that may or may not involve a loss of consciousness (LOC). Duration of symptoms is highly variable and may last from several minutes to days, weeks, months, or longer in some cases.

Sideline Evaluation

Sideline evaluation for concussion is most often completed by the team physician and/or athletic trainer. In the event that neither is available, EMT services may provide this evaluation. Initial evaluation should proceed in accordance with Advance

Trauma Life Support protocols: Primary Survey to Assess Airway, Respiratory/Breathing, Circulatory, and Neurologic Deficit [5]. Assessment while immobilizing the cervical spine is critical, as acute TBI patients should be presumed to have concomitant cervical spine injuries until excluded. Following initial evaluation, a secondary survey may begin, with attention to history of the accident (possible antecedent event like syncope, transient ischemic attack, seizure, etc.), past medical history (especially previous concussions, bleeding diathesis, cardiac disease, etc.), and medications (especially antithrombotic usage). Reversible causes of altered mental status should be considered and rapidly excluded (including hypoperfusion, hypoxemia, hypoglycemia, intoxication, etc.). It is important in the emergency department or medical office that the secondary survey includes details regarding neurologic improvement or deterioration since the time of injury.

Sport-related injuries after which a player displays signs or symptoms of a concussion require immediate removal from play and evaluation onsite by a physician or other licensed healthcare provider, or in some cases urgent transfer to a facility with those services (e.g. emergency department). Evaluation of cognitive function in the sport setting is essential, as standard orientation questions (e.g. time, place, and person) have been shown to be unreliable [6]. Brief sideline assessment tools that evaluate attention and memory function have been shown to be practical and effective. Examples include the Sport Concussion Assessment Tool (SCAT3) [6] and the Standardized Assessment of Concussion (SAC) [7]. These abbreviated tests are intended only for rapid sideline screening and do not replace comprehensive neuropsychological testing performed by trained neuropsychologists which are more sensitive to subtle deficits that may exist beyond the acute episode.

Red flags for activating emergency services and transport to the nearest hospital include GCS <15 (for more than 30 min), deteriorating mental status, potential spinal injury, or progressive/worsening/new neurologic signs. Anyone suspected of suffering a concussion should be evaluated by a medical professional as soon as possible.

Conventional neuroimaging, such as computed tomography (CT) scan and magnetic resonance imaging (MRI) is typically normal following concussive injury, and is thus an adjunct to clinical diagnosis. Importantly, absolute indications for CT scan have been validated and are presented in table 3. Complicated mTBI is a consequential subtype within the TBI spectrum and is defined as an injury with the clinical characteristics of concussion/mTBI and evidence of macroscopic damage (contusion, extra-axial hemorrhage) on the day-of-injury cranial CT scan. Studies have demonstrated 6-month outcomes to be more similar between patients suffering complicated mTBI and those suffering moderate TBI, as opposed to typical concussion only [8]. Table 4 describes GCS scores associated with mild, moderate, and severe TBI.

Table 3. Factors associated with risk of intracranial injury following concussion: CT is required in a patient presenting for minor head injury and GCS 15 with any of the findings below

Low	Moderate	High
Headache	Posttraumatic LOC, amnesia, or confusion	Depressed or decreasing level of consciousness (e.g. GCS <15 two hours after injury)
Vomiting	Progressive headache	≥65 years of age
>60 years of age	Unreliable or inadequate history (including amnesia and deficits in short-term memory)	Focal neurologic abnormalities
Drug or alcohol intoxication	Dangerous mechanism	Penetrating injury or depressed skull fracture
Visible soft-tissue trauma above the clavicle		Any sign of basal skull fracture
Posttraumatic seizure		≥2 episodes of vomiting

Table 4. Classification of head injury severity

mTBI/concussion	GCS = 13–15
Moderate TBI	GCS = 9–12
Severe TBI	GCS = 3–8

Acute Treatment, Disposition, and Follow-Up

The treatment of concussion begins with prompt identification of the injury, and proceeds to the systematic return to daily activities. The clinician initially evaluating the patient must decide if further assessment, neuroimaging, or prolonged observation is indicated based on premorbid clinical characteristics (age, comorbidities, antithrombotic usage, etc.), exam features, concomitant injuries, and social situation. Concussed patients who are admitted to the emergency room may be discharged home if the following conditions are met at 4 h after injury: (1) GCS of 15, (2) normal alertness, behavior, and cognition, (3) improving neurologic status, (4) no indication for CT scan, and (5) a responsible adult is available to observe the patient for 24 h. Importantly, the clinical status of TBI patients may worsen rapidly even after a relatively innocuous presentation. Serial monitoring for deterioration is essential over the initial 24 h following injury. If a concussion does not require transport to another facility, ongoing monitoring is recommended. If the injury occurs during an athletic event, the athlete will be removed from play for the remainder of the game. The most recent consensus statement that arose from the 4th International Conference on Concussion in Sport definitively reported a unanimous agreement among experts that no same-day return to play should occur after concussion, given that symptoms can evolve over time and sideline tests may be insensitive to subtle changes that occur following concussion. Although the athlete may be sitting on the sideline, he/she should be monitored by the physician and/or athletic trainer over time in order to ensure that deterioration does not occur. This monitoring can involve repeated use of a brief sideline evaluation, or it can be a more informal assessment of symptoms and cognitive status.

Narcotics, muscle relaxants, alcohol, recreational drugs, or any other sedating substance should not be consumed during the acute postconcussive phase. If analgesia is necessary, acetaminophen should be recommended; however, NSAIDs and aspirin are to be avoided. There are no contraindications to antiemetic use.

Postinjury Management: Subacute to Chronic Concussion Management

In most cases, patients should rest and refrain from participating in their usual activities (work, study, driving, etc.) for at least 24–48 h, or until they can be appropriately evaluated by a trained professional who can moderate recommendations based upon early recovery. While symptomatic in the subacute phase, strenuous activity should be avoided. In students, this will typically involve restriction from sports, most exercise, and physical education classes. Physical work restrictions for adults will vary based upon symptom severity and occupational demands. For those patients not managed by an institution with a concussion management protocol, it is typically suggested that they should be evaluated by their primary physician if they do not return to normal function (asymptomatic status) within 2–3 days.

Clinical Course following Concussion

Patients may experience diverse physical, cognitive, and emotional symptoms during the initial days to weeks following an injury. These include, but are not limited to, headaches, fatigue, fogginess, drowsiness, dizziness, and difficulty concentrating. Symptomatic recovery typically occurs within 2 weeks in more than 85% of patients [5]. Nearly 100% report symptom resolution by 1 month, and cognitive effects are negligible after 1–3 months [9]. Numerous studies of concussion in high school athletes suggest a wide range of recovery times, with most falling in the 1-month time frame mentioned above. However, symptoms and functional impairment may persist for much longer in a small portion of those injured. Multiple factors are believed to potentially play a role in rate of recovery, including gender, cognitive reserve, preexisting history of learning or attention disorders, current or prior history of psychiatric disorder, genetics, prior history of brain injury/concussion, and history of migraine or other headache disorder. At present, the precise contribution of each risk factor to individual recovery rates remains unknown. It is important to reassure patients that symptoms associated with postconcussion syndrome typically resolve quickly with rest and proper management.

Symptom	None	Mild		Moderate		Severe	
Headache	0	1	2	3	4	5	6
Nausea	0	1	2	3	4	5	6
Vomiting	0	1	2	3	4	5	6
Balance problems	0	1	2	3	4	5	6
Dizziness	0	1	2	3	4	5	6
Fatigue	0	1	2	3	4	5	6
Trouble falling asleep	0	1	2	3	4	5	6
Sleeping more than usual	0	1	2	3	4	5	6
Sleeping less than usual	0	1	2	3	4	5	6
Drowsiness	0	1	2	3	4	5	6
Sensitivity to light	0	1	2	3	4	5	6
Sensitivity to noise	0	1	2	3	4	5	6
Irritability	0	1	2	3	4	5	6
Sadness	0	1	2	3	4	5	6
Nervousness	0	1	2	3	4	5	6
Feeling more emotional	0	1	2	3	4	5	6
Numbness or tingling	0	1	2	3	4	5	6
Feeling slowed down	0	1	2	3	4	5	6
Feeling mentally 'foggy'	0	1	2	3	4	5	6
Difficulty concentrating	0	1	2	3	4	5	6
Difficulty remembering	0	1	2	3	4	5	6
Visual problems	0	1	2	3	4	5	6

Fig. 1. The Post-Concussion Symptom Scale.

Multidisciplinary management of concussion often begins at the subacute phase. It is at this point, in many comprehensive concussion programs, that the physician and/or athletic trainer engage the remainder of the multidisciplinary team in the athlete's care. Early education of patients and families regarding management strategy (typically cognitive and physical rest until asymptomatic, then gradual resumption of activity) and recovery expectations (time course and expected resolution of symptoms) is very important in the management of concussion and for the prevention of persistent symptoms. Patients participating in early intervention programs (including neuropsychological testing, reassurance, and access to a multidisciplinary team) report fewer postconcussion symptoms at 3 and 6 months after injury compared to standard hospital care [10]. Below, we describe the most common professionals who may be involved in management and rehabilitation of concussion in the subacute and chronic phases.

Athletic Trainer

Although athletic trainers are typically involved in concussion management from baseline testing and injury to recovery and return to play, it is important to note the significant role most athletic trainers play in an athlete's recovery from concussion. During the acute recovery phase, the athletic trainer monitors the athlete's symptoms on a regular (often daily) basis and provides feedback to the teachers

Please use the following scale to rate each symptom:							
	None	Mild		Moderate		Severe	
	0	1	2	3	4	5	6

SYMPTOMS	SEVERITY RATING						
	Date:	Date:	Date:	Date:	Date:	Date:	Date:
Headache							
Nausea							
Vomiting							
Balance problems							
Dizziness							
Fatigue							
Trouble falling asleep							
Sleeping too much							
Sleeping too little							
Drowsiness							
Sensitvity to light							
Sensitivity to noise							
Irritability							
Sadness							
Feeling nervous							
Feeling emotional							
Numbness or tingling							
Feeling too slow							
Mentally 'foggy'							
Difficulty concentrating							
Memory problems							
Visual problems							
Total							

Fig. 2. The Post-Concussion Symptom Scale weekly monitoring checklist.

and athletic staff regarding the student's disposition (see fig. 1 and 2 for examples of the Post-Concussion Symptom Scale in a daily and weekly monitoring form [11]). In addition, athletic trainers may complete regular assessments of balance and computerized neuropsychological testing at recommended intervals, usually in consultation with the managing physician or neuropsychologist, in order to understand the progress of the athlete's recovery. Once the athlete is asymptomatic at rest, the graded return to exertion is usually supervised by the athletic trainer. Although there is no universally agreed-upon or mandated return-to-exertion plan, most at the high school level and below involve a 5- to 6-day progression that begins with light exertion and culminates in return to contact sport participation (e.g. McCrory et al. [6]).

Neuropsychologist

When available, a neuropsychologist can provide primary support for concussion management during the subacute phase. A neuropsychologist trained in concussion evaluation and management can provide and interpret postinjury neuropsychological testing, whether through a widely used computerized testing protocol, paper-and-pencil assessment, or a combination of both. Many neuropsychologists who work with athletes have also been trained to perform basic assessments of balance function. Often, once the diagnosis of concussion is made, and the athlete is removed from play, the neuropsychologist can regularly monitor the recovery of an athlete through serial assessments of cognitive function, symptoms, and balance. Neuropsychologists are trained to understand the relation of cognitive function to other factors, such as mood and history of learning problems. In addition, if symptoms are severe and/or persistent, a neuropsychologist can translate the cognitive performance and symptom patterns of a concussed student into academic accommodations that can help the student maximize his or her involvement in academics while minimizing symptom impact. In cases where severe symptoms or cognitive dysfunction are present, the neuropsychologist can offer recommendations for remaining out of school, or transitioning to a more restrictive (temporary) academic setting such as partial days or homebound education. In some states, the neuropsychologist can manage a concussion case from the subacute through return-to-play phase in conjunction with the athletic training staff. In other states, final clearance from an MD or DO is required for return to play, and a few states require physician clearance to begin the noncontact exertion progression after symptoms remit.

School Staff

If a student's concussion symptoms last for more than a few days, it is almost certain that several members of the academic institution will become part of the multidisciplinary management. Typically, a student's guidance counselor, school nurse, and teachers will be involved in the process. The guidance counselor will often be the hub through which academic accommodations are provided to teachers, and will be able to communicate with teachers to monitor progress and identify areas of difficulty before escalation. The school nurse often monitors concussion symptoms as the student moves throughout the day, and can provide a place where the concussed student can rest during the day if symptoms spike. In cases of chronic symptoms and protracted recovery, cognitive difficulties, particularly if not monitored regularly or correctly, can lead to significant declines in academic performance which can affect a student's future academic options (e.g. college acceptance, tracking for accelerated courses, etc.). Thus, early involvement and regular communication with important school staff is critical for the student's short-term and long-term success during the recovery process and beyond.

Physical Therapist

Upper body musculoskeletal injuries can often co-occur with head injuries. Thus, the physician or athletic trainer may identify a collateral injury that requires rehabilitation through a course of physical therapy. There is some evidence that supervised subsymptom threshold exercise training in patients with postconcussion syndrome can lead to improved symptoms [12, 13]. Once a patient is asymptomatic, a physical therapist can supervise the graded return to exertion. At the University of Pittsburgh Medical Center, the Sports Concussion Program designed a 5-stage exertion protocol [14] that incorporates therapeutic exercises while in the symptomatic and asymptomatic phases.

Vestibular Therapist

Dizziness and balance problems are common symptoms following concussion [15]. As with other concussion symptoms, these are most often transient and resolve with rest, requiring no additional intervention. However, when vestibular symptoms are severe or persistent, the patient may benefit from vestibular therapy. This type of therapy is usually performed by specially trained physical therapists. Commonly prescribed exercises involve improving eye-head coordination, standing static balance, and ambulation [16].

Neuro-Optometrist

Visual problems can be caused by head injury. In addition to affecting visual processing, these vision difficulties can exacerbate balance or vestibular difficulties in multiple ways. Difficulties with accommodative convergence, ocular motor control, and other visual functions can lead to difficulty processing visual information which can cause vertiginous symptoms. Reception, integration, and processing of information from visual, vestibular, and somatosensory systems are complex processes that, if interrupted, may cause a variety of symptoms. If these issues are present, the patient may require neuro-optometric (visual) rehabilitation and/or vestibular therapy to maximally reduce or fully resolve symptoms [17].

Psychotherapist or Counselor

Mood changes can occur as acute or chronic symptoms following concussion. In the short term, injured persons may experience transient feelings of depression, anxiety, irritability, or frustration – typically related to being injured and the subsequent losses associated with the injury (e.g. cannot play sports, work restrictions, academic difficulties, and uncomfortable symptoms). However, mood symptoms can become chronic and evolve into clinical disorders like major depression or generalized anxiety. Functional MRI studies of depression in concussed athletes have identified pathophysiological changes consistent with a limbic-frontal model of depression, and have found a relation between the severity of depression symptoms and neural response [18]. Individual psychotherapy can help an injured individual process losses related to the change in health status and provide emotional support throughout the recovery process. A licensed psychologist, counselor, or licensed clinical social worker who has experience with mild brain injury or medical populations can provide this treatment, which usually consists of weekly sessions for a period of up to several months if needed. Of course, when symptoms are severe, treatment may also include psychotropic medication prescribed by a psychiatrist, neuropsychiatrist, or other physician. We typically encourage psychotherapy in most cases so that the individual may learn coping skills, fully process emotions, and better understand the source of their mood difficulties. Counseling is also very useful when an athlete must retire from his or her sport, or an injured person is unable to return to his or her prior occupation because of postconcussion syndrome and/or related injuries.

Neurologist or Physiatrist

If postconcussion symptoms are chronic and cause significant impairment in daily activities or quality of life, medication management may be indicated. The prescribing physician should have knowledge and experience in treating brain injury and postconcussion syndrome. Most often, neurologists and physiatrists with training in managing postconcussion syndrome are called upon to provide this treatment. Common symptoms that are treated with medication include headaches, disordered sleep, cognitive symptoms (concentration/memory problems, mental fogginess, cognitive slowing), and emotional symptoms. Reddy [19] provides a comprehensive overview of medication management of symptoms of postconcussion syndrome.

Return to Play

Once an athlete is symptom free at rest, a graduated return to noncontact, nonrisk exertion is initiated. In typical cases of concussion without protracted recovery, this protocol is often 5–7 days in duration, beginning with light levels of physical exercise and progressing to gradually increasing levels until the athlete is able to maximally exert without a recurrence of symptoms. The Consensus Statement on Concussion in Sport, originating from the 4th International Conference on Concussion in Sport [6] offers an example of a general graded return to exertion protocol, and Johnston et al. [20] offer examples of sport-specific protocols. Athletes should not progress through more than one level every 24 h, and if any level of activity causes a return of symptoms, the athlete should stop immediately. Once asymptomatic again for 24 h, they will usually restart exertion at the level at which they were previously asymptomatic, though some institutions' protocols require the athlete to begin at stage 1 again.

Most often, the return to exertion is supervised by an athletic trainer, though in some cases physical therapists or team physicians may be involved. In addition to being asymptomatic at rest and with exertion, the athlete must have also returned to baseline levels of function on neurocognitive testing and balance evaluation, as well as any other preinjury testing that has been completed. If the athlete has received treatment or rehabilitative care from other providers, they must demonstrate clearance from those providers as well. The neuropsychologist (or other professional trained to interpret pre- and postinjury testing) will be involved at this phase as well. Ideally, the athlete will complete a final neurocognitive testing session after he/she has completed or almost completed the exertion protocol without symptoms. This allows the care team to ensure cognitive function is at baseline levels, and also allows a final check of symptom reporting, as many cognitive testing platforms include symptom checklists. In rare cases, an athlete may hide mild lingering symptoms throughout the exertion protocol, and experience a subsequent decline in function when completing the 'final' cognitive test. Also, having the athlete report symptoms to the care team as well as on a self-report checklist allows multiple assurances that the athlete is indeed symptom free. It has been the case that an athlete will report asymptomatic status to parents, coaches, physicians, etc., and then disclose mild lingering symptoms on a checklist.

Conclusion

Although concussion is deemed a 'mild' brain injury, the lack of structural findings and the diversity of presentation and recovery of symptoms make this injury one of the most complex to properly manage, particularly in cases of protracted recovery. Often, as described in the literature through analysis of group statistics, the injured person will recover within hours or days without complication, with little disruption to the person's usual life patterns, and with rest, avoidance of injury, and observation as the only 'treatment'. In cases of student-athletes, management of this type of injury will typically require a small multidisciplinary team that involves the physician, athletic trainer, and perhaps consulting neuropsychologist. In this chapter, we have reviewed components of a successful concussion management program and team-based management approach. Figure 3 provides a basic outline of the management approach from pre-injury screening and education to clinical recovery from simple and more chronic concussion.

As medical providers, athletic staff, student-athletes, and parents have become more aware of the signs and symptoms of injury and the consequences of repeated concussion or premature return to play, more cases of protracted recovery (which may have previously gone untreated or misdiagnosed) are being evaluated and managed. When managed well, cases of protracted recovery will often require a larger team that communicates frequently throughout the recovery. If symptoms do not resolve within a few weeks, or seem atypical, evaluation and treatment of the most problematic symptoms will help the injured person function better and experience a reduction in the type or intensity of symptoms as they recover. Because concussion symptoms vary among individuals and among injuries, no single treatment or treatment plan will be appropriate for the management of every complex or protracted case. In addition, even in cases of protracted recovery, the intensity and presentation of symptoms can change over time and with changes in activity (e.g. returning to school or work, etc.). Thus, proper man-

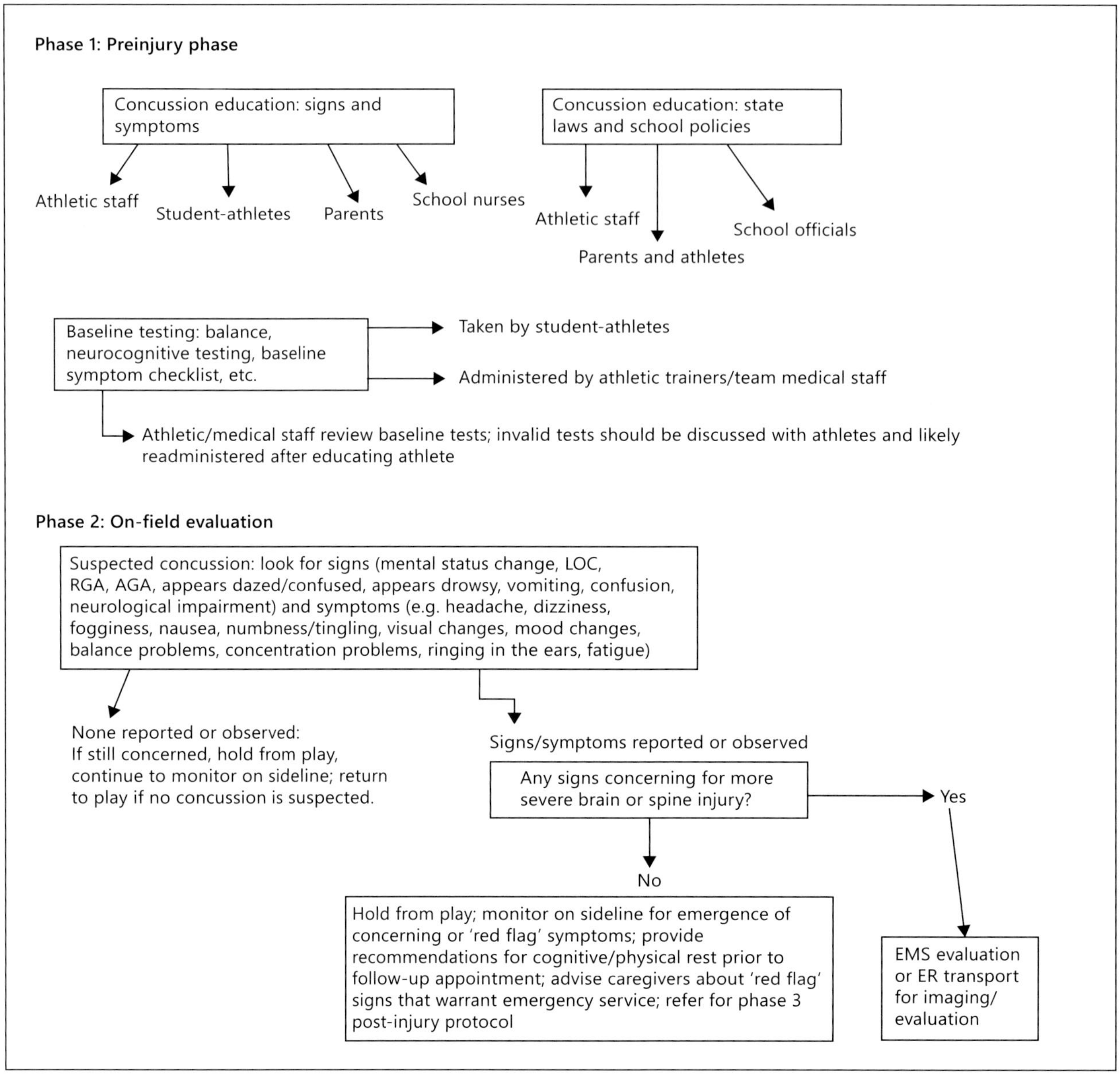

Fig. 3. Model management tree for sports concussion. RGA = Retrograde amnesia; AGA = anterograde amnesia; PM&R = physical medicine and rehabilitation.

agement requires *regular* and *detailed* follow-up of the injured person through the duration of their recovery. This careful follow up requires input from a variety of healthcare providers and other sources who will work together and communicate frequently to provide the most expeditious recovery and best outcomes for the concussed individual, both during their recovery and as they reintegrate into their regular athletic, academic, occupational, and social activities.

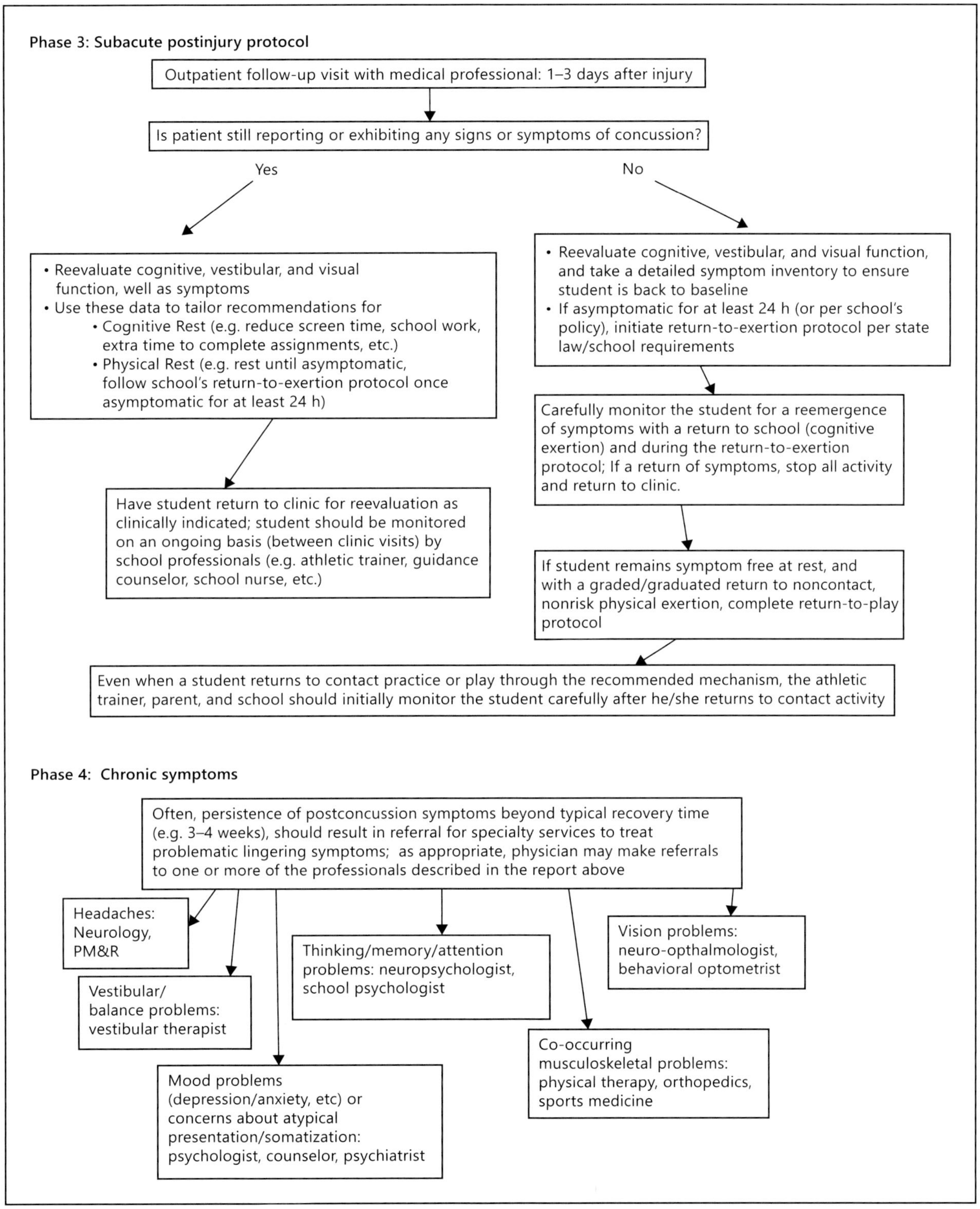

Fig. 3. Continued.

References

1 McCrea M, Guskiewicz KM, Marshall SW: Acute effects and recovery time following concussion in collegiate football players. Br J Sports Med 2004;38: 369–371.

2 Practice parameter: the management of concussion in sports (summary statement): report of the Quality Standards Subcommittee. Neurology 1997;48:581–585.

3 Mild Traumatic Brain Injury Committee, ACoRM, Head Injury Interdisciplinary Special Interest Group: Definition of mild traumatic brain injury. J Head Traum Rehab 1993;8:86–87.

4 Centers for Disease Control and Prevention: Heads up: facts for physicians about mild TBI (mTBI). 2007. http://www.cdc.gov/concussion/headsup/pdf/Facts_for_Physicians_booklet-a.pdf.

5 Scorza KA, Raleigh MF, O'Connor FG: Current concepts in concussion: evaluation and management. Am Fam Physician 2012;85:123–132.

6 McCrory P, Meeuwisse WH, Aubry M, Cantu B, Dvorak J, Echemendia RJ, Turner M: Consensus statement on concussion in sport: The 4th International Conference on Concussion in Sport held in Zurich, November 2012. Br J Sports Med 2013;47: 250–258.

7 McCrea M: Standardized mental status testing on the sideline after sport-related concussion. J Athl Train 2001;36:274.

8 Williams DH, Levin HS, Eisenberg HM: Mild head injury classification. Neurosurgery 1990;27:422–428.

9 Snell DL, Surgenor LJ, Hay-Smith EJ, Siegert RJ: A systematic review of psychological treatments for mild traumatic brain injury: an update on the evidence. J Clin Exp Neuropsychol 2009;31:20–38.

10 Comper P, Bisschop SM, Carnide N, Tricco A: A systematic review of treatments for mild traumatic brain injury. Brain Inj 2005;19:863–880.

11 Lovell MR, Collins MW: Neuropsychological assessment of the college football player. J Head Trauma Rehabil 1998;13:9–26.

12 Baker JG, Freitas MS, Leddy JJ, Kozlowski KF, Willer BS: Return to full functioning after graded exercise assessment and progressive exercise treatment of postconcussion syndrome. Rehabil Res Pract 2012; 2012:705309.

13 Leddy JJ, Kozlowski K, Donnelly JP, Pendergast DR, Epstein LH, Willer B: A preliminary study of subsymptom threshold exercise training for refractory post-concussion syndrome. Clin J Sport Med 2010; 20:21–27.

14 Collins M, Anderson K, Fedor S, Kegel N, Kontos A, Mucha A, Troutman-Enseki C: The science of concussion: advancements in assessment, management, and rehabilitation. http://www.upmcphysicianresources.com/files/dmfile/S725-UPMC_Restore_Concussion_SpecEd_11.pdf.

15 Lovell MR, Iverson GL, Collins MW, Podell K, Johnston KM, Pardini D, Pardini J, Norwig J, Maroon JC: Measurement of symptoms following sports-related concussion: reliability and normative data for the post-concussion scale. Appl Neuropsychol 2006;13: 166–174.

16 Alsalaheen BA, Whitney SL, Mucha A, Morris LO, Furman JM, Sparto PJ: Exercise prescription patterns in patients treated with vestibular rehabilitation after concussion. Physiother Res Int 2013;18: 100–108.

17 Cohen AH: Vision rehabilitation for visual-vestibular dysfunction: the role of the neuro-optometrist. Neurorehabilitation 2013;32:483–492.

18 Chen JK, Johnston KM, Petrides M, Ptito A: Neural substrates of symptoms of depression following concussion in male athletes with persisting postconcussion symptoms. Arch Gen Psychiat 2008;65:81–89.

19 Reddy CC: Postconcussion syndrome: a physiatrist's approach. PM R 2011;3:S396–S405.

20 Johnston KM, Kissick J, Chen JK: Current concepts in concussion rehabilitation. Curr Sports Med Rep 2004;3:316–323.

21 Holm L, Cassidy JD, Carroll LJ, Borg J, Neurotrauma Task Force on Mild Traumatic Brain Injury of the WHO Collaborating Centre: Summary of the WHO Collaborating Centre for Neurotrauma Task Force on Mild Traumatic Brain Injury. J Rehabil Med 2005; 37:137–141.

Jamie E. Pardini, PhD
Department of Neurosurgery, University of Pittsburgh Medical Center
200 Lothrop Street Suite B-400
Pittsburgh, PA 15213 (USA)
E-Mail pardinij@upmc.edu

Niranjan A, Lunsford LD (eds): Concussion. Prog Neurol Surg. Basel, Karger, 2014, vol 28, pp 213–225
DOI: 10.1159/000358785

Vulnerability in Speed of Visuomotor Ability

Ann B. Shuttleworth-Edwards[a] · Sarah E. Radloff[b] ·
Victoria J. Whitefield-Alexander[a]

Departments of [a]Psychology and [b]Statistics, Rhodes University, Grahamstown, South Africa

Abstract

The aim of this report is to illustrate the utility of neurocognitive testing as an investigative method to establish the presence of persistent effects of concussive brain injury amongst players of a contact sport with high risk of such injury. The report reviews the outcomes of three previously published neuropsychological studies on South African Rugby Union (hereafter 'rugby') from school through to the national adult level. The diagnostic utility of differential effects per se, as well as differential *practice* effects on visuomotor function, as a means of distinguishing poorer neurocognitive outcome for rugby versus demographically equivalent noncontact sports players, is described. From various methodological angles, at each level of play, the reviewed studies attest to the presence of long-term vulnerability in visuomotor speed in association with participation in rugby, in turn implicating diffuse frontotemporal dysfunction due to repetitive concussive and subconcussive injury amongst rugby players. As visuomotor speed is a prime function called upon for optimal scholastic and occupational performance, the robustly demonstrated decrement is of immediate clinical importance. Of critical heuristic relevance, however, is evidence of residual brain dysfunction in association with rugby as early as school level, which may ultimately be the precursor of chronic traumatic encephalopathy.

© 2014 S. Karger AG, Basel

Concussive brain injury is a common feature characterizing the field contact sports [1, 2]. Alongside the growing popularity of these sports at both child and adult levels, optimal management of the injury has evolved as a major area of concern among the medical and neuropsychological community [3, 4]. It has long been acknowledged that boxing is associated with repeated head insults resulting in structural neurological damage, permanent neurocognitive deficits, and the possible long-term outcome of chronic traumatic encephalopathy [5, 6]. However, it is only more recently that permanent effects of the injury have been raised as an issue of concern in field contact sports. The disquiet has arisen in the wake of multiple neuropsychological studies of American football, soccer, and Rugby Union (hereafter 'rugby') that reveal lingering deleterious psychometric test outcome for players of these sports [7]. In light of the interpretive nature of such investigations, which involves measurement of brain output as distinct from direct examination of the brain, as well as the cross-sectional nature of many of the studies, there has been a tenacious reserve, if not skepticism expressed amongst some about the validity of these findings [8].

In very recent times, however, potent cross-validation of the repeated psychometric indications of residual brain dysfunction is being achieved from more direct evidence of structural brain damage from neuroimaging and autopsy studies for older, and even in some instances for younger, participants of these sports [9–12]. In other words, the new relatively 'hard' evidence makes it more difficult to ignore or dismiss as alarmist the long history of psychometric test outcome presented over the past two decades similarly in support of residual effects on brain function of cumulative concussive injury [7]. Added impetus in this regard is being derived from the media frenzy around a multimillion dollar legal settlement by the National Football League (NFL) for suppressing the dangers of the injury [13]. Such cross-validation in turn ratifies the use of psychometric testing, when contextualized appropriately within the formal conceptual parameters of clinical neuropsychology, as a critically important investigative method in this area. Importantly, while the imaging and autopsy studies in question have used samples predominantly of players of American football or ice hockey, on logical grounds the disturbing implications can clearly be extrapolated beyond these convenience populations within the USA and Canada to other contact sports including rugby [13]. In other words, there is the compelling indication from these imaging and autopsy studies, supported indirectly by psychometric evidence, for developing neurodegenerative disease in association with long-term participation in *any* sport where player-to-player and player-to-ground collisions are intrinsic to the sport, thereby resulting in subconcussive (microtrauma) and concussive events being incurred on a repetitive basis.

Of the at risk field contact sports, rugby (played extensively in the UK, New Zealand, Australia, and South Africa) is considered to be the most dangerous, and reveals a higher incidence of reported concussion than American football [2]. Participants of rugby, therefore, are a highly suited population on which to evaluate concussion sequelae per se, and especially the hotly debated issue of whether or not there are damaging long-term effects of repetitive concussive and subconcussive brain injury. To this end, specifically using psychometric testing as an investigative method, a number of studies and/or collation of various studies have been completed and published by the present first author and colleagues [14–16], the key features of which will be reviewed below. Prior to embarking on the review, however, it is important to provide a synthesis of key conceptual parameters relevant to using neuropsychological evaluation in particular as an investigative tool in the concussion arena, as distinct from other investigative techniques, and to define other key concepts as applied in the three research studies.

Conceptual Issues

Clinical neuropsychology is defined as 'an applied science concerned with the behavioural expression of brain dysfunction' [17]. Intrinsic to the science is a vast body of research starting in the first half of the 20th century with screening of brain-injured servicemen during the First World War that has linked various alterations and limitations of cognitive function with disturbances in specific parts of the brain and/or more complex neuropathological presentations. The critical point about this form of investigation is that it is an indirect measure of the brain, and therefore is necessarily interpretive and hypothetical to a much greater extent than the more direct examinations of brain structure and function enabled by autopsy and/or neuroimaging investigative methods. Nevertheless, the crucial contribution of neuropsychological research to neurological knowledge in general resides in the need to establish the behavioral effect of brain changes in addition to the concrete indication of brain alteration in and of itself.

Specifically, neuropsychological investigation can be defined as a specialist level of inquiry about brain output rather than straight brain observation, which can only be established on the basis of cognitive, emotional, and behavioral testing, clinical observation, and inquiry, as this is a relatively noninvasive and cost-effective mode of investigation. Importantly, expense aside, it is not always possible to identify brain changes by means of other more direct investigative techniques despite massive technological advances in those fields, especially when anomalous brain function is in the early stages, and of a diffuse nature such as with concussive brain injury [4, 17]. In contrast, evidence of behavioral change, especially on probing neurocognitive examination, has the power to identify early signs of critical brain alterations in advance of their subsequent confirmation via other more direct modes of examination. In turn this knowledge may provide crucial clues as to etiological links and stage of onset of a particular pathology.

Finally, for the conceptual clarity in this report, it is noted that the term 'concussive brain injury' will be alternatively referred to in this report as 'mild traumatic brain injury' such as is conventionally applied in the sports literature, although it is acknowledged that some use the terms separately to refer to different types of injury. In their research protocols, all the studies to be reported on below [14–16] use the term concussion to refer to a relatively low-velocity injury that causes brain 'shaking', being a subset of traumatic brain injury [4]. Operationally, the research studies in question define a concussion as any event following a head or body collision where there was any loss of consciousness or period of amnesia, or any changes in mental and physical status implicating postconcussion symptoms as typically described in the literature [18]. The focus of the three studies to be reviewed is on the long-term, i.e. chronic, outcome of concussion, as distinct from acute and subacute effects. In these studies, the term 'chronic' has been operationally differentiated from more immediate acute sequelae that typically resolve within 3 months after the injury, with effects which persist for longer than this being viewed as chronic, i.e. relatively intractable [19].

A review of the three designated studies on rugby follows below [14–16], the full methodological details are available in the original reports and will not be replicated here.

Study 1: Shuttleworth-Edwards et al., 2004 [14]

In an early research investigation, using paper-and-pencil psychometric testing in a relatively exploratory fashion with a wide-ranging test battery, it was decided to investigate the additive effect of repetitive sports concussion by conducting a comparative analysis of the percentages of players of South African rugby with objective test deficit [14]. The mode of psychometric test score evaluation took the form of a separate personalized analysis of every score within an individual's test profile, in each case evaluated in comparison with a demographically appropriate norm, thereby tapping the full extent of deficit in a clinically relevant manner that is not possible in a group analysis. On this basis it was hypothesized that due to the aggregation effect of repeated concussion via participation in rugby, in association with longer or more exposed positional play, and/or in association with a prior cognitive vulnerability, rugby players would show more impairment than noncontact sport controls, more at risk forward players would show more impairment than backline players, older and higher level players would show more impairment than younger players, and players who had a recorded history of a learning problem would show more impairment than noncontact sport controls without a recorded history of a learning problem.

Study Participants

Exclusion criteria for the study were a history of substance abuse, neurological or psychiatric condition, prior moderate or severe head injury for any reason (i.e. loss of unconsciousness >30 min), any prior grade failure, and/or a recorded learning problem. The final sample of predominantly white English- and Afrikaans-speaking adults consisted of 26 national open rugby players (15 forwards and 11 backs), 19 national under-21 rugby players (11 forwards and 8 backs), and 47 school rugby players (28 forwards and 19 backs), with control groups being made up, respectively, of 21 national open cricketers, a younger group of 21 national open field hockey players, and 34 schoolboy field hockey players. Cricket (as with baseball) and field hockey (in contrast to ice hockey) are sports which are not characterized by multiple concussions due to collisions between players or players to ground [20], which renders them highly suitable to call upon when making up noncontact sport control groups. Six school boys with a prior history of a learning problem, excluded from the main study, formed two subgroups for further comparative purposes, consisting of 3 rugby players with a learning problem, and 3 field hockey players without a learning problem.

All comparative groups in the main study were equivalent for age, education, and estimated IQ ($p > 0.05$ in all instances) with the exception of the national under-21 rugby players who were significantly lower than field hockey controls with respect to all these variables ($p < 0.05$ in all instances). Since each level of play was analyzed separately, the outcome of the national open and school cohorts would not be contaminated due to the demographic differences exclusively in the under-21 group. In the subgroup analysis, the rugby group with a learning disability had a lower IQ estimate than the field hockey control group with a learning disability (mean IQ: 113.5 vs. 101.0, respectively), so that any deleterious effects in the rugby group could not be accounted for by lower intellectual ability.

Procedure and Outcome

Participants were assessed individually by psychology interns using standardized test formats, at the rugby preseason juncture following a 5-month rugby playing break, in order to exclude the acute and subacute effects of concussion. A wide spectrum of commonly employed paper-and-pencil neuropsychological measures, across a comprehensive spectrum of functional modalities known to be sensitive to impairments following mild traumatic brain injury, viz. attention and concentration, visuoperceptual processing speed, memory, verbal fluency, and hand motor dexterity, were used. Deficit was defined as a score greater than 1 SD from the best available normative data in the direction of poorer performance.

Taken overall, the outcome of the main group test comparisons, in which percentages of individuals with cognitive deficit were compared via χ^2 analyses, was in support of all the hypotheses with rugby players showing more deficit than controls, forward players exhibiting more deficit than backline players, and older players demonstrating more problems than younger school boy players in each of the functional areas of speed of information processing, memory, verbal fluency, and hand motor dexterity. The function that most frequently differentiated these groups significantly in the direction of the hypotheses was in visuospatial processing speed, incorporating outcome from the Wechsler Intelligence Adult Scale Digit Symbol Substitution subtest and the Trail Making Test as described in the source article [14]. The outcome for the subset of school boys with a learning disability was again in the hypothesized direction, with much more impairment for rugby players than controls in the areas of attention, processing speed, and visual memory, despite having a higher estimated IQ than the field hockey subgroup with a learning problem. The percentage of cognitive deficit for these cognitively vulnerable rugby players in both verbal and nonverbal attentional tasks clustered around 67–100% of cases, compared with close on zero indication of deficit across tests for the similarly cognitively vulnerable field hockey players. Although the subgroup sample numbers were small, the descriptive findings are commensurate with the research of Collins et al. [21], who demonstrated significantly increased cognitive deficit in football players with repeated concussions and a learning disability compared with concussed football players without a learning disability.

A heuristic strength of this early study using paper-and-pencil testing is its exploratory nature of using a wide battery that allowed for a comparative view on which tests served best to differentiate between the at risk rugby groups and the control groups. Further, the mode of investigation was based on an analysis of the proportion (i.e. number) of rugby players who showed neuropsychological deficits on tests relative to appropriate norms in areas known to be susceptible to damage in association with mild traumatic brain injury. In that this is a mode of analysis typically applied in clinical situations, the outcome can be seen to have clinical as well as statistical relevance. A limitation of the study that might be cause for challenging the validity of the outcome, however, is the very fact of its having such a wide test battery with multiple comparisons calling for Bonferroni's correction to guard against the chance of a type 1 error (finding erroneous significance by chance). These were not applied thereby opening the study to the criticism of possibly inflating effects [22, 23]. On the other hand, the relatively subtle nature of the findings in respect to the small sample numbers might have served to obscure relevant effects [22, 23]. These criticisms call for more focused hypothesis-testing research in terms of test modality for larger sample numbers, and provided the incentive for further investigation of the study data, to be described below.

Study 2: Shuttleworth-Edwards and Radloff, 2008 [15]

Typically in many of the early neuropsychological studies on contact sports, an expansive battery of tests was used with a view to enhancing sensitivity to subtle mild brain injury effects [7], such as was also applied in the earlier series of South African rugby studies described above [14]. However, as also alluded to above, the use of multiple measures in the research context calls for substantial adjustments towards statistical stringency in order to guard against type I errors. In order to circumvent the problem it has been suggested that data derived from collections of smaller exploratory studies should be combined to gain the increased statistical power that becomes available in a larger sample [22, 23]. Further, the employment of a restricted neurocognitive variable with a view to focused hypothesis testing (rather than the application of a wide-ranging exploratory test battery) is considered the more appropriate methodological route to follow [22, 23].

Accordingly, the aim of this new study [15] was to provide a focused neurocognitive investigation into outcome for the single functional modality of visuomotor processing speed, using data that were available from the earlier wide-ranging investigation described above [14] that explored a spectrum of functional modalities on rugby players at the first team high school, under-21 national, and open national levels. Data selection for the new analysis pertained to all rugby participants and noncontact sport controls in the prior study from each of the three levels of play, and was exclusively in respect of the two tests of visuomotor speed that were identified as being the most discriminatory of possible brain injury effects within the wide battery employed in that study series, viz. Digit Symbol Substitution Test and Trail Making Test parts A and B, as described by Lezak et al. [17]. Specifically, the Digit Symbol Substitution Test calls upon visual scanning, motor persistence, sustained attention, response speed, and visuomotor coordination, and is consistently more sensitive to brain damage than the other Wechsler Intelligence Scale subtests [17]. The Trail Making Test similarly taps visual scanning, motor persistence, sustained attention, and response speed, as well as visuomotor tracking, divided attention, and cognitive flexibility [17]. As with Digit Symbol Substitution, the test is highly sensitive to the effects of even mild brain injury.

It was hypothesized that there would be clinically relevant signs of diminished performance in visuomotor processing speed for the cerebrally at risk rugby players compared with a noncontact sport group, and amongst cerebrally more at risk forward players compared with backs, due to a history of cumulative concussive and subconcussive events sustained in association with years of participation in the sport. It was expected that synergistically these concussive events would have cumulative effects on rugby players during many years of exposure to the game and predispose them to neuropsychological vulnerability in the prototypically sensitive area of visuomotor processing speed.

Study Participants

Participants for the newly combined analysis were top team South African male rugby players (n = 124) versus top team South African noncontact sport controls including a mixture of cricket and field hockey athletes (n = 102), across the three participant stages of play of the earlier study. The total rugby group was divided for comparison between forward positional players who are more exposed to cerebral injury, and backline players who are less exposed to cerebral injury (n = 71 and 53, respectively). As indicated for the original three studies, exclusion criteria were a history of alcohol or substance abuse, neurological or psychiatric disease, a prior failed grade or learning disability, or moderate to severe TBI (loss of consciousness >30 min). All comparative groups were statistically equivalent for age, level of education, and estimated IQ, as well as performance on the Finger Tapping Preferred and Non-Preferred Hand Tests ensure that none of these variables, including physical hand injury, did not account for slowing on visuomotor tracking tasks ($p > 0.05$ in all instances). Finally, there was a highly significant difference in the percentage of rugby players with a history of 2+ concussions compared with controls (53 vs. 17% respectively, $p < 0.0001$), but no significant difference in the percentage of forwards with a history of 2+ concussions compared with backs (49 vs. 53% respectively, $p > 0.05$).

Procedure and Outcome

As indicated above, from the original wide-ranging battery, only two tests within the single functional modality of visuomotor processing speed were isolated in light of their demonstrated superior sensitivity. These included the Digit Symbol Substitution Test with the score representing the number of pairings of symbol and numbers com-

Table 1. t test comparisons of rugby vs. controls and forwards vs. backs for the Digit Symbol Substitution Test, Trail Making Test (TMT) A and B, and Processing Speed (PS) factor

	Rugby (n = 124) mean ± SD	Control (n = 102) mean ± SD	t value	Effect size, δ	95% CI	p value	Forwards (n = 71) mean ± SD	Backs (n = 53) mean ± SD	t value	Effect size, δ	95% CI	p value
Digit Symbol	49.98±9.20	53.41±8.28	2.92	0.39	0.13 to 0.65	0.004**	47.99±9.00	52.63±8.85	2.86	0.52	0.16 to 0.88	0.005**
TMT A	27.86±7.98	24.87±6.78	–3.00	–0.40	–0.66 to –0.13	0.003**	27.76±7.42	28.00±8.75	0.16	0.03	–0.32 to 0.38	0.872
TMT B	58.57±19.68	53.00±14.53	–2.38	–0.32	–0.58 to –0.05	0.018*	60.26±20.99	56.33±17.73	–1.10	–0.20	–0.55 to 0.16	0.273
PS factor	–0.21±1.06	0.25±0.85	3.51	0.47	0.20 to 0.74	0.0005**	–0.33±1.02	–0.04±1.11	1.54	0.28	–0.08 to 0.64	0.127

Reproduced from Shuttleworth-Edwards and Radloff [15], with kind permission from Oxford University Press, publishers of *Archives of Clinical Neuropsychology*.
* $p < 0.05$; ** $p < 0.01$.

pleted in 90 s, and the Trail Making Test parts A and B, which are scored according to the time needed to complete the task, as described in well-known neuropsychological texts [17]. As described earlier in respect of the original series of studies from which the data were taken, the tests were administered individually in the standardized formats by psychology interns at preseason following the 5-month break to identify residual rather than acute effects.

The test data were submitted to factor analysis, correlational analyses of test scores with age, and independent samples t test analyses to test for differences in performance on the tests and the mean factor scores between the comparative groups. The factor analysis revealed a single dominant factor with an eigenvalue greater than 1 (λ = 1.88; hereafter termed 'processing speed factor'), accounting for 62.6% of the variation in the data. This finding confirmed the legitimacy of targeting a single neurocognitive function as the dependent variable via the use of the two designated neurocognitive tests, on the basis of which Bonferroni's adjustments were not considered indicated. With reference to table 1, it is evident that t test comparisons of the total rugby group versus controls and forwards versus backs revealed highly significant differences in the direction of poorer performance for the rugby group compared with controls on the Digit Symbol Substitution Test, Trail Making Test parts A and B, and the processing speed factor, and for forwards compared with backs on the Digit Symbol Substitution Test ($p < 0.001$ in most instances), all with clinically relevant effect sizes. Finally, correlations between age and rugby test scores were not significant ($p > 0.05$ in all instances).

Overall, taking significant outcome into account, it was considered that the results implicated depressed performance for the rugby players relative to controls and for the forwards versus backs, and is of clinical relevance due to years of exposure to cumulative concussive and subconcussive events. The absence of significant correlations between age and test scores for rugby participants implicated the presence of deleterious effects on processing speed at all levels of play. In that the comparative groups were well matched for age, education, and IQ, the presence of preexisting differences due to sports affiliation (rugby vs. noncontact sport) does not appear likely. Further, the presence of pre-existing sports group differences does not provide a satisfactory explanation for the *within* rugby group findings of the study, which revealed poorer performance on the Digit Symbol Substitution subtest for more at risk forward players compared with backline players. Rather, the substantive differentiating feature of the rugby group from controls was the presence of a significantly higher number of reported concussions for rugby players, without even taking into consideration the known high tendency for underreporting of this injury and an overlay of necessarily unreported subconcussive incidents that are likely to have occurred over a long rugby playing career. It was concluded that this composite study provided compelling support to the growing evidence across a number of studies of lowered performance on speeded visuomotor tasks for participants of rugby at all levels of play starting already at the end of the high school years, being a phenomenon worthy of on-going investigation.

Study 3: Shuttleworth-Edwards et al., 2014 [16]

The series of cross-sectional South African rugby studies described above, using paper-and-pencil instruments for preseason testing alone, were followed by three new prospective rugby studies employing computerized testing for pre- and postseason testing. These three new studies, the details of which are summarized elsewhere [16], employed the Immediate Post-Concussion Assessment and Cognitive Testing (ImPACT) computerized test [24, 25], and were specifically targeted at high school and university levels of play. A common feature of note when perusing the outcome of these new studies was that the noncontact sports groups improved on the computerized ImPACT Visual Motor Speed (VMS) composite between the pre- and postseason test intervals, whereas the rugby players did not. It is well documented that brain damage populations typically fail to learn with practice on cognitive tests where there is an expected practice effect [17, 26], and therefore it was considered that this feature had important investigative potential as a possible diagnostic indicator of residual cerebral impairment in association cumulative concussive events sustained in rugby.

Accordingly, for the purposes of a new analysis, it was decided to combine the prospective pre- versus postseason outcome data available from these three new South African rugby studies on the single functional modality of visuoperceptual speed as tapped by the ImPACT VMS composite. It was hypothesized that cognitive vulnerability would be apparent in the contact sport groups compared to equivalent noncontact sport controls due to failure to benefit from practice on this task, as a consequence of a long-term history of many years of participation in a sport with a high risk of concussive insults, in interaction with the effects of any unrecognized concussive and subconcussive event sustained during the most recent season of participation in the sport (i.e. hidden within season effects), none of which would be characteristic of the

Table 2. Combined sample: dependent t test comparisons of ImPACT Visual Motor Speed (VMS) scores at the pre- vs. post-season intervals for the rugby and noncontact sports groups

Source	Sample size, n	Preseason mean ± SD	Postseason mean ± SD	t value	Effect size δ-value	95% CI	p value
Rugby VMS	145	36.57±6.80	36.77±6.62	–0.393	–0.03	–0.20 to 0.13	0.695
Noncontact VMS	106	36.65±7.24	38.39±6.70	–3.967	–0.39	–0.58 to –0.19	<0.001***

Reproduced from Shuttleworth-Edwards et al. [16], with kind permission from Oxford University Press, publishers of *Archives of Clinical Neuropsychology*. *** $p < 0.001$.

controls. Importantly, it was considered that the overall postseason outcome would reflect the cognitive status of high school and university rugby players, none of whom would have been formally identified as recently concussed, shortly before the onset of their end of year examinations.

Study Participants

Exclusion criteria were the same as for the earlier paper-and-pencil studies, with the critical added exclusion criterion for the prospective study of any individuals concussed over the season, to ensure the presence of an ostensibly symptom-free group. The final sample was made up of rugby (n = 145) versus noncontact sport controls (n = 106) who were considered equivalent for age, education, and estimated intellectual ability; however, there was a highly significant difference in the entire past history of number of concussions reported between the pooled rugby and noncontact sports groups ($p < 0.001$), in the direction of more concussions for rugby players, accompanied by a high effect size of clinical relevance (d = 0.82, CI: 0.56, 1.08).

Procedure and Outcome

In the case of all three base studies, ImPACT was administered in groups by psychology interns in its standard automated form in computer laboratories under suitably controlled conditions. Dependent t test comparisons of the ImPACT VMS scores at pre- versus postseason for the newly combined sample (table 2) revealed a highly significant improvement for the noncontact controls ($p < 0.001$), in contrast to the absence of significant improvement for rugby players ($p = 0.695$), and a significant interaction effect for sport ($p = 0.028$; table 2; fig. 1).

It was concluded that in contrast to the improvement shown by the controls on the ImPACT VMS, the total absence of a practice effect for rugby players when it is expected, supported by a significant group-by-season interaction effect (table 2; fig. 1), may be considered clinically meaningful. This implicates the presence of persistent deleterious effects on the ImPACT VMS composite that might be attributable to brain injury sustained over years of playing rugby in combination with an overlay of any

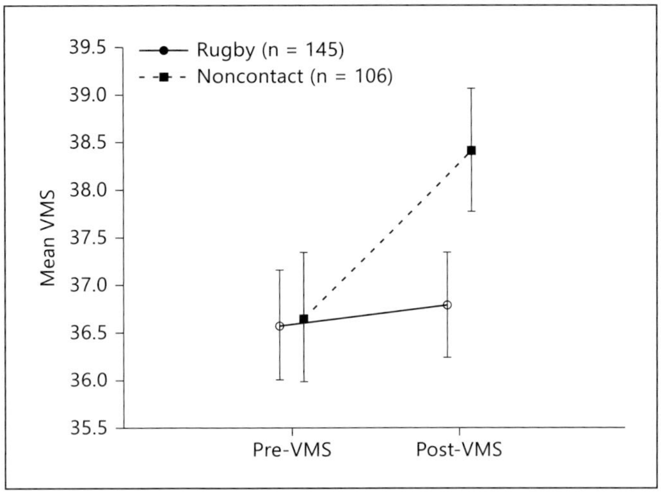

Fig. 1. Combined study: pre- vs. postseason ImPACT Visual Motor Speed (VMS) scores (±SE) for university and high school rugby players vs. noncontact sport controls. Figure reproduced from Shuttleworth-Edwards et al. [16] with kind permission of Oxford University Press, publishers of *Archives of Clinical Neuropsychology*.

such effects sustained by players over the most recent rugby season. Again, as with the previously described studies, the comparative groups were well matched for age, education, and estimated IQ, with the obvious differentiating feature between the two groups of the newly combined sample being the clinically relevant, significantly higher number of reported concussions for rugby players relative to controls. Accordingly, from a neuropsychological perspective there is a compelling implication arising out of the present research of neurocognitive vulnerability amongst a significant proportion of the rugby playing group due to the effects of brain-related insults that typically occur over years of participation in the sport, and/or the effects of undisclosed insults sustained over the season and/or a combination of both factors.

Conclusions

A review of three studies on the effects of repetitive concussion in association with participation in South African rugby has served to illustrate the diagnostic potential of neurocognitive testing in the evaluation of this injury, specifically in the area of visuomotor processing speed. The research studies have been undertaken at school, university, and professional levels of play, using first paper-and-pencil testing in a series of studies with a wide exploratory test battery. This was followed by more focused hypothesis-testing research targeting visuomotor speed alone, after it was identified routinely across these earlier studies as the most discriminating task to demonstrate the presence of long-term deleterious effects of the repetitive concussive injury in association with participation the sport. The vulnerability in visuomotor processing that was so evident across all the reviewed studies, regardless of mode of evaluation or level of play, serves to implicate executive dysfunction and/or slowed processing speed in association with the frontotemporal diffuse brain damage that typically accompanies the acceleration-deceleration closed head injury, and accounts for a deleterious outcome per se, or a smaller than normal practice effect in the rugby group.

Overall these repeated findings within the discipline of neuropsychological science, based on the *indirect* examination of brain function, from a variety of methodological stances, are given substantial credence by recent imaging and autopsy studies that provide more concrete evidence via direct examination of brain structure and function of residual brain anomalies amongst long-term players of such sports. The critical contribution of the neuropsychological investigative route is that it is sensitive to very subtle signs that may not be visible, or even ethically open to investigation via more direct methods of examining the brain, thereby providing important pointers to the likely time of onset of the subsequent more advanced brain impairment in evidence from the imaging and autopsy studies. From the review of these three broad neuropsychological research investigations, which were each based in turn on a composite analysis of a series of smaller studies, it is clear that clinically relevant brain dysfunction is apparent as early as the high school level in learners who would otherwise be considered clinically normal in terms of harboring any current concussion sequelae. The mode of investigation needs to be taken seriously as a necessary arm in unraveling the long-term outcome of the concussive brain injury, the age of clinically relevant onset, and the moderating variables in its behavioral presentation.

References

1 Cassidy JD, Carroll LJ, Peloso PM, Borg J, von Holst H: Incidence, risk factors and prevention of mild traumatic brain injury: results of the WHO Collaborating Centre Task Force on Mild Traumatic Brain Injury. J Rehabil Med 2004;Suppl 43:28–60.

2 Shuttleworth-Edwards AB, Noakes TD, Radloff SE, Whitefield VJ, Roberts CO, Clark SJ, Essack FB, Zoccola D, Boulind MJ, Case SE, Smith IP, Mitchell JL: The comparative incidence of reported concussions for follow-up management in South African Rugby Union. Clin J Sport Med 2008;18:403–409.

3 Schatz P, Moser RS: Current issues in pediatric sports concussion. Clin Neuropsychol 2011;25: 1042–1057.

4 McCrory P, Meeuwisse W, Aubry M, Cantu R, Dvorak J, Echemedia RJ, Engebretsen M, Johnston K, Kutcher J, Raftery M, Sills A: Consensus statement on concussion in sport – the 4th International Conference on Concussion in Sport Held in Zurich, November 2012. Clin J Sport Med 2013;23:89–117.

5 Lundberg GD: Brain injury in boxing. Am J Forensic Med Pathol 1985;6:192–198.

6 Jordan BD: Chronic traumatic brain injury associated with boxing. Semin Neurol 2000;20:179–185.

7 Shuttleworth-Edwards AB, Whitefield VJ: Ethically we can no longer sit on the fence: a neuropsychological perspective on the cerebrally hazardous contact sports. S Afr J Sports Med 2007;19:32–38.

8 Solomon G, Ott D, Lovell M: Long-term neurocognitive dysfunction in sports: what is the evidence? Clin Sports Med 2011;30:165–177.

9 De Beaumont L, Theoret H, Mongeon D, Messier J, Leclerc S, Tremblay S, Ellemberg D, Lassonde M: Brain function decline in healthy retired athletes who sustained their last sports concussion in early adulthood. Brain 2009;132:695–708.

10 Tremblay S, De Beaumont L, Henry L, Boulanger Y, Evans A, Bourgouin P, Poirier J, Theoret H, Lassonde M: Sports concussions and aging: a neuroimaging investigation. Cereb Cortex 2013;23:1159–1166.

11 McKee A, Stein T, Nowinski C, Stern R, Daneshvar D, Alvarez V, Lee HS, Hall G, Wojtowicz S, Baugh C, Riley D, Kubilus C, Cormier K, Matthew A, Martin B, Abraham C, Ikezu T, Reichard R, Wolozin B, Budson A, Goldstein L, Kowall N, Cantu R: The spectrum of disease in chronic traumatic encephalopathy. Brain 2013;136:43–64.

12 Omalu B, Bailes J, Hamilton R, Kamboh M, Hammers J, Case M, Fitzsimmons R: Emerging histomorphologic phenotypes of chronic traumatic encephalopathy in American athletes. Neurosurgery 2011; 69:173–183.
13 Rugby union could face NFL-style lawsuit on concussion – neuroscientist. 2013. http://www theguardian com/sport/2013/oct/17/rugby-union-nfl-lawsuit-concussion.
14 Shuttleworth-Edwards AB, Border M, Reid I, Radloff S: South African Rugby Union; in Lovell MR, Echemendia RE, Barth JT, Collins MW (eds): Traumatic Brain Injury in Sports: An International Neuropsychological Perspective. Leiden, Swets & Zeitlinger, 2004, pp 149–168.
15 Shuttleworth-Edwards AB, Radloff SE: Compromised visuomotor processing speed in players of Rugby Union from school through to the adult national level. Arch Clin Neuropsychol 2008;23:511–520.
16 Shuttleworth-Edwards A, Radloff S, Whitefield-Alexander V, Smith I, Horsman M: Practice effects reveal visuomotor vulnerability on school and university rugby players. Arch Clin Neuropsychol 2014;29: 86–99.
17 Lezak M, Howieson D, Bigler E, Tranel D: Neuropsychological Assessment, ed 5. Oxford, Oxford Univesity Press, 2012.
18 Lovell M, Collins M, Bradley J: Return to play following sports-related concussion. Clin Sports Med 2004; 23:421–441.
19 Reitan RM, Wolfson D: The two faces of mild head injury. Arch Clin Neuropsychol 1999;14:191–202.
20 Powell JW, Barber-Foss KD: Traumatic brain injury in high school athletes. JAMA 1999;282:958–963.
21 Collins MW, Grindell SH, Lovell MR, Dede DE, Moser DJ, Phalin BR, Nogle S, Wasik M, Cordry D, Daugherty KM, Sears SF, Indelicato P, McKeag DB: Relationship between concussion and neuropsychological performance in college football players. JAMA 1999;282:964–970.
22 Frencham KA, Fox AM, Maybery MT: Neuropsychological studies of mild traumatic brain injury: a meta-analytic review of research since 1995. J Clin Exp Neuropsychol 2005;27:334–351.
23 Demakis GJ: Meta-analysis in neuropsychology: basic approaches, findings, and applications. Clin Neuropsychol 2006;20:10–26.
24 Lovell MR, Collins MW, Podell K, Powell J, Maroon J: ImPACT: Immediate Post-Concussion Assessment and Cognitive Testing. Pittsburgh, NeuroHealth Systems LLC, 2000.
25 Shuttleworth-Edwards A, Whitefield-Alexander V: The ImPACT neurocognitive screening test: a survey of South African research, current and projected applications; in Cockcroft K, Laher S (eds): Psychological Assessment in South Africa: Research and Applications. Johannesburg, Wits Press, 2013, pp 443–460.
26 Duff K, Beglinger L, Schultz S, Moser DJ, McCaffrey RJ, Haase RF, Westervelt H, Langbehn D, Paulsen J: Practice effects in the prediction of long-term cognitive outcome in three patient samples: a novel prognostic index. Arch Clin Neuropsychol 2007;22:15–24.

Prof. Ann B. Shuttleworth-Edwards, PhD
Department of Psychology, Rhodes University
Grahamstown 6139 (South Africa)
E-Mail a.edwards@ru.ac.za

Niranjan A, Lunsford LD (eds): Concussion. Prog Neurol Surg. Basel, Karger, 2014, vol 28, pp 226–233
DOI: 10.1159/000358786

Detecting Eye Movement Abnormalities from Concussion

Jun Maruta[a] · Jamshid Ghajar[a, b]

[a]Brain Trauma Foundation, and [b]Department of Neurosurgery, Stanford University School of Medicine, Stanford, Calif., USA

Abstract

An attention-based biomarker may be useful for concussion screening. A key role of attention is to generate time-based expectancies of specific sensory information, and it is postulated that postconcussion cognitive impairments and symptoms may stem from a primary deficit in this predictive timing mechanism. There is a close relationship between gaze and attention, but in addressing predictive timing, there is a need for an appropriate testing paradigm and methods to quantify oculomotor anomalies. We have utilized a continuous predictive visual tracking paradigm because human visual tracking requires predicting the temporal course of a stimulus and dynamically synchronizing the required action with the stimulus. We have shown that concussion patients often show disrupted gaze-target synchronization characterized by large gaze position error variability and overall phase advancement. Various attention components interact with visual tracking, and thus there is a possibility that different neurological and physiological conditions produce identifiable visual tracking characteristics. Analyzing neuromotor functions, specifically oculomotor synchronization, can provide a fast, accurate, and reliable assessment of cognitive functions. © 2014 S. Karger AG, Basel

Eye Movement and Eye Movement Recording

Detecting eye movement abnormalities may provide a fast, accurate, and reliable way to screen for concussion. Eyes move for different reasons and purposes. For example, eyes may move to stabilize or optimize vision when there is a relative movement of the visual world, e.g. during head movements. This class of eye movements is phylogenetically old and largely under reflexive control. Another important goal of eye movement is to foveate, i.e. to orient the eyes to capture the image of a specific object within the fovea.

Not all animals have a fovea, but it is highly developed in humans, allowing for highly specific image analysis by the brain. On the other hand, the central allocation of this specialized function entails sharp vision to be limited only within a small selected part of the captured image, and redirecting this locus of sharp vision requires

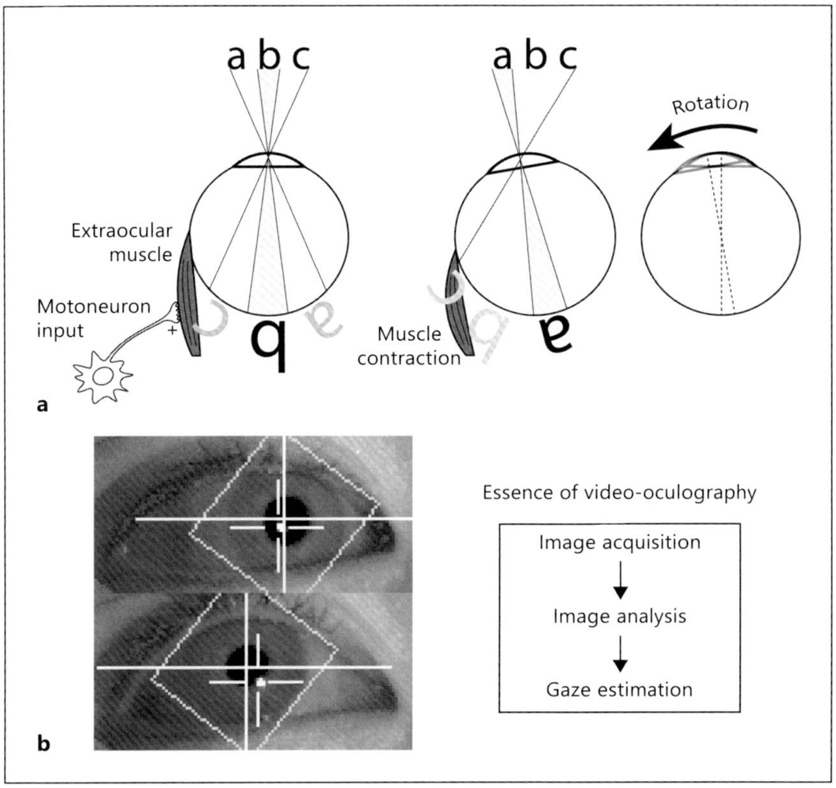

Fig. 1. Eye movement measurement. **a** Specific objects are brought into the line of sight through eye rotation. **b** Video-oculography reconstructs angles of eye rotation from two-dimensional images. The crosshairs indicate centers of the pupil and the reflection of an infrared light source.

movement of the eye, i.e. foveation. Afoveate animals, such as rabbits, do not move the eyes around to examine objects [1].

Although visual acuity is determined by foveal vision, the relationship between the ability to see clearly and to orient the gaze accurately tends to be overlooked. However, the relationship is most easily described in terms of attention, as inherently suggested by selective allocation of resources for information processing. The neural basis of the overlap between gaze and attention networks has been demonstrated using functional magnetic resonance imaging [2].

Eye movements are rotation controlled by a set of muscles attached to the eyeball and the skull (fig. 1a). Eye movements can be described in terms of angles of rotation in specific coordinate planes or axes. There are different classes of eye movement, which include visual fixation, saccade, and smooth pursuit. *Visual fixation* holds the image of a stationary object on the fovea when the head is stationary. It is not a nonmovement, but is under active neural control. A *saccade* causes a rapid change in the eye orientation and can bring the image of the object of interest onto the fovea. *Smooth pursuit* aids continuous stabilization of the image of a moving target on the fovea. There are other classes of movements including vergence and ocular reflexes, as well as those resulting from a failure to hold a steady gaze, such as tremor, drift, and spontaneous nystagmus. Visual fixation, smooth pursuit, saccades, and vergence are elements of eye movement that can support foveal vision and thus can be purposive. However, different classes of eye movements can co-occur or interact with one another. Quantification of eye movements can provide valuable clues related to the working of the brain.

One way to measure eye movement is to analyze sequential images of the eye (fig. 1b). Recent technological advances in image processing and miniaturization have produced noninvasive video-oculography units capable of recording eye positions with high spatial and temporal resolutions, and appropriate for clinical settings. Three-dimensional rotation of the eye is captured as changes in the locations of specific landmarks within two-dimensional images, from which the angle of eye rotation that physically took place is estimated. The pupil is usually very dark and has an elliptical shape. These features can be quickly identified, frame-by-frame, using a computer, which makes the pupil a good landmark for tracking. Another good landmark is a bright spot on the cornea produced by the reflection of a light source, the location of which also moves within the image frame in relation to eye rotation.

The coordinates related to image pixels must be mapped to physical coordinates. Without this calibration process, the locations of landmarks in the acquired images have no physical meaning. With proper calibration, combined tracking of the pupil and corneal reflection can produce a very precise measurement. Ideally, the physical relationship between the head and the camera should be stable; however, there are head-free video-oculography techniques, which involve compensating for head movement artifacts with complex computational algorithms.

Predictive Visual Tracking

Visual tracking (also known as ocular pursuit) is a combination of smooth pursuit and saccadic eye movements and supports perceptual stability of the object of interest that is in motion. While saccadic tracking, i.e. an alternating sequence of saccades and fixations, allows only for temporally isolated observations of the target, the integration of smooth pursuit in tracking reduces slipping of the image to allow for a continuous observation of the target.

Generating and maintaining time-based expectancies of specific sensory information requires allocation of neural resources. It is postulated that attention plays a key role in this process and that various cognitive impairments and symptoms of concussion patients may stem from a primary deficit in this mechanism [3]. Human visual tracking provides an ideal model for studying the ability to predict the temporal course of a stimulus and then dynamically synchronize the required action with it: were we to direct the gaze to where the target was detected, even a short delay could mean that the target had moved away from the location (fig. 2). *Although visual sci-*

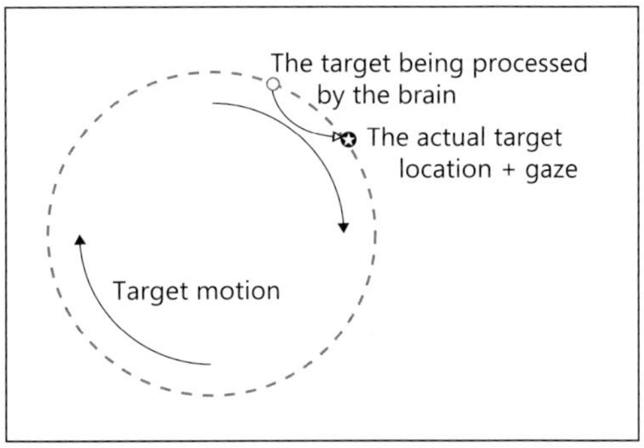

Fig. 2. Prediction and visuomotor synchronization. Maintaining the gaze on the target requires synchronization of the motor output with predicted target motion, rather than the incoming sensory information.

ence has extensively exploited the relative constancy of the visual world, scientific inquiry into dynamic foveation, or visuomotor synchronization, has been limited.

Predictive timing is critical for offsetting the constraint posed by the sensorimotor processing delay. This capacity prepares a motor outcome to intercept the forthcoming events. For example, predictive timing allows for balance to be maintained when turning a corner and for information to be derived from a continuously changing stimulus such as a visually moving object. In abnormal states of the brain, however, predictive timing may be compromised. We posit that the functional integrity of the predictive timing capacity can be assessed with quantification of predictive visual tracking performance.

Performance Assessment of Circular Visual Tracking

The use of a circular target trajectory [4, 5] is exceptionally well suited for assessing the maintenance of predictive visual tracking. With a target traveling at a constant angular velocity with a fixed radius, the motion is highly predictable as it can be described with only two constants. In addition, unlike a one-dimensional tracking paradigm, there is no endpoint; thus, the periodic movement can continue indefinitely within the orbital range of the eye.

Visual tracking performance may be quantified with parameters such as smooth pursuit velocity gain, phase error, and root-mean-square error (fig. 3). One metric for visuomotor synchronization is gaze positional error variability [6, 7]. Quantifying performance variability is essential since a dysfunction in predictive timing should increase performance variability. In a circular tracking paradigm, the gaze error variability in the direction parallel (tangential) to the target trajectory has a specific relevance to the precision of predictive timing.

Although adult humans have normally developed extraordinary visuomotor coordination skills, there are interindividual variations in visual tracking performance. There is also stability of individuals' performance over time, implying that interindi-

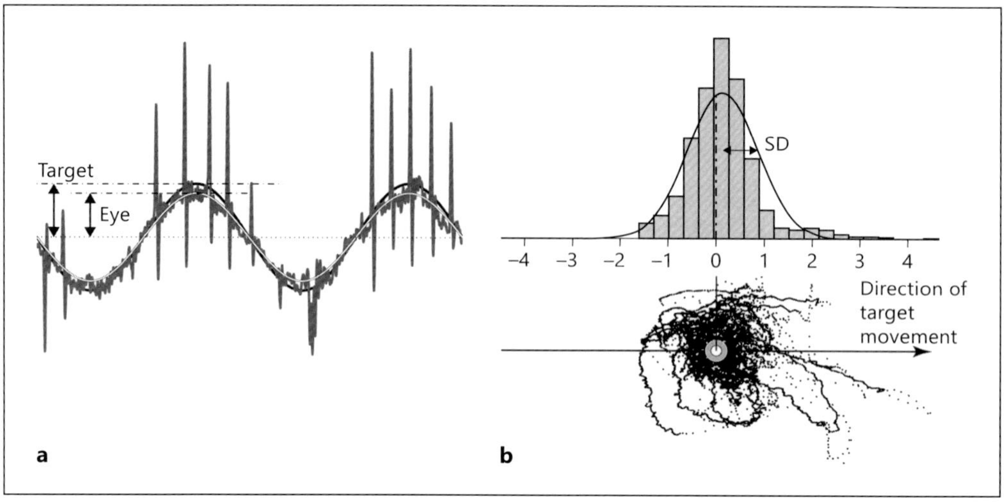

Fig. 3. Quantification of visual tracking performance. **a** Smooth pursuit velocity gain. The target velocity is shown with the smooth black trace, and the eye velocity with the jagged gray trace. Only the vertical components are shown in this example. The spikes in the eye velocity trace represent saccades, and the white trace superimposed on the eye velocity trace represents a sinusoidal fit of the smooth pursuit velocity. The smooth pursuit velocity gain is calculated as the ratio of the amplitudes of modulations of smooth pursuit eye and target velocities. **b** Position error variability. Top: histogram of instantaneous gaze positional error in the direction parallel (tangential) to the target movement, corresponding to the scattergram below; the variability of the distribution can be described with the standard deviation. Bottom: scattergram of the gaze positional error with the target trajectory straightened (arrow); each dot represents a sample taken at 500 Hz.

vidual variations characterize personal cognitive traits. Indeed, the performance indices of circular visual tracking show good test-retest reliability with intraclass correlation coefficients larger than 0.6 over a 2-week period [7]. Thus, the performance scores and their variations can provide insights into the spectrum of neurological differences and cognitive functioning, and each measurement allows for a single individual to be contrasted with a normative data set. In contrast, when the expected stability of the test outcome is not observed within an individual, a change in the person's neurological or physiological state may be suspected. The ordinary stability of visual tracking indices hints at the possibility of monitoring of disease or cognitive states by means of comparisons to baseline standards.

Concussion

Attention impairment is a key symptom of concussion [8, 9]. Although attention can be impaired in other conditions, and thus measures of attention cannot provide a biomarker specific for concussion, measuring and monitoring the attentional states of pa-

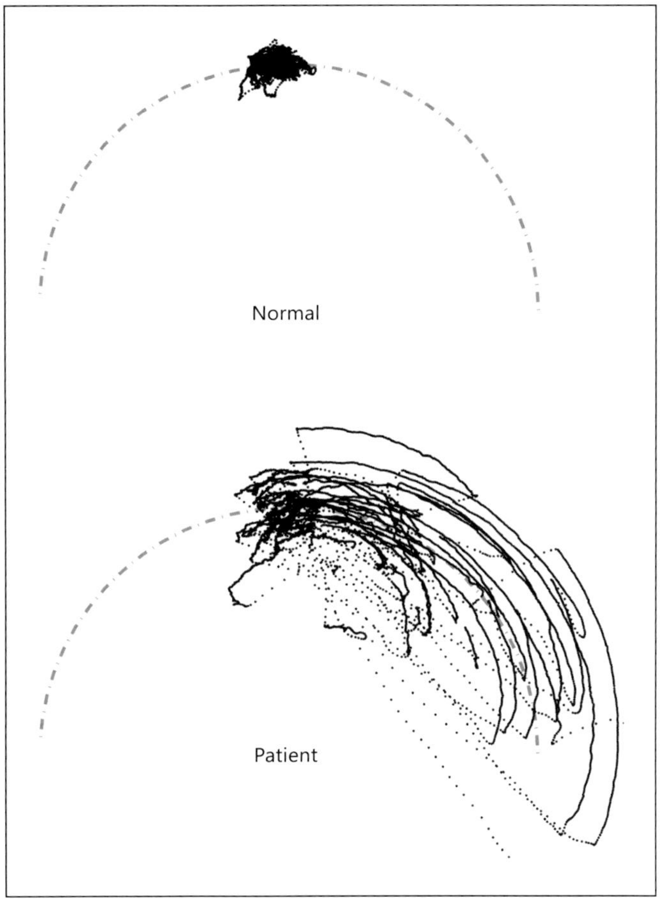

Fig. 4. Scattergram of gaze positions relative to the target. The coordinates are transformed so that the target is fixed at the 12 o'clock position. The dot-dashed line indicates the target trajectory with a 10° radius in visual angle. Each dot represents a sample taken at 500 Hz, and those displaced clockwise from the 12 o'clock position represent gaze positions ahead of the target. The patient was a 16-year-old student athlete who was injured 8 days prior to testing. Adapted from [11].

tients are important for preventing reinjury and assessing recovery. Circular visual tracking measures are proposed as a biomarker for anticipatory neural activity [6, 7, 10].

Figure 4 illustrates disrupted visuomotor synchronization in a concussion patient indicated by large gaze position error variability and overall phase advancement. This pattern is associated with large anticipatory saccades [6, 7]. It is noteworthy that the gaze should land along the circular path ahead of the target. The behavior demonstrates preserved spatial prediction as well as precision of oculomotor control (as opposed to accuracy), and draws a distinction between the abilities to direct the gaze where the target will eventually be and to direct the gaze there in time for the target's arrival.

Similar behavior can be seen within the normal spectrum, in keeping with the often subtle nature of concussion consequences. Still, the visual tracking performance of a group of acute concussion patients with postconcussive symptoms was found to be worse than that of a normal control group (fig. 5) [11]. In addition, when the patients were retested 1 month after the injury, most showed improvement, contrasting with

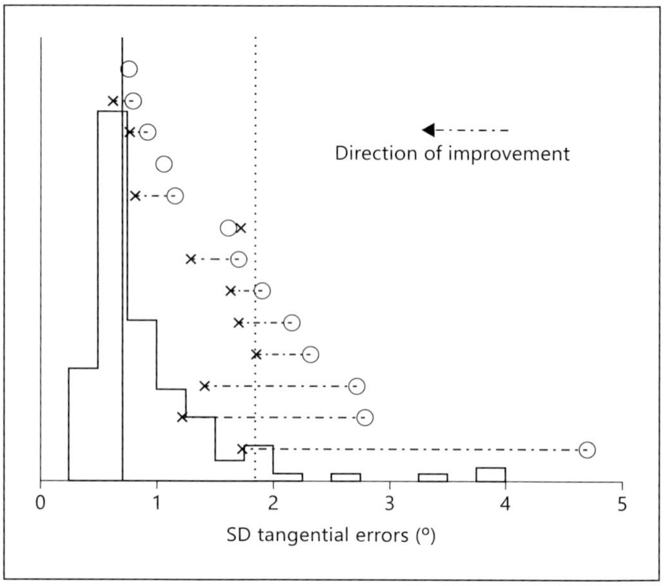

Fig. 5. Changes in a visual tracking index compared against a normative histogram. The change in the scores at the acute stage (○) and 1-month follow-up (×) for each concussion subject is indicated by horizontal dot-dashed lines. The concussion subjects are arranged based on their acute stage SD tangential error values. Two subjects dropped out of the study after the initial testing. The solid vertical line running through the histogram indicates the median, and the dotted vertical line separates the worst 5% of the normal population from the rest. Adapted from [11].

performance stability observed in normal individuals [11]. Thus, both group and interindividual comparisons are useful for monitoring progress after concussion.

Many factors, such as fatigue, intoxication, and psychiatric illnesses, can affect attention and interfere with visual tracking performance. However, attention is not a unitary cognitive process. Challenges lie in identifying how physiological, neurological, or psychiatric conditions influence specific components of attention. Different conditions may produce different patterns of changes in visual tracking indices, and these patterns may uniquely identify concussion.

Conclusion

The myriad cognitive impairments and symptoms associated with concussion are postulated to be secondary consequences of a primary deficit in attention, specifically in the ability to synchronize with external events [3, 10, 11]. Sensorimotor synchronization is quantified best by visual tracking of a predictably moving target; thus, we have focused on characterizing eye movements during predictive visual tracking. Experimental results indicate that the visual tracking indices allow for comparison of performance to a normative standard as well as for monitoring within-individual changes. In addition to predictive visual tracking, oculomotor anomalies associated with concussion also include deficits in vergence [12], antisaccade [13], and memory-guided saccades [13]. Further advances in analytics and eye-tracking technology will allow a broad application of oculomotor assessment for concussion and other cognitive impairments.

References

1 Hughes A: Topographical relationships between the anatomy and physiology of the rabbit visual system. Doc Ophthalmol 1971;30:33–159.

2 Corbetta M, Akbudak E, Conturo TE, Snyder AZ, Ollinger JM, Drury HA, Linenweber MR, Petersen SE, Raichle ME, Van Essen DC, Shulman GL: A common network of functional areas for attention and eye movements. Neuron 1998;21:761–773.

3 Ghajar J, Ivry RB; Cognitive and Neurobiological Research Consortium: The predictive brain state: timing deficiency in traumatic brain injury? Neurorehabil Neural Repair 2008;22:217–227.

4 Umeda Y, Sakata E: The circular eye-tracking test. I. Simultaneous recording of the horizontal and vertical component of eye movement in the eye-tracking test. ORL J Otorhinolaryngol Relat Spec 1975;37: 290–298.

5 van der Steen J, Tamminga EP, Collewijn H: A comparison of oculomotor pursuit of a target in circular real, beta or sigma motion. Vision Res 1983;23: 1655–1661.

6 Maruta J, Suh M, Niogi SN, Mukherjee P, Ghajar J: Visual tracking synchronization as a metric for concussion screening. J Head Trauma Rehabil 2010;25: 293–305.

7 Maruta J, Heaton KJ, Kryskow EM, Maule AL, Ghajar J: Dynamic visuomotor synchronization: quantification of predictive timing. Behav Res Methods 2013;45:289–300.

8 Binder LM, Rohling ML, Larrabee GJ: A review of mild head trauma. Part I: meta-analytic review of neuropsychological studies. J Clin Exp Neuropsychol 1997;19:421–431.

9 Bernstein DM: Recovery from mild head injury. Brain Inj 1999;13:151–172.

10 Maruta J, Lee SW, Jacobs EF, Ghajar J: A unified science of concussion. Ann NY Acad Sci 2010;1208: 58–66.

11 Maruta J, Tong J, Lee SW, Iqbal Z, Schonberger A, Ghajar J: EYE-TRAC: monitoring attention and utility for mTBI. Proc SPIE 2012;8371:83710L-1

12 Thiagarajan P, Ciuffreda KJ, Ludlam DP: Vergence dysfunction in mild traumatic brain injury (mTBI): a review. Ophthalmic Physiol Opt 2011;31:456–468.

13 Heitger MH, Jones RD, Macleod AD, Snell DL, Frampton CM, Anderson TJ: Impaired eye movements in post-concussion syndrome indicate suboptimal brain function beyond the influence of depression, malingering or intellectual ability. Brain 2009; 132:2850–2870.

Jun Maruta, PhD
Brain Trauma Foundation
7 World Trade Center, 34th Floor
250 Greenwich Street, New York, NY 10007 (USA)
E-Mail jmaruta@braintrauma.org

Niranjan A, Lunsford LD (eds): Concussion. Prog Neurol Surg. Basel, Karger, 2014, vol 28, pp 234–242
DOI: 10.1159/000358787

Neurodegenerative Changes after Mild Traumatic Brain Injury

Saeed Fakhran · Lea Alhilali

Division of Neuroradiology, Department of Radiology, University of Pittsburgh School of Medicine, Pittsburgh, Pa., USA

Abstract

A link between mild traumatic brain injury (mTBI) and neurodegenerative diseases, specifically Alzheimer's disease and chronic traumatic encephalopathy (CTE), has long been suspected. Shared clinical symptomology – most notably the prominent role of central auditory dysfunction and sleep-wake disturbances in both disease states – and similar findings on postmortem pathological examination has further reinforced suspected commonality between these seemingly disparate entities. However, conventional imaging techniques, including computed tomography and anatomic magnetic resonance, are unable to detect the symptomatic injuries in mTBI patients and therefore detection of neurodegenerative changes in vivo has previously not been reported. Recent research using diffusion tensor imaging, a novel imaging technique, and focused on patient-reported symptoms has for the first time demonstrated imaging findings in mTBI patients in vivo that are strikingly similar to Alzheimer's dementia and CTE. Moving forward, research will focus on identifying what renders certain patients with mTBI susceptible to developing full-fledged Alzheimer's disease and CTE later in life.

© 2014 S. Karger AG, Basel

It has long been suspected that repeated episodes of concussive and subconcussive injury are associated with both cognitive and behavioral impairments later in life. As early as 1928, medical manuscripts started using the term 'punch drunk' to refer to behavioral impairments suffered by boxers after their careers were over [1]. Subsequent papers referred to terms such as 'dementia pugilistica' [2], and a case series in 1973 sought to distinguish this particular dementia from other neurodegenerative disorders [3].

Unfortunately, the 85 years since the term 'punch drunk' was first coined have only confirmed the suspicions of those initial researchers, as an ever-increasing body of medical research has revealed a variety of links between even a single episode of mild traumatic brain injury (mTBI) and neurodegenerative diseases later in life.

The term 'dementia pugilistica' today has been replaced with the term 'chronic traumatic encephalopathy (CTE)', as the body of evidence has grown to show that it affects not only boxers, but also a multitude of patients with repetitive mTBI. CTE is now felt to be a neurodegenerative disease caused by any type of repetitive mild brain trauma, and has recently gained widespread media attention, in large part due to the unexpected deaths of high-profile former National Football League (NFL) players suffering from the condition. The recent settlement of a lawsuit between the NFL and current and former players worth in excess of USD 700,000,000 relating to treatment and prevention of the condition brought even greater media attention and focus upon the treatment of concussion and prevention of its potential long-term sequelae.

However, CTE is not the only neurodegenerative disease linked to brain trauma. A link between traumatic brain injury and Alzheimer's dementia has long been postulated, although it has received significantly less attention than the link between trauma and CTE. While this link remains controversial in some circles, multiple epidemiological studies have linked TBI as a major risk factor in the later development of Alzheimer's dementia [4, 5]. Unlike CTE, Alzheimer's disease (AD) is a major epidemiological health problem and perhaps the most well-known neurodegenerative disease, currently affecting over 3 million Americans [6]. A devastating and mind-robbing condition, the impact of AD on society is only growing as it is projected to affect over 100 million people worldwide by 2050 [6].

In the following pages, we will review clinical and pathological links among mTBI, CTE, and AD, and then explore recent striking similarities between imaging findings in young concussion patients and pathologic findings in CTE and AD.

Links between Mild Traumatic Brain Injury and Alzheimer's Dementia

Clinical Symptomology

Despite the fact that Alzheimer's dementia and mTBI seem to resemble two disparate disease processes – one affecting older people toward the end of life, and the other afflicting younger people in the prime of life – they in fact share some strikingly common clinical symptoms.

Central auditory dysfunction, defined as the inability to properly filter out background noise, is one of the shared symptoms seen prominently in both disease processes. Amongst the most burdensome of postconcussion symptoms, this seemingly innocuous problem often leads to difficulty concentrating, frustration on the part of both the patient and their parents, and a decline in academic performance.

Following mTBI, neurological mechanisms implicated in various auditory processes, including low-redundancy speech recognition, tone pattern recognition, and dichotic listening, may be disrupted [7]. The mechanism thought to underlie this dysfunction is impaired auditory sensory gating – the inability to filter out background sensory information – and is identified electrophysiologically via an elevated P50 ratio. Simply stated, the P50 ratio is an electrophysiological metric based on middle latency auditory cortical evoked potential occurring 50 ms after presentation of paired auditory stimuli presented 500 ms apart, and is believed to reflect auditory gating [8].

Similarly, auditory dysfunction is a frustrating symptom in patients suffering from AD. Multiple researchers have now shown that an elevated P50 ratio is not only seen in the setting of mild cognitive impairment, but in fact larger P50 amplitudes can predict which patients with mild cognitive impairment will progress to develop full-fledged AD [9, 10].

Similar to central auditory dysfunction, sleep-wake disturbances (SWDs) – a broad set of abnormalities related to difficulties initiating and maintaining a normal quality and length of sleep – are another symptom class shared by both Alzheimer's dementia patients and mTBI patients. SWDs can be particularly frustrating after mTBI, as the inability to obtain quality rest often exacerbates other postconcussion symptoms and impedes a proper recovery.

Multiple authors have provided both subjective and objective evidence of SWDs following mTBI [11, 12], with subjective patient complaints of difficulty falling asleep, early-morning awakening, and nonrestorative sleep, as well as objective evidence of sleep dysfunction including abnormal polysomnographic and actigraphic monitoring findings. In fact, SWDs have been estimated to affect up to 28% of adolescents following minor brain trauma [11].

Similarly, disruption of normal circadian rhythms and SWDs feature prominently in the pathology of AD. Although there are well-known and researched changes of circadian activity associated with aging, several authors have started explicitly examining the temporal relationship between circadian activity disruption and dementia onset. Much like an elevated P50 ratio, it has been found that disrupted circadian rhythm, measured on actigraphy, can predict both future development of mild cognitive impairment in cognitively normal patients, as well as progression to full-fledged AD in patients with mild cognitive impairment [13, 14].

Pathology

Amyloid-β plaques and neurofibrillary tangles (NFTs), identified on postmortem microscopic examination of the brain, are well-known hallmarks of AD. While NFTs have also been described in the brains of individuals exposed to repetitive mild concussive or subconcussive injuries, such as boxers [15] and former professional football players [16], until recently such findings had not been seen following only a single episode of mTBI in humans.

However, it has recently been demonstrated that both NFTs and amyloid-β plaques are present at both a higher density and a wider distribution in patients surviving greater than 1 year following a single episode of mTBI compared with age-matched controls [17]. In fact, widespread and extensive NFTs were seen in over 30% of individuals under 60 years of age, following a single mTBI, compared to minimal pathology noted in age-matched controls. This naturally led to the rather worrisome and somewhat disturbing conclusion that pathologic evidence of neurodegenerative disease, similar to that seen in AD, may be initiated or accelerated in the chronic pathologic milieu following survival after a single episode of mTBI, even in young adults [17].

Imaging Similarities between Mild Traumatic Brain Injury and Neurodegenerative Diseases

Novel Imaging Techniques

Conventional imaging methods [i.e. magnetic resonance imaging (MRI) and computed tomography] have had relatively little to contribute in the evaluation of patients with mTBI. Traditionally, only a small minority of mTBI patients underwent imaging evaluation, which typically was reserved for patients with atypical symptoms and performed in order to exclude a more serious brain injury. Occasionally, conventional MRI would demonstrate microhemorrhages, which were felt to be the sequelae of diffuse axonal injury, but of unclear clinical significance. In the vast majority of cases, however, not even microhemorrhages are seen. Therefore, the sine qua non of mTBI has come to be normal conventional brain imaging, with the causative white matter injury thought to be beyond the resolution of conventional imaging.

However, the advent of diffusion tensor imaging (DTI), a relatively novel MR technique to noninvasively assess the microstructural integrity of white matter, has helped to elucidate an imaging correlate to the cognitive impairments that often result from mTBI. DTI examines the molecular diffusion of water, described by its fractional anisotropy [18]. In normal white matter, water diffuses readily along the orientation of axonal fibers, and any change in the microstructure of white matter and coherence of the white matter fiber tract – as may be seen after mTBI – will reduce the fractional anisotropy, making DTI a prime tool in mTBI assessment [18].

The role of DTI versus conventional MRI after mTBI was tested in an important study that sought to compare the importance of abnormalities on conventional MR (namely microhemorrhages seen on T2*-GRE sequences) with abnormalities seen on DTI by attempting to correlate both with postconcussion cognitive symptoms. Abnormalities on DTI strongly correlated with cognitive symptoms, cementing the role of DTI as a valuable tool in post-mTBI analysis. The presence or absence of microhemorrhages, however, had no correlation with patient symptoms, validating the relatively limited role of conventional MR in the evaluation of mTBI patients [18].

Mild Traumatic Brain Injury and Alzheimer's Disease on Imaging

Despite the shared clinical and pathologic features seen in both AD and mTBI, until recently no imaging similarities between these disease processes had been demonstrated. This is in part due to the difficulties imaging the actual white matter injury in mTBI patients. To begin, even when white matter injuries are detected in mTBI patients, it is difficult to discern which of the abnormalities are truly related to the acute

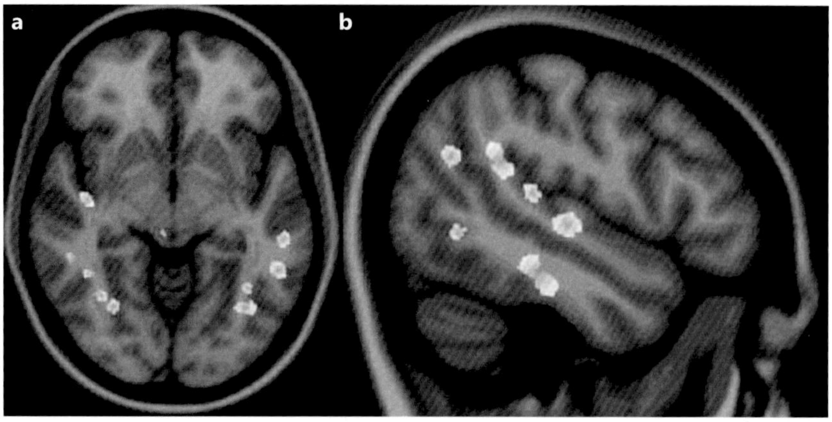

Fig. 1. Symptomatic white matter abnormalities in mTBI patients prominently involve the auditory cortex, correlating with clinical central auditory dysfunction. Images derived from tract-based spatial statistics results and rendered on T1-weighted images from the Montreal Neurological Institute atlas show symptomatic white matter abnormalities resemble those in Alzheimer's dementia. Regions of white matter abnormality that significantly correlate with patient-reported postconcussion symptoms are most prominently seen in the auditory cortices in the axial (**a**) and sagittal (**b**) planes.

traumatic event, and which are sequelae of a prior injury. While numerous studies have demonstrated white matter abnormalities on DTI in mTBI patients relative to controls [19], given that many white matter injuries may be clinically silent or chronic injuries (in a population with a prior concussion history), the significance of these abnormalities has been difficult to discern.

As a result, it has been difficult to determine from imaging which of the many observed white matter injuries are truly related to postconcussion symptoms. In an attempt to elucidate the symptomatic white matter injuries, further studies have sought to correlate postconcussive cognitive dysfunction with observed white matter abnormalities. However, in the absence of a baseline cognitive function for comparison, and given inherent baseline differences in cognitive function across a given population, it is difficult to place these findings in a proper clinical context.

While abnormalities found on cognitive testing may be affected by baseline cognitive function, patient-reported symptoms are more likely to be the result of the trauma itself. A recent and novel study correlated white matter abnormalities in mTBI patients with postconcussion symptoms based on patient-reported symptoms rather than clinically deduced cognitive deficits [20]. As in prior studies, these patients demonstrated diffuse white matter abnormalities relative to controls, but of these, only those at the gray-white junction posteriorly correlated with symptoms, including a significant cluster around the primary and association auditory cortices (fig. 1).

The auditory cortex is one of the earliest regions where abnormalities are seen in Alzheimer's dementia, with imaging abnormalities seen in this region in patients with the Presenilin gene mutation (familial AD) prior to symptom onset [21]. Simi-

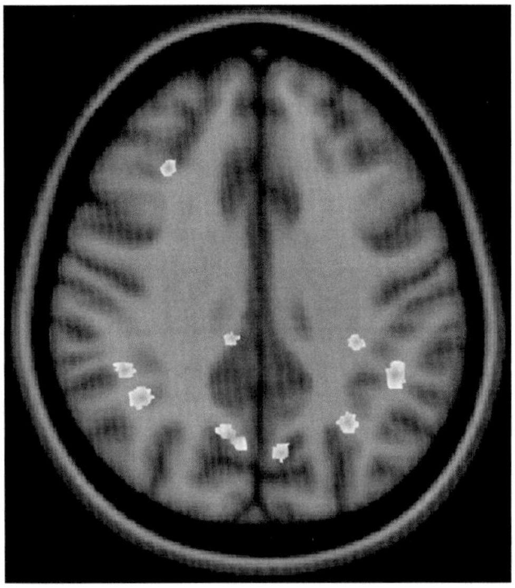

Fig. 2. Symptomatic white matter changes in mTBI patients resemble regions of wallerian degeneration seen in AD patients. Images derived from tract-based spatial statistics results and rendered on T1-weighted images from the Montreal Neurological Institute atlas show symptomatic white matter abnormalities in predominantly subcortical white matter in the posterior parietal regions, where regions of wallerian degeneration are seen in AD patients.

larly, the distribution of the white matter abnormalities at the gray-white junction seen on DTI in mTBI patients mirrors the wallerian degeneration that occurs with AD. When AD affects the neocortex, loss of large pyramidal neurons is seen, which have prominent subcortical projections [22]. The resulting wallerian degeneration is thus seen predominantly in the subcortical white matter in the posterior parietal, temporal, and occipital regions, with this distribution distinguishing these wallerian-related white matter abnormalities in AD from age-related chronic microvascular ischemic findings, which tend to involve deep white matter and do not have a predominantly posterior distribution [23]. The symptomatic white matter abnormalities in mTBI in this study closely mirrored this distribution of large pyramidal neuron loss in AD, with wallerian-type changes in the posterior subcortical white matter (fig. 2).

The distribution of the injuries at the gray-white junction was at the depth of sulci and at points of geometric inflection (fig. 3). This is also the distribution of NFTs and αβ-plaques in CTE, a distribution felt to reflect the regions of greatest stress during compression and subsequent reexpansion of the brain after a traumatic impact [24].

It is interesting that although prominent differences in white matter integrity were seen between mTBI patients and controls in previously reported regions of interest, notably the corpus callosum, these did not correlate with patient-reported symptoms (fig. 4).

Given the strong similarity between the distribution of symptomatic white matter injuries in mTBI patients and the known pathologic findings in both AD and CTE, this study went further to evaluate mTBI patients presenting with one of the most common clinical symptoms in mTBI and AD: SWDs. Evaluating this subset

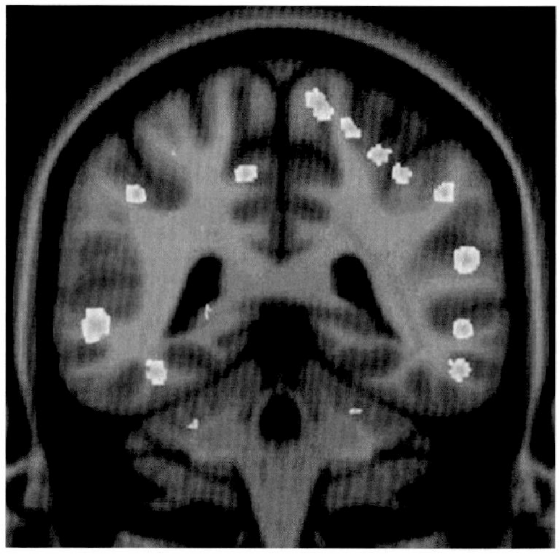

Fig. 3. Distribution of symptomatic white matter changes in mTBI patients mirrors the distribution of plaques and NFTs in CTE. Images derived from tract-based spatial statistics results and rendered on T1-weighted images from the Montreal Neurological Institute atlas show symptomatic white matter abnormalities resemble those in CTE. Regions of white matter abnormality, predominantly along the depths of sulci and points of geometric inflection, similar to the pattern of NFT and amyloid-β plaque deposition in CTE, correlate with patient-reported postconcussion symptoms.

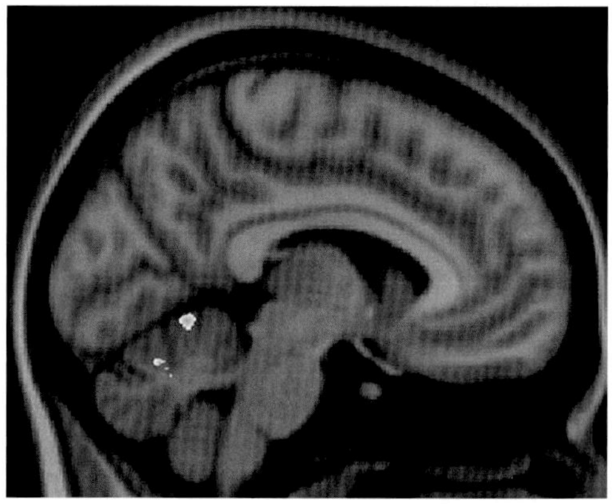

Fig. 4. Although abnormalities have previously been reported in the corpus callosum, these do not correlate with postconcussion symptoms. Images derived from tract-based spatial statistics results and rendered on T1-weighted images from the Montreal Neurological Institute atlas show no symptomatic white matter abnormalities in the region of the corpus callosum.

of patients, it was found that abnormalities in the parahippocampus were seen in mTBI patients with SWDs compared to those without sleep symptoms (fig. 5). Intriguingly, the parahippocampus is among the first regions to be involved in early Alzheimer's dementia and is among the regions of greatest involvement in CTE [25].

This study was the first to demonstrate imaging findings of mTBI which strongly resemble the distribution of findings in AD and CTE. This finding may open new research opportunities, with greater collaboration between mTBI and AD research. Obviously not all patients with mTBI will go on to develop neurodegenerative disease later in life. Unfortunately, at this point it remains unclear which subset of patients will suffer from AD or CTE later in life and what predisposes them to develop these debilitating neurodegenerative diseases. Currently, the focus has been on a genetic predisposition in a subset of patients, specifically those with abnormalities in the apo-

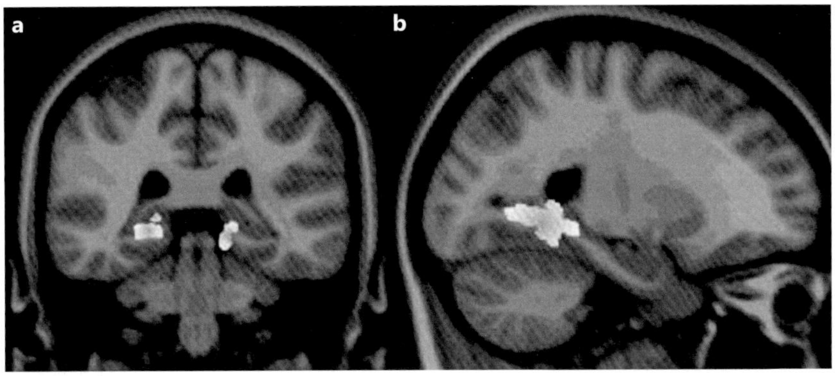

Fig. 5. White matter abnormalities in mTBI patients with SWDs involve the parahippocampus, similar to Alzheimer's dementia. Images derived from tract-based spatial statistics results and rendered on T1-weighted images from the Montreal Neurological Institute atlas show white matter abnormalities associated with SWDs are similar to findings in early Alzheimer's dementia. Voxels with significantly decreased fractional anisotropy for patients with mild TBI and SWDs relative to those without sleep symptoms involve the parahippocampal regions in the coronal (**a**) and sagittal (**b**) planes, paralleling the first changes in Alzheimer's dementia, when SWDs are among the heralding symptoms.

lipoprotein E allele [26]. This continued search for the factor that renders certain mTBI patients vulnerable to future neurodegenerative changes should bring hope to those suffering from mTBI, as the devastating changes associated with AD and CTE may not be from damage already done, but from a secondary neurodegenerative cascade that may be prevented.

References

1 Martland HS: Punch drunk. JAMA 1928;91:1103–1107.
2 Millspaugh JA: Dementia pugilistica. US Naval Med Bull 1937;35:297–303.
3 Corsellis JA, Bruton CJ, Freedman-Browne D: The aftermath of boxing. Psychol Med 1973;3:270–273.
4 Guo Z, Cupples LA, Kurz A, Aurebach SH, Volicer L, Chui H, Green RC, Sadovnick AD, Duara R, Decarli C, Johnson K, Go RC, Growdon JH, Haines JL, Kukull WA, Farrer LA: Head injury and the risk of AD in the MIRAGE study. Neurology 2000;54:1316–1323.
5 Plassman BL, Havlik RJ, Steffens DC, Helms MJ, Newman TN, Drosdick D, Phillips C, Gau BA, Welsh-Bohmer KA, Burke JR, Guralnik JM, Breitner JC: Documented head injury in early adulthood and risk of Alzheimer's disease and other dementias. Neurology 2000;55:1158–1166.
6 Breunig JJ, Guillot-Sesiter MV, Town T: Brain injury, neuroinflammation and Alzheimer's disease. Front Aging Neurosci 2013;5:1–10.
7 Nölle C, Todt E, Seidl R, Ernst A: Pathophysiological changes of the central auditory pathway after blunt trauma of the head. J Neurotrauma 2004;21:251–258.
8 Arciniegas D, Olincy A, Topkoff J, McRae K, Cawthra E, Filley CM, Reite M, Adler LE: Impaired auitory gating and P50 nonsupression following traumatic brain injury. J Neuropsychiatry Clin Neurosci 2000;12:77–85.
9 Idrizbegovic E, Hederstierna C, Dahlquist M, Kämpfe Nordström C, Jelic V, Rosenhall U: Central auditory dysfunction in early Alzheimer's disease and in mild cognitive impairment. Age Ageing 2011;40:249–254.

10 Golob E, Irimajiri R, Starr A: Auditory cortical activity in amnestic mild cognitive impairment: relationship to subtype and conversion to dementia. Brain 2007;130:740–752.
11 Pillar G, Averbooch E, Katz N, Peled N, Kaufman Y, Shahar E: Prevalence and risk of sleep disturbances in adolescents after minor head injury. Pediatr Neurol 2003;29:131–135.
12 Kaufman Y, Tzischinsky O, Epstein R, Etzioni A, Lavie P, Pillar G: Long-lasting sleep patterns of adult patients with minor traumatic brain injury (mTBI) and non-mTBI subjects. Sleep Med 2008;9:481–487.
13 Schlosser Covell GE, Dhawan PS, Lee Iannotti JK, Hoffman-Snyder CR, Wellik KE, Caselli RJ, Woodruff BK, Wingerchuk DM, Demaerschalk BM: Disrupted daytime activity and altered sleep-wake patterns may predict transition to mild cognitive impairment or dementia: a critically appraised topic. Neurologist 2012;18:426–429.
14 Tranah GJ, Blackwell T, Stone KL, Ancoli-Israel S, Paudel ML, Ensrud KE, Cauley JA, Redline S, Hillier TA, Cummings SR, Yaffe K: Circadian activity rhythms and risk of incident dementia and mild cognitive impairment in older women. Ann Neurol 2011;70:722–732.
15 Tokuda T, Ikeda S, Yanagisawa N, Ihara Y, Glenner GG: Re-examinnation of ex-boxers' brains using immunohistochemistry with antibodies to amyloid beta-protein and tau protein. Acta Neuropathol 1991; 82:280–285.
16 Omalu BI, DeKosky ST, Hamilton RL, Minster RL, Kamboh MI, Shakir AM, Wecht CH: Chronic traumatic encephalopathy in a national football league player: part II. Neurosurgery 2006;59:1086–1092.
17 Johnson VE, Stewart W, Smith DH: Widespread tau and amyloid-beta pathology many years after a single traumatic brain injury in humans. Brain Pathol 2012;22:142–149.
18 Niogi SN, Mukherjee P, Ghajar J, Johnson C, Kolster RA, Sarkar R, Lee H, Meeker M, Zimmerman RD, Manley GT, McCandliss BD: Extent of microstructural white matter injury in postconcussive syndrome correlates with impaired cognitive reaction time: a 3T diffusion tensor imaging study of mild traumatic brain injury. AJNR Am J Neuroradiol 2008;29:967–973.
19 Hulkower MB, Poliak DB, Rosenbaum SB, Zimmerman ME, Lipton ML: A decade of DTI in traumatic brain injury: 10 years and 100 articles later. AJNR Am J Neuroradiol 2013;34:2064–2074.
20 Fakhran S, Yaeger K, Alhilali L: Symptomatic white matter changes in mild traumatic brain injury resemble pathologic features of early Alzheimer dementia. Radiology 2013;269:249–257.
21 Ginestroni A, Battaglini M, Della Nave R, Moretti M, Tessa C, Giannelli M, Caffarra P, Nacmias B, Bessi V, Sorbi S, Bracco L, De Stefano N, Mascalchi M: Early structural changes in individuals at risk of familial Alzheimer's disease: a volumetry and magnetization transfer MR imaging study. J Neurol 2009;256:925–932
22 Viswanathan A, Gray F, Bousser MG, Baudrimont M, Chabriat H: Cortical neuronal apoptosis in CADASIL. Stroke 2006;37:2690–2695.
23 Yoshiura T, Mihara F, Koga H, Ohyagi Y, Noguchi T, Togao O, Ogomori K, Miyoshi K, Yamasaki T, Kaneko K, Ichimiya A, Kanba S, Honda H: Mapping of subcortical white matter abnormality in Alzheimer's disease using diffusion-weighted magnetic resonance imaging. Acad Radiol 2006;13:1460–1464.
24 Romito-DiGiacomo RR, Menegay H, Cicero SA, Herrup K: Effects of Alzheimer's disease on different cortical layers: the role of intrinsic differences in Abeta susceptibility. J Neurosci 2007;27:8496–8504.
25 Huang Y, Potter R, Sigurdson W, Santacruz A, Shih S, Ju YE, Kasten T, Morris JC, Mintun M, Duntley S, Bateman RJ: Effects of age and amyloid deposition on Aβ dynamics in the human central nervous system. Arch Neurol 2012;69:51–58.
26 Mahley R, Huang Y: Apolipoprotein E sets the stage: response to injury triggers neuropathology. Neuron 2012;76:871–885.

Saeed Fakhran, MD
Departments of Radiology, Division of Neuroradiology University of Pittsburgh School of Medicine
200 Lothrop St., Presby South Tower, 8th Floor, 8 North
Pittsburgh, PA 15213 (USA)
E-Mail fakhrans@upmc.edu

Niranjan A, Lunsford LD (eds): Concussion. Prog Neurol Surg. Basel, Karger, 2014, vol 28, pp 243–250
DOI: 10.1159/000358788

Future Directions in Brain Injury Research

Thomas A. Gennarelli

Emeritus Professor of Neurosurgery, Medical College of Wisconsin, Milwaukee, Wis., and Clinical Professor of Neurosurgery, George Washington University, Washington, D.C., USA

Abstract

This paper reviews the potential future directions that are important for brain injury research, especially with regard to concussion. The avenues of proposed research are categorized according to current concepts of concussion, types of concussion, and a global schema for globally reducing the burden of concussion.
© 2014 S. Karger AG, Basel

In order to propose a rational approach to the future directions of head injury research we must first ask, 'What is the goal of future research?' The shortsighted, but incorrect answer might be 'to improve survival and quality of survival after traumatic brain injury (TBI)'. A more universal goal, however, might be 'to decrease the societal, economic, social, and personal burden of TBI and to eradicate TBI as much as possible ... like smallpox, polio, and plague'. The latter, being broader in scope, transcends conventional biomedical research. Figure 1 was a paradigm once used by the Centers for Disease Control and Prevention (CDC) to define the needs of TBI research. Five interrelated modules are required for a comprehensive approach to the problem. While the current trend in biomedical research has focused on the clinical care module by trying to develop a single modality treatment based on understanding the changes in brain function at the genetic or molecular level, this has resulted in no practical advances in treatment in the past several decades. Rather, the number of TBI patients, confirmed by epidemiology, has been decreased by advances in prevention and biomechanical protection. This has decreased the overall burden of TBI (and its mortality), while rehabilitation efforts have markedly improved for survivors. Thus, we must broaden our concepts of TBI research and no longer search for treatment with a single magic bullet. What is most important in this five-module paradigm is that there must be an interdisciplinary and

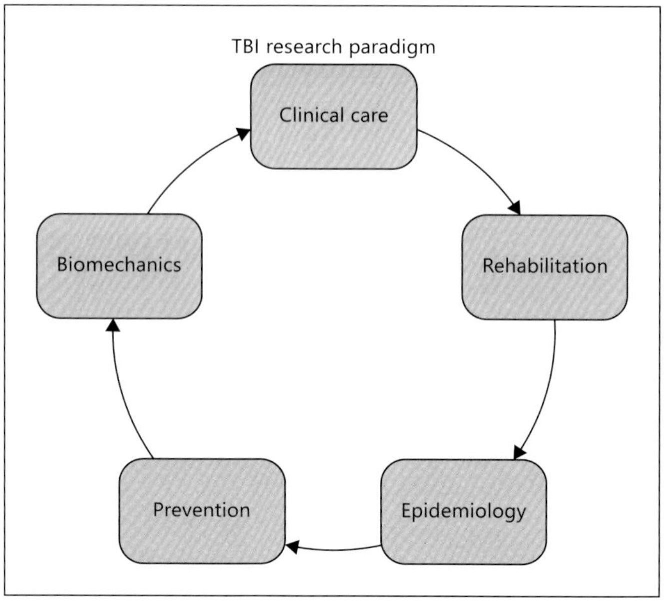

Fig. 1. TBI research paradigm.

transdisciplinary approach as well as a coordination of efforts between the modules. It is disappointing that, to date, no governmental agency has sought a coordinated effort regarding TBI research.

Nonetheless, there has been a dramatic fall in mortality from approximately 75% to 20% due to severe TBI since 1950 in the USA and other high-income countries. This improved survivability did not result from a magic bullet, but rather from improved vehicular safety, improved delivery of injured trauma victims to medical facilities that are prepared to care for them, and improved neurocritical care. We cannot, however, be complacent with these results because the non-high-income countries will continue to contribute to a worldwide increase in trauma and TBI over the next few decades. The World Health Organization (WHO) estimates that 90% of nonintentional deaths will occur in low- and middle-income countries and that the death rate will be almost double that of high-income countries (65 vs. 35 deaths per 100,000 population) [1]. Overall, the number of injury deaths will be 8.4 million by 2020, up by 65% from 5.1 million in 1990. Regarding traffic fatalities, despite a decrease of mortality in industrialized countries, the world traffic fatalities are estimated to increase 54% from 1.3 million currently to nearly 2.0 million by 2020 [2]. One half to two thirds of these fatalities involve TBI. Thus, we should anticipate the need for subsequent TBI research in all five modalities aimed at severe and survivable TBI.

This being the case, a comprehensive analysis of all the avenues of future research in head injury is unrealistic here. Certainly each module of research has its own avenues to pursue and each type of traumatic head injury requires further research on its own. Thus, this review will focus on the general research needs for concussion.

The Concussion Syndromes

Concussion has been of medical interest for most of the 20th century, and even much earlier with observations going back to antiquity. In 1935, Sir Charles Symonds declared, 'Of all the effects of head injury, the most interesting is … concussion' [3]. Early debates centered on whether concussion was due to the direct effects of head injury (i.e. mechanical energy), brief cerebral ischemia, or a rapid rise in intracranial pressure [4]. The classical experiments of Denny-Brown and Russell in the 1940s [5], Ommaya and Gennarelli [6] in the 1970s, and others paved the way for most of our current knowledge regarding concussion. Initially, concussion was focused on what is now viewed as the more severe end of concussion, namely when temporary unconsciousness or coma occurs. However, as early as the 1960s it was recognized that transient disturbances of brain function could occur after trauma without coma [7, 8], resulting in the definition being expanded. Over the years, the conceptual background of concussion has changed. These changes have driven research to date and will continue to stimulate future research.

Prior to the 1960s, concussion was considered to be temporary traumatic unconsciousness with no anatomical abnormality. The diagnosis of anatomic abnormality was somewhat loose since prior to computed tomography scanning a direct diagnosis could only be made by surgery or autopsy, and an indirect diagnosis could only be made by cerebral angiography. It was then recognized that transient disturbances of brain function could occur without coma and, thus, concussion without coma was defined.

In 1974, Ommaya and Gennarelli [6] proposed a hypothesis for concussion, which is still in use today. Their hypothesis consisted of several parts: (1) concussion has a series of gradations of injury severity (caused by mechanical energy, e.g. trauma), (2) the severity of the clinical alterations is related to the severity of the mechanical input to the brain that produced the mechanical strains in the brain in different regions and in different amounts, (3) the sequence of concussion severity results from a centripetal sequence of disruptive effects on brain function and structure, and (4) that rotational components of accelerative trauma to the head produce a graded centripetal progression of diffuse cortical-subcortical disconnexion phenomena which is always maximal at the periphery and enhanced at sites of structural inhomogeneity.

This has subsequently become known as the 'centripetal theory'. These observations on concussion were based on theoretical [9], experimental [3, 4], and clinical data. The clinical data most observed dealt with civilian assaults, falls, and motor vehicle crashes, and to a much lesser extent sports injuries; however, this concept became the basis for subsequent gradations of sports concussion [10].

Further research [11, 12] demonstrated that prolonged traumatic coma was associated with axonal injury and coined the term 'diffuse axonal injury (DAI)' for it. This research also showed that DAI is at the far end (most severe) of a spectrum of injuries that begins with concussion (fig. 2; table 1). Therefore, it is reasonable to assume that

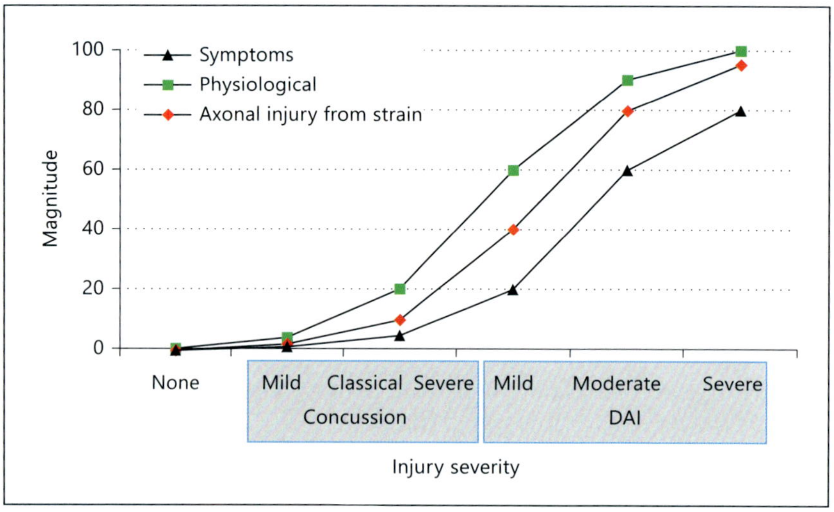

Fig. 2. The continuum of diffuse brain injury.

Table 1. Definitions of diffuse brain injury categories

Abbreviation	Description	AIS	Ommaya and Gennarelli concussion grade	LOC, h
MC	mild concussion	1	1–3	0
CC	classical concussion	2	4	<1
SC	severe concussion	3	4	1–6
Mild DAI	mild DAI	4	5	6–24
Mod DAI	moderate DAI	5	5	>24[a]
Sev DAI	severe DAI	5	5	>24[b]

AIS = Abbreviated Injury Scale; LOS = loss of consciousness. [a] No brainstem abnormality. [b] With decerebration, decortication.

concussion could also be associated with axonal injury, albeit at a lesser degree than DAI [13]. Similarly, it was assumed that the mechanisms of cellular dysfunction that were thought to be associated with DAI are also involved in concussion. These mechanisms, as well as others to be identified, have and will continue to provide areas for research. These areas could include ionic disequilibrium, oxidative dysfunction, receptor changes, inflammation, and gene regulation changes; however, a full discourse on the future research needs of these large areas is beyond the scope of this review.

The concept that concussions were usually associated with full recovery was challenged by Rimel et al. [14]. They established that not all persons with concussion have only temporary symptoms, which stimulated a large amount of research documenting persisting concussion symptoms (also known as postconcussion

Table 2. Types of traumatic head injury

- Scalp lacerations
- Skull fractures
- Focal brain injuries
  - Contusion, laceration
  - Hemorrhage: EDH, SAH, SDH, ICH
- Diffuse brain injuries
  - Concussion syndromes
    - Civilian nonsport concussion
    - Civilian sport concussion
    - Combat concussion
  - Diffuse axonal injury
  - Brain swelling
    - Unilateral
    - Bilateral
- Penetrating injuries
- Blast/explosive injuries

EDH = Extradural hematoma; SAH = subarachnoid hemorrhage; SDH = subdural hematoma; ICH = intracerebral hematoma.

syndrome). Currently, the understanding of the causes of persisting concussion symptoms is incomplete in subsets of the concussion population, but future research will hopefully elucidate differences in individual susceptibilities in civilian, sport, and military concussion.

Further research has shown that the constellation of concussive and postconcussive symptoms and outcome may vary with the cause of concussion. Thus, we now distinguish between at least three different types of concussion (table 2). The first type is civilian nonsport concussion, which is generally the classical definition of concussion, i.e. a transient disturbance of neurological function due to falls, assaults, and motor vehicle-related sources. This type of concussion tends to come from singular rather than repetitive events and typically has few if any sequelae. The second type is civilian sport concussion. This newly defined entity can be repetitive and multiple, and although most have few symptoms after 10 to 45 days, there is fear that long-term effects may occur and lead to chronic traumatic encephalopathy, dementia, behavioral abnormalities, amyotrophic lateral sclerosis, parkinsonism, or Alzheimer's disease. The third type is combat-related concussion. These concussions occur either in association with causes similar to civilian concussions (falls, motor vehicle crashes, etc.) or with causes unique to military life, namely blast, fragment, and ballistic environments. In addition, these injuries often occur to more than one individual in a socially tightly structured group where one can witness several friends being subjected to the same traumatic event. This may be one reason why this group of concussion seems to be more highly associated and co-related with posttraumatic stress disorder, the symptoms of which often intersect with those following concussion so much that future research will be undertaken to separate the two.

The possibility of anatomical abnormalities associated with concussion has been recently opined using sophisticated magnetic resonance imaging methods after concussion. Although some studies have supported the concept that the primary locus of injury in mild concussion (without coma) is in the axon, others, particularly involving blast-related concussion, have challenged that concept. Also, the possibility that the neuronal soma, dendrites, synapse, mitochondria, or glia could be involved in mild concussion is consistent with the centripetal theory where cortical injury would be expected to be more prevalent than deep brain, white matter, diencephalic, or brain stem injury. Hence, because the density of axon bundles is less than in the white matter, other structures are liable to be injured.

Future Research Needs

The paradigm shown in figure 1 can be used to further predict the research needs for concussion, i.e. biomechanics, prevention, epidemiology, rehabilitation, and clinical care.

Biomechanics
This module is important for defining the qualitative and quantitative mechanisms involved in the various types of concussion. It has been known for several decades that angular head motions are important for concussion. Experimental concussion has shown that angular, but not translational (linear), acceleration of the head can produce the entire spectrum of diffuse brain injury from mild concussion to severe DAI [4, 10]. More recently, large volumes of quantitative data have been generated from instrumented helmets (mostly American football and more recently hockey). Unfortunately, the bulk of these observations are from nonconcussed players; some data exist from mild concussion, but relatively few data are available for coma-producing concussion. Therefore, it is difficult to relate injury thresholds in a helmeted sports situation from those scaled from experimental animal data or generated by mathematical modelling. Thus, injury thresholds and injury risk functions are not yet agreed upon and there is a critical need to resolve these issues.

Furthermore, it has become unclear whether the mechanics of concussion symptoms are the same for all concussion types. For a long time, mechanical energy that produced shear strain in the brain or tensile strains in axons has been the predominant theory for concussion symptoms. However, new experimental data involving the response of the brain or neural tissue suggests that a blast may involve much lower levels of strain than previously thought to be injurious and so another physical factor, perhaps stress or pressure, may be the cause of symptoms involving blast. A search for cellular and tissue injury thresholds for dysfunction at high and low frequencies is necessary to better understand how mechanical energy from different sources affects neural tissue. Studies are required to define the effect of multiple exposures to mechanical energy to understand the cumulative effects of subinjurious energy and the potential mechanisms of long-term symptoms or chronic traumatic encephalopathy from mild concussions or subconcussive exposure.

Biomechanics is also important for the generation of devices that mitigate concussion protection. The vehicular environment has and will continue to be a fertile ground for the development of newer and improved protective devices to mitigate head and extracranial injury. This has already been done to a large degree for frontal crashes with crash-absorbing structures, laminated windshields, padded dashboards, and airbags. Similar side- and rear-impact protective devices are less well developed, but research is being pursued in this area.

Prevention

Governmental agencies and the WHO need to continue to monitor the causes and incidence of concussion. Regulatory and educational efforts must be improved and strengthened so that continued public awareness regarding concussion and its prevention are highly visible. Some government agencies must get more active in regulatory efforts that will diminish concussion. In particular, test procedures and injury risk curves for concussion using angular head motion variables, after decades of discussion, must be incorporated into vehicle safety. Nongovernmental agencies such as professional, academic, and club sport leagues must provide real-time feedback status of the incidence of concussion and openly endorse rule and equipment changes that may improve safety. Finally, low-income countries must be supported to follow the same public awareness and safety measures as high-income countries.

Epidemiology

Efforts to collect, analyze, and make public data regarding concussion must take the highest priority in sports, military, and vehicular environments. National and international agencies need to specifically collect concussion data so that rational preventive measures can be implemented. In addition, better systems to define and categorize concussion based on physiological, structural, or imaging should be identified.

Rehabilitation

Concerning rehabilitation, the emergence of neuropsychologists, sports medicine physicians, athletic trainers, and physiatrists from testers to investigators should be strengthened and fostered. Furthermore, current studies in biologically based therapies should be supported and better study designs of physiologically and image-based cohorts should continue. Moreover, the definition of outcome measures should be expanded and continued.

Clinical Care

This arena provides the largest area for improvement in understanding the pathobiology of concussion. It includes conventional biomedical research techniques, such as the continued search for the best biomarkers for concussion, and the elucidation of deleterious, as well as reversible, neural pathways of cellular and network injury. Furthermore, the current focus on concussion and repetitive subconcussive injury must be expanded by more sophisticated biological and mathematical models.

Conclusion

Efforts to diminish the global burden of concussion will require a coordinated multidisciplinary and transdisciplinary effort of medical, engineering, and public health disciplines, and the coordinated collaboration of multiple national and international health agencies.

References

1 WHO World Report on Violence and Injury. Geneva, WHO, 2002, p 7 of Summary.
2 Mohan D, Tiwari G: Injury Prevention and Control. London, Taylor & Francis, 2003.
3 Symonds CP: Disturbance of cerebral function in concussion. Lancet 1935;225:486–488.
4 Scott WW: Physiology of concussion. Arch Neurol Psychiatry 1940;43:270–283.
5 Denny-Brown D, Russell WR: Experimental cerebral concussion. Brain 1941;64:93–164.
6 Ommaya AK, Gennarelli TA: Cerebral concussion and traumatic unconsciousness: correlation of experimental and clinical observations on blunt head injuries. Brain 1974;97:633–654.
7 Symonds CP: Concussion and its sequellae. Lancet 1962;1:1–5.
8 Ward AA: The physiology of concussion. Clin Neurosurg 1966;12:95–111.
9 Holbourn AHS: Mechanics of head injury. Lancet 1943;2:438–441.
10 Bailes JE, Cantu RC: Head injury in athletes. Neurosurgery 2001;48:26–46.
11 Adams JH, Graham DI, Murray LS, Scott G: Diffuse axonal injury due to nonmissile head injury in humans: an analysis of 45 cases. Ann Neurol 1982;12: 557–563.
12 Gennarelli TA, Thibault LE, Adams JH, Graham DI, Thompson CJ, Marcincin RP: Diffuse axonal injury and traumatic coma in the primate. Ann Neurol 1982;12:564–574.
13 Adams JH, Doyle D, Ford I, Gennarelli TA, Graham DI, Mclellan DR: Diffuse axonal injury in head injury: definition, diagnosis and grading. Histopathology 1989;15:49–59.
14 Rimel RW, Giordani B, Barth JT, Boll TJ, Jane JA: Disability caused by minor head injury. Neurosurgery 1981;9:221–228.

Thomas A. Gennarelli, MD
822 Grist Mill Lane
West Chester, PA 19380 (USA)
E-Mail tgennarelli@att.net

Author Index

Subject Index